PEDIATRIC BRAIN DEATH AND ORGAN/TISSUE RETRIEVAL

Medical, Ethical, and Legal Aspects

PEDIATRIC BRAIN DEATH AND ORGAN/TISSUE RETRIEVAL

Medical, Ethical, and Legal Aspects

EDITED BY

HOWARD H. KAUFMAN, M.D.

West Virginia University Health Sciences Center
Morgantown, West Virginia

PLENUM MEDICAL BOOK COMPANY
NEW YORK AND LONDON

Library of Congress Cataloging in Publication Data

Pediatric brain death and organ/tissue retrieval: medical, ethical, and legal aspects /
edited by Howard H. Kaufman.
  p.   cm.
Based on a conference held in March 1987.
Includes bibliographies and index.
ISBN-13: 978-1-4684-5534-2   e-ISBN-13: 978-1-4684-5532-8
DOI: 10.1007/978-1-4684-5532-8
  1. Brain death in children—Moral and ethical aspects—Congresses. 2. Donation of
organs, tissues, etc.—Moral and ethical aspects—Congresses. I. Kaufman, Howard H.
  [DNLM: 1. Brain Death—in infancy & childhood—congresses. 2. Ethics, Medical—
congresses. 3. Organ Procurement—Congresses. 4. Transplantation, Homologous—in
infancy & childhood—congresses. W 820 P371 1987]
RA1063.3.P43   1989
174′.25—dc 19
DNLM/DLC   88-38893
for Library of Congress   CIP

© 1989 Plenum Publishing Corporation
Softcover reprint of the hardcover 1st edition   1989
233 Spring Street, New York, N.Y. 10013

Plenum Medical Book Company is an imprint of Plenum Publishing Corporation

CONTRIBUTORS

LUIS A. ALVAREZ, M.D.
Department of Neurology
Albert Einstein College of Medicine and Montefiore
  Medical Center
Bronx, New York 10467

NANCY ASCHER, M.D.
Department of Surgery
University of California at San Francisco
San Francisco, California 94143-0780

HELEN LEVINE BATTEN, M.A.
Bigel Institute for Health Policy
Brandeis University
Waltham, Massachusetts 02254

JOHN BAXTER, M.D.
Department of Special Procedures
Division of Radiology
Geisinger Clinic
Geisinger Medical Center
Danville, Pennsylvania 17822

DONALD R. BENNETT, M.D.
Department of Neurology
University of Nebraska College of Medicine
Omaha, Nebraska 68105
Department of Neurology
Creighton University School of Medicine
Omaha, Nebraska 68105-1065

H. RICHARD BERESFORD, M.D., J.D.
Department of Neurology
North Shore University Hospital
Manhasset, New York 11030
Cornell University Medical College
New York, New York 10021

PETER McL. BLACK, M.D., PH.D
Neurosurgical Service
Brigham and Women's Hospital and The Children's Hospital
Department of Surgery
Harvard Medical School
Boston, Massachusetts 02115

DAVID BRILL, M.D.
Department of Nuclear Imaging
Division of Radiology
Geisinger Clinic
Geisinger Medical Center
Danville, Pennsylvania 17822

KELVIN G. M. BROCKBANK, PH.D.
Research and Development
CryoLife, Inc.
Marietta, Georgia 30067
Department of Pathology
Medical University of South Carolina
Charleston, South Carolina 29425

DEREK BRUCE, M.B., CH.B.
International Pediatric Neurosurgery Institute
Humana Advanced Surgical Institutes
Medical City Hospital
Dallas, Texas 75230

ARTHUR L. CAPLAN, PH.D.
Center for Biomedical Ethics
University of Minnesota
Minneapolis, Minnesota 55455

ALEXANDER MORGAN CAPRON, LL.B.
The Law Center and the School of Medicine
University of Southern California
Los Angeles, California 90089-0071

JAMES F. CHILDRESS, B.D., M.A., PH.D.
*Departments of Religious Studies and Medical
  Education*
University of Virginia
Charlottesville, Virginia 22903

RONALD E. CRANFORD, M.D.
Department of Neurology
Hennepin County Medical Center
Minneapolis, Minnesota 55415

T. FORCHT DAGI, M.D., M.P.H., M.T.S.
Department of Neurosurgery
Brown University
Providence, Rhode Island 02903

Kennedy Institute of Ethics
Georgetown University Law Center
Washington, D. C. 20016

BEVERLY A. DAVIDOFF
Administration
Bronx Municipal Hospital
Bronx, New York 10461

JOHN F. EDMONDS, M.D., B.S.,
  F.R.C.P.(C)
Intensive Care Unit
The Hospital for Sick Children
Toronto, Ontario M5G 1X8
Canada

NORMAN FOST, M.D., M.P.H.
Department of Pediatrics
University of Wisconsin
Madison, Wisconsin 53792

JULIE FULTON
Department of Sociology
University of Minnesota
Minneapolis, Minnesota 55455

ROBERT FULTON, PH.D.
Department of Sociology
University of Minnesota
Minneapolis, Minnesota 55455

SUSAN GLEESON
Technology Management
Blue Cross and Blue Shield Association
Chicago, Illinois 60611

JULIUS M. GOODMAN, M.D.
Indianapolis Neurosurgical Group
Neuroscience Section
Methodist Hospital of Indiana
Division of Neurosurgery
Indiana University Medical Center
Indianapolis, Indiana 46202-1206

LARRY L. HECK, M.D.
Section of Nuclear Radiology
Methodist Hospital of Indiana
Indianapolis, Indiana 46202-1206

ALBERT R. JONSEN, PH.D.
Department of Medical History and Ethics
University of Washington School of Medicine
Seattle, Washington 98105

HOWARD H. KAUFMAN, M.D.
Department of Neurosurgery
West Virginia University Health Sciences Center
Morgantown, West Virginia 26506

CARL H. LISMAN
Private Law Practice
Burlington, Vermont 05402

JOANNE LYNN, M.D., F.A.C.P.
ICU Research and Geriatrics
George Washington University Medical Center
Washington, D.C. 20037

J. GORDON MCCOMB, M.D.
Division of Neurosurgery
Childrens Hospital of Los Angeles
Department of Neurosurgery
*University of Southern California School of
  Medicine*
Los Angeles, California 90027

DAVID C. MCCULLOUGH, M.D.
*Department of Neurological Surgery and Child
  Health and Development*
George Washington University School of Medicine
Washington, D. C. 20037

Department of Neurosurgery
Children's Hospital National Medical Center
Washington, D. C. 20010

ROBERT T. MCNALLY, PH.D.
Research and Development
CryoLife, Inc.
Marietta, Georgia 30067

Department of Pathology
Medical University of South Carolina
Charleston, South Carolina 29425

JOEL E. MILLER
*Insurance, Managed Care, and Provider Relations
  Division*
Health Insurance Association of America
Washington, D. C. 20036

SOLOMON L. MOSHÉ, M.D.
Departments of Neurology and Pediatrics
Albert Einstein College of Medicine and Montefiore
  Medical Center
Bronx, New York 10467

STEPHEN K. NUGENT, M.D.
Pediatric Intensive Care Unit
Methodist Hospital of Indiana
Indianapolis, Indiana 46202-1206

MARK O'BRIEN, M.D.
Departments of Surgery and Pediatrics
Emory University School of Medicine
Neurosurgical Section
Henrietta Egleston Hospital for Children
Atlanta, Georgia 30322

JOHN J. PARIS, S.J., PH.D.
Department of Ethics
College of the Holy Cross
Worcester, Massachusetts 01610

Department of Community Medicine
Tufts Medical School
Boston, Massachusetts 02111

R. JOHN C. PEARSON, M.B., M.P.H.
Department of Community Medicine
West Virginia University Medical Center
Morgantown, West Virginia 26506

STEPHANIE G. PRATT, M.M.
Office of Health Services Research
West Virginia University Medical Center
Morgantown, West Virginia 26506

JEFFREY M. PROTTAS, PH.D.
Bigel Institute for Health Policy
Brandeis University
Waltham, Massachusetts 02254

JOHN C. ROBERTS, M.D.
Department of Internal Medicine
Abbott–Northwestern Hospital
Minneapolis, Minnesota 55404

JOHN A. ROBERTSON, J.D.
School of Law
University of Texas at Austin
Austin, Texas 78705

SANFORD SCHNEIDER, M.D.
Department of Pediatrics and Neurology
Division of Child Neurology
Loma Linda University School of Medicine
Loma Linda, California 92350

BERNADETTE SCHUMAKER
Division of Dialysis and Transplant Payment
  Policy
Health Care Financing Administration
U. S. Department of Health and Human Services
Baltimore, Maryland 21207

JAN ARTHUR SCHWARTZ, M.D.
Departments of Anesthesiology and Pediatrics
Geisinger Clinic
Geisinger Medical Center
Danville, Pennsylvania 17822

LINDA D. SHEAFFER
Office of Organ Transplantation
Bureau of Resources Development
Health Resources and Services Administration
Rockville, Maryland 20857

ROBERTA G. SIMMONS, PH.D.
Department of Sociology
University of Minnesota
Minneapolis, Minnesota 55455

DAVID A. STUMPF, M.D., PH.D.
Department of Pediatrics and Neurology
Northwestern University Medical School
The Children's Memorial Hospital
Chicago, Illinois 60614

DAVID N. SUNDWALL, M.D.
U. S. Department of Health and Human Services
Rockville, Maryland 20857

RABBI MOSHE TENDLER, PH.D.
Yeshiva University
New York, New York 10033

I. DAVID TODRES, M.D.
Pediatric Intensive Care Unit
Massachusetts General Hospital
Boston, Massachusetts 02114

Department of Pediatrics and Anesthesiology
Harvard Medical School
Boston, Massachusetts 02115

MICHAEL S. TURNER, M.D.
Indianapolis Neurosurgical Group
Neuroscience Section
Methodist Hospital of Indiana
Department of Neurosurgery
Indiana University Medical Center
Indianapolis, Indiana 46202-1206

CHARLES T. VAN BUREN, M.D.
Division of Immunology/Organ Transplantation
University of Texas Medical School at Houston
Houston, Texas 77030

ROBERT M. VEATCH, PH.D.
Kennedy Institute of Ethics
Georgetown University
Washington, D. C. 20057

SIK-NIN WONG, M.D., B.S. (H.K.)
Intensive Care Unit
The Hospital for Sick Children
Toronto, Ontario M5G 1X8
Canada

PREFACE

The death of a child, one whose vulnerability and unfilled promise compounds the tragedy of any death, touches us deeply. When that death occurs due to the generally unexpected and sudden loss of brain function, it is particularly poignant. And yet, when death comes, it should be diagnosed expeditiously. The professional responsibilities of the physician require that he both recognize brain death and inform the family of its occurrence. In addition, since recent advances in transplantation provide the possibility of using the organs of a brain-dead child to save the lives of other children, the concepts of beneficence and charity further compel physicians to facilitate such transplantations by informing the family about this possibility.

Criteria of brain death have been refined over about 30 years since the term *coma dépassé* (beyond coma) was coined by Mollaret and Goulon in 1957 (Kaufman and Lynn, 1986). The last major criteria evolved on a national level were those of the President's Commission in 1981. However, studies to date have concentrated on adults, and relatively little work has been reported about developing brain death criteria for the young. Indeed, the advisors to the President's Commission suggested that there are significant—although not well defined—differences in the ability of the brains of those under five years of age to recover from clinical states that would be accepted as indicative of complete and irreversible loss of brain function in adults.

The determination of brain death in children has assumed increased importance for two reasons. First, with improvements in resuscitation techniques, cardiac activity can be supported for many days in children whose brains have irreversibly ceased all function. However, doing so ignores the reality of the situation, keeps the family in a kind of limbo, does not fulfill the physician's obligation to society to recognize death, requires health care workers to treat a dead body, expends resources to no benefit for the child or family, and in the minds of some is actually abusing the body. In addition, ongoing developments in transplantation have provided the opportunity to use organs from victims of brain death to improve and even save the lives of others (Table I). The use of cyclosporin beginning in 1983–1984 eliminated the devastating side effects of impairment of mental and physical development by the high-dose steroids that had been used previously and thus made transplantation more attractive for children. In many circumstances, organs must be size-matched. Therefore, when the needy patients are small children, young donors must be identified and their organs retrieved if these recipients are to survive. Thus, it is important to consider how to diagnose death by neurologic criteria in children and how to transcend the tragedy of these circumstances by using organs from such children to restore health in other children.

In 1984, a project was initiated to gather information about work being done to define brain-based criteria for death and to study organ retrieval in young children in the United States and Canada, to hold a conference on the subject, and to publish the papers presented at that confer-

TABLE I.   Transplantation in the United

Organ or tissue	Transplants performed in the U.S.						
	1981	1982	1983	1984	1985	1986	
Kidney	4,885	5,358	6,162	6,968	7,695	8,973	6
Heart	62	103	172	346	731	1,368	3
Heart/lung	5	7	20	22	30	45	1
Liver	26	62	164	308	605	924	2
Pancreas	—	35	61	87	133	140	4
Cornea	—	18,500	21,250	24,000	26,326	31,000	2
Bone marrow	475	800	990	1,000	1,200	1,160	5

[a] Medicare coverage for ESRD began July 1, 1973.
[b] Cadaver donor patient.
[c] Cadaver donor graft.
[d] Living related patient.
[e] Living related graft.

ence. It soon became apparent that a number of individuals and groups were thinking about these issues and had been studying them. Indeed, in the interim, comprehensive reviews about pediatric brain death have been published (Ashwal and Schneider, 1987; Drake et al., 1986), a national task force including pediatricians and neurologists has developed guidelines (Task Force for the Determination of Brain Death in Children, 1987), and a national study on the use of isotope blood flow studies has been carried out (see Chapter 16). At the same time, as transplantation has become more successful, the need for organs has increased. The controversial subject of retrieving organs from anencephalics is being discussed more, as are many other aspects of organ retrieval. With the aid of the American Council on Transplantation and a generous grant by the Sandoz Corporation, the conference was held in March 1987, and included discussions about these and other subjects. The speakers and their associates have expanded and updated their presentations for this book.

In the first chapter of Part I, Background: Including Historical, Ethical, Legal, and Practical Considerations, Dr. Dagi discusses the historical, religious, philosophical, and ethical background of the consideration of brain death. A religious perspective on brain death and organ retrieval is provided in the next three articles in which Jewish, Catholic, and Protestant thinking is described. Professor Capron reviews the legal status of brain death. Dr. Lynn recounts her development of the criteria of the President's Commission and the issues to be considered in developing any new criteria, particularly in regard to infants.

In Part II, Criteria for the Declaration of Brain Death in Children, several neurosurgeons, pediatric neurologists, and pediatric intensivists discuss their experience with brain death in children, including how they evolved their criteria and what these are, the number of cases they have seen and in what disease entities, and their experience in requesting and obtaining organ donation. In addition, Dr. Stumpf presents a consensus document of a national task force. Discussions of cerebral blood flow testing, including the results of a national survey, and EEG considerations follow. Clearly there is not yet unanimity on criteria for the diagnosis of brain death in the pediatric population. But many criteria have been developed and are being used on a day-to-day basis. Considering for how short a period this subject has been studied and the increasing information being gathered about brain death in adults as well as in children, I suspect that within a few years it will be possible to assemble representatives of all interested parties to evolve a consensus similar to that arrived at by the President's Commission.

In Part III, Issues in Brain Death Related to Organ Donation, Dr. Pearson and Stephanie Pratt estimate the organ and tissue donor pool in the United States using various data bases. After explaining anencephaly, Drs. Cranford and Roberts suggest that anencephalics should become organ donors. Dr. Robertson presents alternative arguments in opposing relaxing the brain death standard. Dr. Veatch discusses another entity, the "higher-brain-oriented concept of death," with the proviso that the patient or his surrogate should have the right to individually elect the use of such criteria for death.

In Part IV, Needs and Possibilities in Transplantation, Dr. Van Buren elucidates the developments in immunosuppression which have been the most critical factor in the explosion in transplantation successes. Dr. Ascher enumerates the needs for transplants in the young and projects the numbers of human donors available as well as some other alternatives. Drs. Brockbank and McNally catalogue the tissues, including corneas, pancreatic cells, heart valves, blood vessels, bone marrow, cartilage and bone, and ligaments and tendons, which are now or will soon be transplanted.

In Part V, Other Topics in Organ Retrieval and Donation, Dr. Jonsen reviews the ethical bases of organ donation, pointing out that at this time charity rather than justice is the dominant consideration. Dr. Prottas and Ms. Batten analyze neurosurgeons' and ICU nurses' attitudes toward organ retrieval, highlighting the social and interpersonal issues that are current impediments to increased procurement. Drs. Simmons and Fulton and Julie Fulton describe their interviews with donor families and the generally positive effect that donation had. Dr. Beresford discusses legal aspects of organ transfer and possibilities for increasing the number of organs available by altering current laws. Mr. Lisman describes the National Conference of Commissioners on Uniform State Laws and its efforts to update the Uniform Anatomical Gift Act. Dr. Caplan discusses required request laws and their effects, in terms of both successes and failures. Dr. Fost points out problems in allocation in our health care system and offers arguments favoring allowing sale of organs.

In Part VI, Funding of Transplantation, Ms. Schumaker of the Health Care Financing Administration, Ms. Gleeson of Blue Cross/Blue Shield, and Mr. Miller of the Health Insurance Association of America discuss funding for transplantation. Dr. Sundwall presents federal activities which have encouraged and are promoting transplantation on a national level.

This book was conceived as a collection of essays dealing with a variety of issues concerning pediatric brain death and organ retrieval being currently discussed. Both subjects have many controversial areas, and people who are involved with one tend to be involved with the other and to have had experience with and opinions about both. For this reason, the authors were encouraged to reflect beyond the specific issue of their chapters. Although this approach has introduced some redundancy into the book, it seemed appropriate to let people who feel deeply about these problems express thoughts which may help shed light on the issues.

During production of the book several encouraging developments have occurred. Required request laws have been passed in most of the states (although their full effect has not yet been determined), government funding is being increased in a variety of areas, and technical improvements have been reported which now may make isolated lung transplantation a successful endeavor (Baldwin, 1988; Toronto Lung Transplant Group, 1988). A recent issue of *The Hastings Center Report* (October/November, 1988) was largely devoted to the topic of anencephalics as donors.

ACKNOWLEDGMENTS. I would like to thank Sandoz for funding the conference that was the inspiration for this book, and particularly Dean Work and Larry Bauer for their assistance; Larry Hunsicker, President, Nancy Holland, Executive Director, and Arthur Harrell, Staff Director for Professional Education of the American Council on Transplantation, for their help; my own staff members, Mrs. Robin Metheny and Ms. Joyce Herschberger; my wife, Romaine; and my sons, Ezekiel and Zachary, who I hope will never need the knowledge summarized in this book.

HOWARD H. KAUFMAN, M.D.

Morgantown, West Virginia

REFERENCES

Ashwal, S., Schneider, S., 1987, Brain death in children, *Pediatric Neurol.* **3:**5–11, 69–77.
Baldwin, J. C., 1988, Lung transplantation, *JAMA* **259:**2286–2287.
Drake, B., Ashwal, S., Schneider, S., 1986, Determination of cerebral death in the pediatric intensive care unit, *Pediatrics* 78:197–112.
Kaufman, H. H., Lynn, J., 1986, Brain death, *Neurosurgery* **19:**850–856.
Task Force for the Determination of Brain Death in Children: Guidelines for the determination of brain death in children, 1987, *Pediatric Neurol.* **3:**242–243.
Toronto Lung Transplant Group, 1988, Experience with single-lung transplantation for pulmonary fibrosis, *JAMA* **259:**2258–2262.

CONTENTS

ISSUES IN BRAIN DEATH RELATED TO ORGAN DONATION

NEEDS AND POSSIBILITIES IN TRANSPLANTATION

OTHER TOPICS IN ORGAN RETRIEVAL AND DONATION

FUNDING OF TRANSPLANTATION

I

BACKGROUND: INCLUDING HISTORICAL, ETHICAL, LEGAL, AND PRACTICAL CONSIDERATIONS

1

Death-Defining Acts
Historical and Cultural Observations on the End of Life

T. Forcht Dagi

1. INTRODUCTION

For the past two decades, physicians, philosophers, attorneys, legislators, and the public at large have been forced to confront a number of controversies engendered by the Harvard Ad Hoc Committee to Examine the Definition of Brain Death (hereinafter called the Ad Hoc Committee). The voluminous literature that has arisen has concentrated on three areas: the meanings of death and the implications of redefining death in terms of cerebral function, the development of satisfactory criteria for diagnosing brain death, and the establishment of uniform codes for the declaration of death. Despite intensive efforts on the part of many segments of the professional, academic, and policy-making communities, the controversies have not been resolved, nor has the public become reconciled to all aspects of accepted practice.

The literature on brain death may have fixed on the wrong questions. It is not sufficient to redefine death or achieve a consensus regarding the criteria upon which death is to be declared: the problem is first to determine when it becomes permissible to treat people as if they were dead, however death may be defined; and second, how the changes that are contemplated in the management of death will affect accepted standards of behavior. The redefinition of death is only one part of a complex process that results in attitudinal and behavioral changes. If this process is circumvented or abbreviated, the resulting societal dissonance will only heighten the level of controversy. In many ways, this is what has occurred over the past 20 years. Brain death—more precisely, brain-based criteria for the declaration of death—has become widely, although not universally accepted. But as society has reached into the idea of brain death in order to resolve other problems in the management of death, the limits of cultural acceptability have been tested and, quite often, strained.

The purpose of this chapter is to shift the focus of the literature from its preoccupation with

T. Forcht Dagi • Department of Neurosurgery, Brown University, Providence, Rhode Island 02903; Kennedy Institute of Ethics, Georgetown University Law Center, Washington, D. C. 20016.

definitional issues and technical criteria to a consideration of some more fundamental problems. To this end, I shall explore the concept of brain death by reexamining its historical, religious, philosophical and ethical provenance. It is best to begin with a review of the conclusions of the Ad Hoc Committee and why they were criticized.

2. THE HARVARD AD HOC COMMITTEE

In 1968, the *Journal of the American Medical Association* published a report from the Harvard Ad Hoc Committee to Examine the Definition of Brain Death, a group mandated to "define irreversible coma as a new criterion for death." This report profoundly affected the treatment of comatose and hopelessly ill (Beecher, 1968):

> From ancient times down to the recent past it was clear that, when the respiration and heart stopped, the brain would die in a few minutes; so the obvious criterion of no heart beat as synonymous with death was sufficiently accurate. In those times, the heart was considered to be the central organ of the body; it is not surprising that its failure marked the onset of death. This is no longer valid when modern resuscitative and support measures are used. These improved activities can now restore "life" as judged by the ancient standards of persistent respiration and continuing heart beat. This can be the case even when there is not the remotest possibility of an individual recovering consciousness following massive brain damage.

In the words of the Committee (Beecher, 1968), the basis for seeking a new criterion of death originated in the perception that

> (1) Improvements in resuscitative and supportive measures have led to increased efforts to save those who are desperately injured. Sometimes these efforts have only partial success so that the result is an individual whose heart continues to beat but whose brain is irreversibly damaged. The burden is great on patients who suffer permanent loss of intellect, on their families, on the hospitals, and on those in need of hospital beds already occupied by these comatose patients. (2) Obsolete criteria for the definition of death can lead to controversy in obtaining organs for transplantation.

Thus, three factors motivated the Ad Hoc Committee: the fate of patients for whom the application of advanced means of life support resulted prolonged vegetative existence rather than in a cure; the needs of organ transplantation programs; and a sense of critical shortfall in intensive care unit (ICU) beds.

This report engendered considerable controversy. First, the Ad Hoc Committee was criticized for its claim to have redefined death (Beecher, 1968). Many commentators pointed out that the Committee had merely refined techniques for diagnosing death (Capron and Kass, 1982; Veatch, 1976; Walton, 1979; Jonas, 1982) and had redefined very little. Second, the Committee was criticized for polluting its empathy for the patient with utilitarian concerns.* For example, Hans Jonas commented:

---

*The Ad Hoc Committee was motivated to change the definition of death based on two principles that can be described as *empathic* and *instrumental*. Both principles are derived from fundamental philosophical beliefs concerning both the value of life and the scope of entitlement to scarce benefits that are restricted either by physical availability, like well-matched organs for transplantation, or by the character and the limitations of the health care system.

The empathic argument contends that permanent loss of intellect evokes great suffering both in the smitten individual and in those close to him. This argument originates in a dualist view of mankind that is discussed in more detail elsewhere in this essay. Briefly, dualism perceives the human organism to have two parts. The first component, the Divine, noble, or "higher" component, has been called many things, in-

Can I take this as corroborating my initial suspicion that this *interest* [the "transplant interest"], in spite of its notably muted expression in the Committee Report, was and is the major motivation behind the definitional effort? . . . I contend that, pure as this interest, viz., to save other lives, is in itself, its intrusion into the *theoretical* attempt to define death makes the attempt impure; and the Harvard Committee should never have allowed itself to adulterate the purity of its scientific case by baiting it with the prospect of this *extraneous*—though extremely appealing gain" (1982, originally published in 1974). Third, the Committee was accused of failing to distinguish between three sets of overlapping issues: (1) the meanings of death at different levels; (2) the techniques of diagnosing death and the criteria on which such techniques relied; (3) the ethical implications of redefining death. Frazer had identified these issues as determinants of the cultural context of death a generation earlier (1933).

Nonetheless, the Ad Hoc Committee brought the idea of redefining death to public attention. The philosophical literature seemed firmly convinced that a satisfactory analysis of the literal and figurative meanings of death would eliminate most of the controversy, and lead to logical changes in the management of death (Veatch, 1976; Korein, 1978; Walton, 1979; Walters, 1982; Bernat *et al.*, 1982). The medical literature argued with equal fervor that the definition of death was a medical and a scientific issue, rather than a philosophical one,* and that the controversial points could be resolved empirically.

Neither the original criteria formulated by the Ad Hoc Committee nor the various modifications that have arisen ever achieved the universal acceptance to which the Committee had aspired. For example, there has been only limited support for the establishment of a national brain-based standard for the declaration of death (Black and Zervas, 1984). Many physicians continue to require familial consent before declaring brain death (Pinkus, 1984). While the hesitation to diagnose brain death in children can be ascribed to the absence of satisfactory technical standards, (Ad Hoc Committee on Brain Death, Children's Hospital, 1987; Coulter, 1987; President's Commission, 1981), the misgivings surrounding the application of brain-based criteria to adults cannot be explained on this basis alone.

Why the continuing resistance to brain-based criteria? It is important to remember that the

---

cluding "soul," "mind," "reason," and "psyche." Though these entities are quite separate in the history of ideas, they seem to stand for the same thing in one respect: in the dualist paradigm, they are always esteemed and always preferred. They also tend to be metaphysical. The second component, base, material, and more "animal," is generally deprecated, often disdained, and sometimes scorned. Typically, but not exclusively, it refers to the body or its representation.

Behind the perception that the loss of intellect (loss of the "higher" part) constitutes such profound suffering that continuation of life is no longer required, there is a scale of values that derives from the dualist tradition. In this hierarchy, anoesis (consciousness with sensation but without thought) is a less worthy state than confusion (consciousness with sensation and addled thought) because the higher functions of which man is capable, those that distinguish him from animals and vegetables, and have been seen by some to represent the Divine spark, are more deficient. The "suffering" imputed to the true vegetative state must be philosophical rather than physical, because this suffering is independent of neurophysiological sensation.

A more blatantly dualistic argument would have been that the absence of the intellect is equivalent to death. The Ad Hoc Committee did not go this far; others, however, have.

The instrumental argument reflects the frankly utilitarian point of view that the continued institutional support of these individuals *unnecessarily* burdens the health care system while depriving other less "desperately" injured, potentially more salvageable, and perhaps more worthy patients of lifesaving organs for transplantation. This argument incorporates certain principles derived from the social utilitarian tradition in that it subjugates the fate of an individual to teleological designs couched in terms of greater good.

*The President's Commission, for example, sought to simplify discussions of death by defining the issues exclusively in scientific, as opposed to religious, philosophical, or sociological terms (The President's Commission on Bioethics, 1981).

establishment of a new criterion for the diagnosis of death was not an academic exercise. It was intended to facilitate the declaration of death in certain individuals who previously would have been considered alive, because it meant that, as a matter of social policy, their death was either desirable or at least acceptable: therefore, one wished to treat them as if they were already dead. It was not death, the cessation of terrestrial life, that was redefined: it was the criteria for the declaration of death and the factors that determined when it would be permissible to treat people as if they were dead.

3. EVOLUTION OF BRAIN-BASED CRITERIA FOR DEATH: HISTORICAL OVERVIEW

3.1. Death and the Afterlife in Classical Times and the Early Church

Both the Greeks and the Romans believed in an afterlife, but they held inconsistent beliefs regarding which was preferable: the divine gift of immortality and the prolongation of life on this world, or the Elysian fields of the next. Aristotle, for example, held that there was a proper span of life. To be cheated of this normal span was tragic, but to be invested with immortality in the absence of eternal youth was a curse. The Stoics taught the benefits of determining the venue of one's death: this was euthanasia, a good death. The Epicureans maintained that experience ended with death and that the afterlife was irrelevant.

By contrast, the early Church emphasized the importance of the afterlife almost to the exclusion of any other consideration. The most extreme statement to this effect was made by the various Gnostic sects (Jonas, 1958; Walker, 1983). Although most were dismissed as heretical, their influence did not disappear. The deathbed brought an opportunity to confess and to gain absolution. The final rituals of contrition were far more important than efforts to forestall death, not only because medicine was fundamentally incapable of changing the natural course of illness, but because death held the promise of a reunion with God: "We know that while we are at home in the body we are away from the Lord, and we would rather be away from the body and at home with the Lord" (II Cor. 5:6–8).

3.2. Medieval Medicine and Resignation toward Death

Even so, there are strong indications of at least some ambivalence toward a full and unquestioning resignation to death. Although members of the Church engaged in healing, schools in Byzantium, as well as in Rome, Ravenna, Marseilles, and Vienna, openly taught medicine in a "pagan," i.e., non-Christian, secular, context throughout the Dark Ages. Monasteries were renowned for their herbaria, but lay healers competed successfully with clerics in diagnosis and prognosis and sometimes practiced surgery when clerics would not. Scattered cures of abscesses, wounds and hernias gave credence to pagan knowledge, much to the chagrin of a Church propounding the belief that recovery from illness or injury was a miraculous event and an expression of Divine favor (Gordon, 1959).

Nonetheless, the Church gradually dominated the practice of medicine and intensified the ambiguity surrounding the legitimacy of forestalling death.* A tradition called *Ars Moriendi*, the

---

*There were two reasons why clerical medicine eclipsed pagan healing practices. First, the *archiatri*, the official physicians under Byzantine rule, consistently failed to avert or cure the epidemics that regularly swept through populated areas (Gordon, 1959). While clerics fared no better, they at least had spiritual hope to offer as their medicine failed. Second, the "pagan" schools were gradually replaced by cathedral and monastic schools in which *physic*, or medicine, was taught side by side with the classical *trivium* (grammar,

art of dying, contributed significantly to this ambiguity. According to this doctrine, all one's spiritual energy was to be devoted to a contemplation of the immanence of death and the vision of the salvation of one's immortal soul. Because suffering prepared the way for salvation, the relief of bodily ailments was not particularly important. This was the orthodox point of view.

Elsewhere in society, however, on more popular levels, unorthodox traditions held sway. Stories of immortality and rejuvenation had never really been eliminated from popular lore, for example, and several observations suggest that such ideas were tolerated. First, alchemists who sought the key to immortality and explorers who sought the fountain of youth were not rejected on these grounds alone by the Church. Second, when distillation was introduced into Europe, alcohol, initially thought to embody Aristotle's quintessence,* the vital stuff of life, was widely used as a medication in the form of *aquavitae*, the water of life. As a restorative, or cordial, to stimulate the heart, *aquavitae* was touted for its abilities to "restore the fainting high and mighty" (Gruman, 1977). Third, a lay tradition of resuscitation and of resisting death coexisted with the *Ars Moriendi*. Finally, there was the matter of popular heresies. Religious heresies abounded after Chialism, a tenth-century movement that predicted the end of the world at the turn of the milennium, was proved wrong. A number of well-known heresies challenged the Church by questioning doctrines of salvation and the immortality of the soul. The Church responded by embarking on an Inquisition according to the guidelines proposed by Bernardo Gui. The dimensions of this response attest to the magnitude of unorthodox thought that must have been extant at the time.

3.3. The Rise of Humanism and the Appreciation of Earthly Life

When the chiliasts were proved wrong, many projects that had ground to a halt as the continued existence of the world was called into question were resumed in a flurry of new activity. Cathedrals and other monuments attesting to the permanence of human effort were completed, and new ones were begun. The atmosphere in Europe changed in other ways as well.

The classical tradition re-emerged, and an appreciation for secular perspectives began to unfold. The earliest expressions of secular thought were mostly political† and addressed the balance of power between the Church and the secular authorities. Both Dante's *De Monarchia* and Machiavelli's *The Prince* concluded that secular authority ought to prevail. Machiavelli went so far as to argue that the allegiance to one's ruler might outweigh the concern for one's soul. The preeminence of the afterlife was undermined. Marsilio Ficino, an early Platonist, argued that a knowledge of the Good could be obtained and enjoyed in this life, without regard for what would transpire in the next. Boccaccio's *Decameron*, a description of life during the plague of 1348 in Florence, depicts a fundamentally secular and impious society.

The spiritual domination of the Church was eroded by the humanist movement. Humanism emphasized the importance of the private individual rather than the community; it validated a notion of morality outside of theology; it admitted the virtue of beauty and the good of knowledge for its own sake; and it permitted man to arrogate to himself both the privilege of defining the Good and the ability to recognize it (Kristeller, 1961). The contemplative life was divorced from the cloister; the dignity of man was rendered as important as divine worship, and man's nature was believed to be good, the original sin notwithstanding. By the early sixteenth century, in such

---

logic, and rhetoric) and *quadrivivium* (arithmetic, music, geometry, and astronomy). Lay medicine did survive in the end, but only in the form of lithotomists, oculists, and medical itinerants of relatively low repute. When the great European universities and the School of Salerno arose in the eleventh and twelfth centuries, lay medicine was deprecated even further.

*The fifth element of the world after earth, air, fire, and water, believed to be the essense of life and a rejuvenative.

†Except for collections of novellas like *Chansons de Roland*.

works as Juan-Luis Vives's *De Ratione Studii Puerilis Epistolae Duae* (1523), the human animal was portrayed at the center of the universe, capable of playing the roles of all other creatures, and standing halfway between the animals and the angels (Kristeller, 1961). Death no longer offered the same certainty as before, the fate of the soul ceased to preoccupy society, and the theme of *Ars Moriendi* was eclipsed by more meliorist outlooks.

The threat to the Church was thought to be very grave. In 1513, the Fifth Lateran Council denounced anyone who raised doubts concerning the immortality of the soul (Burns, 1972). At the same time, the Church was imperilled by the Protestant Reformation. Here too, doctrinal differences often involved the soul, and eschatology was a central issue. Whereas most Englishmen, for example, held that the immortality of the soul was the basis of the dignity of man, many abandoned the belief that the soul retained consciousness and substantial existence after death (Burns, 1972). The idea of man continued to change under the influence of such writers as Thomas More, Erasmus, Hobbes, and Locke. The purpose of man's existence was now commonly understood to be predicated on achievements on this earth, such as peace, wealth, probity, and happiness. Gradually, the value of terrestrial life was appreciably raised.

This trend was reflected in scholarly and popular writing. In 1638, Sir Francis Bacon proposed that learned men turn immediately to a study of the prolongation of life, although it must be admitted that he reverted to a theological framework in order to justify his proposal. "Our labours . . . ," he wrote, "should be the assistance of the Author of Truth and Life, consider by what meanes the Life of man may be prolonged. For long life being an increasing heape of sinnes and sorrowes lightly esteemed of Christians aspiring to Heaven, should not be dispised, because it affords longer opportunity of doing good Workes. . . . " Death had become an enemy.

4. TESTING DEATH

Bacon was equally concerned with uncertainties in the signs of death and the problem of premature interment. Despite the significance ascribed by various religions to the afterlife, premature interment had always been feared. This horror, first enunciated in ancient times, led to an obligation to test death. This obligation, in turn, evolved into an obligation to resuscitate and resulted in the problems which the Ad Hoc Committee attempted to resolve. The course of this evolution will now be traced.

4.1. Ancient Times

The Roman author Servius ascribed the practice of anointing the dead to a last attempt at awakening those who only appeared deceased (Preuss, 1978). Myths and legends prompted the ancients to delay burial for up to 1 week in an attempt to avert this tragedy (Gould and Pyle, 1956):

> in the eighty-fourth Olympiad, Empedocles restored to life a woman who was about to be buried, and . . . this circumstance induced the Greeks, for the future protection of the supposed dead, to establish laws which enacted that no person should be interred until the sixth or seventh day. But even this extension of time did not give satisfaction, and we read that when Hephestion, at whose funeral obsequies Alexander the Great was present, was to be buried, his funeral was delayed until the tenth day.

Such resuscitations were apparently quite common in Greece, for special regulations existed with respect to persons who gave the appearance of death but recovered after their funeral rites. They were prohibited from worship or from entering the temples under any circumstances (Ducachet, 1822). The Romans followed Greek custom (Gould and Pyle, 1956):

While returning to his country house, Asclepiades, a physician . . . saw during the time of Pompey the Great a crowd of mourners about to start a fire on a funeral pile. It is said that by his superior knowledge he perceived indications of life in the corpse and ordered the pile destroyed, subsequently restoring the supposed deceased to life. These examples and several others of a similar nature induced the Romans to delay their funeral rites and laws were enacted to prevent haste in burning as well as interment. It was not until the eighth day that the final rites were performed, the days immediately subsequent to death having their own special ceremonies.

4.2. Talmudic Law

Talmudic Law ruled that intervention to preserve life was mandatory whenever the opportunity presented itself. While the Talmud showed an awareness of potential problems in the definitive diagnosis of death, it placed a premium on immediate burial, even at the risk of premature interment. Evidence of respiratory arrest was deemed sufficient to declare death. Certain limited precautions could be taken in individual cases if there were firm grounds on which to suspect premature interment (Preuss, 1978; Soleveichik, 1978; Tendler, 1978; Rosner, 1986; Bleich, 1986; Dagi, 1987).

4.3. Europe Prior to the Seventeenth Century

Scattered accounts indicate that premature interment was a continuing concern in folk medicine but rarely concerned the healing professions. Primitive resuscitation techniques were carried out whenever death was unexpected, undesirable, or uncertain. After hangings, after drownings, after some industrial accidents, and in some cases of sudden death, the appearance of death was not automatically equated with death in fact (Dagi, 1986).

4.4. Europe during the Enlightenment

In his *Historie of Life and Death* (1638), Bacon asserted that some deaths were preventable and reversible: "The doores of Death are Accidents going before, or following after, or coming with Death. . . . " He collected accounts of premature interment: "Many laid forth, conffin'd & buried . . . hath bin discovered by digging them up agayne, and finding their heads beaten and bruised with striving in the Coffin" and demanded that physicians study ways "To rayse and recover to life such as faint and fall into a swond (in which fits many without helpe would expire). . . . " Failing in this endeavor, they would be obliged to establish reliable indicators of death in order to prevent the tragedy of premature burial. Such indicators, Bacon suggested, would include "Convulsions of the Head and Face, with deepe deadly sighing . . . and the extreme quicke beating of the Pulse, the Heart trembling with the pangs of death. . . . " This stands out as one of the earliest formulations of what can be termed the technical problem: What are the reliable signs of death, short of cadaveric putrefaction?

Many of Bacon's ideas were commonly shared. Cerimon of Ephesus in Shakespeare's *Pericles* declares that:

> Death may usurp on nature many hours
> And yet the fire of life kindle again
> The o'epress'd spirits. I heard of an Egyptian
> That had nine hours lain dead
> Who was by good appliance recovered.
> (3.2.82–86)

It was particularly feared that death and sleep would be confused, or else that herbs and drugs could produce, intentionally or by accident, a state indistinguishable from death. This situation was described in *Romeo and Juliet* when Friar Lawrence says to Juliet:

> Take though this vial, being then in bed,
> And this distilling liquor drink thou off,
> When presently through all thy veins shall run
> A cold and drowsy humour—for no pulse
> Shall keep his native progress, but surcease:
> No warmth, no breath shall testify thou livest;
> The roses in thy lips and cheeks shall fade
> To wanny ashes, thy eyes' windows fall
> Like Death when he shuts up the day of life,
> Each part, depriv'd of supple government,
> Shall stiff and stark and cold appear like death,
> And in this borrow'd likeness of shrunk death
> Thou shalt continue two and forty hours
> And then awake as from a pleasant sleep.''
>
> (4.1.93–106)

Specific precautions were taken against such calamities. A will dated 1652 (Aries, 1982) stipulates: "I wish and ordain that *twenty-four hours* after my decease my body be opened, embalmed, placed in a lead coffin. . . ." (emphasis added). The testator wished to delay his funeral to make certain that he was actually dead before entombment. Scarification and autopsy were added as an additional precautions against premature burial. In 1696, Elisabeth d'Orleans required that before burial she "first be scratched twice with a razor on the soles of the feet" (Aries, 1982). Later, "opening the body," a dissection initially performed for the purpose of embalming or dismembering the body prior to transporting it for burial, became a method of testing the appearance of death. The comptesse de Sauvigny, for example, willed that "[I] be opened 48 hours after my death, and during the interval I wish to be left in my bed" (Aries, 1982). Delay before burial, lamentations, anointment, display of the cadaver, and finally the *conclamatio*—hailing the deceased three times by name in a loud voice—were all invested with religious or symbolic value as part of the mourning ritual, while hoping to distinguish those who only appeared dead from those who were.

In Paris, in 1740, Jacques Benigne Winslow published a seminal work entitled *Quaestio Medico-chirurgica . . . An Mortis Incertae Signa Minus Incerta a Chirurgis, Quam ab Aliis Experiments*. Within two years, it was translated by Jacques-Jean Bruhier d'Ablaincourt into French (Winslow, 1742), and then into English as *The Uncertainty of the Signs of Death and the Danger of Precipitate Interments and Dissections . . . with Proper Directions, Both for Preventing Such Accidents, and Repairing the Misfortunes upon the Constitutions by Them* (Winslow, 1746). This became one of the most influential works of the age*:

> Though death come at some Time or other is the necessary and avoidable PORTION of HUMAN NATURE in its present Condition, it is not always certain, that Persons taken for dead are really and irretrievably deprived of Life; since it is evidence from experience, that many apparently dead, have afterwards proved themselves alive arising from their shrowds, their Coffins, and even from their deaths . . . Incontestable Facts evince that some Subjects, too rashly laid open, have upon feeling the Smart of dissecting Instruments, by their mournful Shrieks and Cries, discovered their too certain Marks of Life, and by that lamentable circumstance exposed the unwary Operator to eternal Infamy, and the implacable Indignation of their surviving Friends'' (section I,b).

---

*It is thought that Winslow had been taken for dead as a child, and narrowly missed premature burial.

An inspectorate of the dead was proposèd. A royal decree soon dictated that "Persons who shall find themselves near a sick man at the time of his presumed decease shall in future refrain from covering him and wrapping his face, removing him from his bed and laying him on a straw or horsehair mattress, thereby exposing him to too cold an air" (Aries, 1982). Elsewhere in Europe, "funeral homes" called *vitae dubiae azilia* (havens of doubtful life) were established to provide repositories where bodies could be stored until they began to decompose. They gained early favor in Weimar, in Berlin, in Munich, and in Mainz. Later, a special provision of the code Napoleon stipulated that no interment should take place without a permit from a public officer, and that this officer should visit the corpse within 24 hr after death* (Ducachet, 1822).

In England, *The Uncertainty of Signs of Death* (Winslow, 1746) inspired Hawes, Fothergill, Johnson, and others to establish a resuscitation society under royal patronage, similar to the one that had achieved great success in Amsterdam. Death, wrote Hawes, could not always be distinguished from life and should be the focus of special and vigilant attention. Bruhier,† he concluded, had

> clearly proved, from the Testimonies of various Authors, and the Attestations of unexceptionable Witnesses, that many Persons who have been buried alive, and were providentially discovered in that State, *had been rescued from the Grave,* and enjoyed the *Pleasures of Society* for several Years after. . . .

In 1782, Hawes wrote:

> I am willing, however, to hope, that since it has been of late *so frequently* demonstrated, that the *vital Principle* may exist, where the Characteristics of Death, except Putrefaction, are present, *the rational Part of the Community* are, at length, disposed to pay some Attention to this Subject.

The resuscitation movement spread throughout Europe and England. In America, it was greeted with great enthusiasm, particularly in Boston, New York, and Philadelphia. The degree of contemporary enthusiasm can be appreciated in the following address by Dr. Benjamin Say to the Philadelphia Humane Society (Say, 1799):

> The Royal Humane Society of London have enlarged and greatly improved the plan of resuscitation, and have extended relief to all sudden cases of apparent death; and aggreably to their reports, several *hundred* lives are preserved by their rewards and drags every year, and since the establishment of that Society, more than *two thousand* persons have been rescued from death.
>
> Previously to the establishment of Societies on their excellent plan, *thousands* of our fellow creatures have been consigned to the tomb, with the unextinguished sparks of life remaining in them, and perhaps many of them in an unprepared state to meet their Creator in a world of spirits.
>
> Where then can we draw the line between life and death? How shall we determine that our fellow mortal laying before us motionless is dead or not? Shall we hastily close his eyes and

---

*"Aucune inhumation ne sera faite sans une autorization, sur papier libre et sans frais, de l'officier de l'état civil, qui ne pourra la délivre qu'après s'être transporte auprès de la personne décédée, pour s'assurer du décès, et que vingt-quatre heures après le décès, hors les cas prévus par les réglements de police (Art. 77). L'act de décès sera dressé par l'officier de l'état civil, sur la déclaration de deux témoin. Ces deux témoins seront, s'il est possible, les deux plus proches, parents ou voisins, ou, lorsqu'une personne sera decédée hors de son domicile, la personne chez laquelle elle sera decedée, et un parent ou autre. (Art. 78)"

†Although Bruhier was only Winslow's translator, authorship of the English text was often mistakenly ascribed to him.

consign him to the grave, without any exertion for his restoration, even though his life has been suspended for two or three hours? no, let us not display such pusillanimity, such inhumanity! Let us rather make use of our best endeavours to put in motion the precious tide of life, and, if we should have the gratification of succeeding, in one influence out of a great number, it will fully repay us for all our exertions.

Initially, the humane societies concentrated on resuscitating those who drowned. Soon, their purview widened to all cases of sudden death, regardless of cause or age (Hawes, 1782):

Even in old age, where life seems to have been gradually drawing to a close the appearances of death are often fallacious.

In 1780, Hawes wrote:

Not many years since, a lady in Cornwall, more than 80 years of age, who had been a considerable time declining, took to her bed, and come a few days, seemingly expired in the morning. As she had often desired not to be buried, till she had been two days dead, her request was to have been regularly complied with by her relations. All that saw her looked upon her as dead, and the report was current through the whole place; nay, a gentleman of the town actually wrote to his friend in the island of Sicily, that she was deceased. But one of those who were paying the last kind office of humanity to her remains, perceived some warmth about the middle of the back, and acquainting her friends with it, they applied a mirrour to her mouth; but after repeated trials, could not observe it in the least gained. Her under jaw was likewise falling, as the common phrase is, and, in short, she had every appearance of a dead person. All this time she had not been stripped or undressed, but the windows were open, as is usual in the chamber of the deceased. In the evening, the heat seemed to increase, and at length she was perceived to breathe. . . .

In 1819, Whiter proposed that the obligation to test the veracity of death be extended to all maladies:

It is recommended that the same Remedies of the Resuscitative Process should be applied to cases of Natural Death, As they are to cases of Violent Death, Drowning, &c. under the same hope of sometimes succeeding in the attempt.

He continued,

The great discovery, which has been made by the Humane Societies does not consist in supplying any new principles, by which we can infallibly decide, that the powers of life are totally and irrecoverably annihilated. On the contrary, they have taught us, that those ordinary signs of Death, which have ever been regarded as infallible criterions of the absolute extinction of the vital principle are all doubtful and fallacious, and that they afford us no evidence whatever on which our decisions can be formed. They have proclaimed to mankind in the most express and unequivocal manner, at least from the force and spirit of their discoveries, that the only evidence on the total extinction of Life is to be found in that mode of decision, to which they have themselves resorted in those peculiar instances, which they have undertaken to examine. This evidence consists in actual experiment on every case, which is presented to the attention; and we are not authorised to pronounce our sentence on the question of absolute and irremediable Death, till all the arts of resuscitation have been applied without effect, which are at present to be found within the sphere of our knowledge. . . . The absence of apparent motion and sensation still continues in these times as in all the past, to be regarded in our ordinary practice as an infallible criterion of the annihilation of life; and on this conclusion at this moment, through the whole extent of the globe, we consign our fellow creatures to their graves, without reflection or remorse.

This proposal marks the acknowledgment of a new imperative, to which religion was soon accommodated. Initially, these ideas were cautiously presented. Dr. Say (1799), for example, closed his address to the Philadelphia Humane Society with a scriptural proof test supporting the prolongation of life:

> Yes, this idea has been most forcibly and happily expressed by our Saviour in the following words: "For what shall it profit a man if he gains the whole world and loses his own life? or what shall he give in exchange for his life?"

Soon these ideas evolved into an eschatology that distinguished accidental or unintended death from the true end of life and proclaimed Divine sanction to overcome the former (Bosworth, 1814):

> In concluding these addresses I would take occasion to remind you of your obligations to Him who hath hitherto preserved you. . . . Cherish towards him the most lively gratitude; and . . . embrace, with all your hearts, the Gospel of Sons; and then you need not doubt that he will not only be your God and your Guide even unto death, but will also at length raise you to the happy place where you shall be out of reach of *accident and calamity* in every form; where "there shall be no more pain," neither sickness nor death; and whence "sorrow and sin" shall flee away, 'to return no more for ever (emphasis added).

Finally, these ideas were cast as a moral responsibility, a Christian duty second only to religion as the subject most fit for man's atttentions (Snart, 1824):

> preservation from the *horrors of the grave by premature interment* . . . A subject (next to *religion*) paramount to all others, and the result of many years serious reflection of a son of sorrow and adversity, conscientiously stimulated to this most imperious moral duty by *humanity*.

> If the author's feeble efforts to convince you of the necessity of interfering in this momentous affair should excite a disposition to see its importance, and your benevolence should impel you to give it full effect, it will satisfy him that having justified his existence . . . he will leave the world better then he *found* it; and, in due time, quietly resign himself to his parent earth, persuaded he was not born or lived in vain.

Life is in the hands of man: neither fixed, nor preordained, and certainly not inferior to the afterlife.* Life was seen as good, nature as rational and benign (Ford, 1961), and prolonged earthly existence a self-evident good.

From this point onward, a failed resuscitation attempt would be taken, in all critical discussions, as the only definitive proof of death (Ducachet, 1822). All that remained was to determine how to resuscitate; the answer evolved from advances in cardiorespiratory physiology over the next century and a half.

5. TECHNICAL ISSUES AND THEORIES ABOUT LIFE AND DEATH

By the first quarter of the eighteenth century, it was widely accepted that external signs of death did not necessarily correspond to death in fact. Many unanswered technical questions about the signs of death were debated in anecdotal reports published under the auspices of resuscitation societies and in the scientific literature. Experimenters sought to define the nature of death by discovering the essence of life and determining when and how that essence was irrecoverably lost.

The background of this endeavor is not widely appreciated. For many centuries, there were two competing beliefs about the nature of death. Death was either perceived to be a sudden event, the result of the loss or separation of some essential quality or substance from the body or was

---

*Three works contributed to the intellectual atmosphere in which this point of view could flourish: Descartes' *Discourse on Method* (1635); La Mettrié's *Man a Machine* (1748), which denied the existence of both God and the soul; and Helvétius' *On Man*, which depicted a God denying His own existence.

understood to be a gradual process, with intermediate stages resembling sleep intervening between life and death (Aries, 1981). Both models allowed for the notion of latent life—a window of time during which the soul (or its equivalent) could be recalled or restored, but they differed significantly in may other ways. Uncertainty about the nature of death went hand in hand with uncertainty about the signs of death; both issues were now perceived as acutely pressing.

One of the most influential works on the nature of death was written by Xavier Bichat, a respected nineteenth century Parisian surgeon (1809). Bichat adhered to the dynamist school of physiology that was in vogue at the time. The "principles of animation" were described in terms of movement that was either spontaneous or irritable, i.e., provokable by external (usually galvanic) stimuli. While acknowledging that the absence of spontaneous movement was not necessarily the same as death, experimenters sought the origins of spontaneity in "a certain something [that] does constantly pervade the whole system, and give life and activity to every fibre" (Adams, 1799). According to some scientists, oxygen, then newly discovered, was the most likely candidate. Others were less certain. In any event, two conclusions reached by Bichat had enormous import: (1) a rejection of the brain as the locus of death, on the grounds that the severence of nerves and the disconnection or removal of the brain from body parts had failed to impede irritability or to impair heartbeat*; and (2) an inference that death was a gradual process rather than a single sudden event, the result of a slow, inexorable deterioration of body systems.†

---

*Bichat considered whether the death of the brain constituted death of the organism. Spontaneous movement was the paradigmatic proof of life. He conducted experiments on decapitated corpses to determine whether movement of the heart could be instigated by galvanic stimulation between the heart and an element of the nervous system.

> I had authority, during the winter of the year 7 [after the Revolution] (1798) to make different experiments upon the bodies of those *guillotined*. They were at my disposal thirty or forty minutes after the execution. In some every species of *mobility* was extinct; and in others this property was restored with greater or less facility in all the muscles, by common agents. It was developed, particularly in the muscles of animal life, by galvanism. But it was in all impossible to produce the slightest motion by arming, [placing electrodes upon and stimulating] either the spinal marrow and the heart, or this last organ and the nerves which it receives from the ganglions by the sympathetic, or from the brain by the *par vagum*. Mechanical *exertants* however directly applied to the fleshy fibres, produced contraction in them. Was this occasioned by the nervous filaments of the heart having been for some time without connexion with the brain? But then, why should the voluntary muscles, equally removed from the connexions, yield to galvanic phenomena?

> . . . Thus have I offered a sufficient number of proofs drawn from observation of diseases as well as from experiments, to answer, I trust, the question proposed in this section, and to justify the assertion that the brain exercises no direct influence on the heart; and that consequently when the first ceases to act, it is indirectly only that the functions of the second are interrupted.

†Bichat posited that human life consisted of animal and organic elements or functions that achieved a homeostasis between synthesis and degeneration, without which the body would decompose as it did after death. "Life," he wrote, "is the totality of those functions which resist death."

In the classical tradition, Bichat distinguished between animal life, representing the sensations, all voluntary motion, and the totality of human experience and communication, and organic life, representing the processes of alimentation and excretion that were shared by all "organized beings, vegetable or animal." Natural death would occur through the gradual extinction of animal life, long before organic life had ceased:

> Observe the man who sinks under extreme old age: he dies gradually; his external functions cease the one after the other; all his senses are closed in succession; the ordinary causes of sensation pass over them without affecting them. . . .

> Thus isolated in the midst of nature, already partly deprived of the functions of the sensitive organs, the old man is soon destined to experience the extinction of thoe of the brain also. Perception no longer exists, inasmuch as there remains nothing on the part of the senses, to produce its exercise; imagination grows dull and is soon altogether lost.

In the end, "the *whole* of the functions cease only because each is successively extinguished . . . the heart is the last to finish its contractions: it is, as has been said, the *ultimum moriens.*"

Neither the work of Bichat nor that of his contemporaries provided satisfactory answers to the fundamental questions that were being asked about the principles of life. Nonetheless, the bureaucratic process of declaring death increasingly relied upon physicians in the hope of preventing misdiagnosis (Ducachet, 1822; Snart, 1824; Aries, 1982). The failure of resuscitation to restore breathing and heartbeat became, *de facto,* the strictest criterion for determining death. Death was reformulated not simply as the *lack* of "vital signs" (literally, "signs of life"), but as the *irreversible loss* of vital signs.

5.1. The Modern Era of Resuscitation and Intensive Care

Throughout the nineteenth and early twentieth centuries, advances in cardiorespiratory physiology were immediately applied to resuscitation techniques. The general imperative to preserve life came to be coupled with a perceived duty to apply the most sophisticated technology to all situations.* There were some cautionary voices: Sir William Osler described pneumonia as the "old man's friend," implying that it was not always necessary to prolong life. On the whole, however, the "miracles of modern medicine" were viewed without ambivalence until the mid-1960s and the crisis of the intensive care unit (ICU).

The extent of the enthusiasm for resuscitation and related aspects of the technological imperative can be sensed from the classic report describing cardiopulmonary resuscitation (CPR) without operative exposure of the heart or the use of external machinery (Kouwenhoven *et al.,* 1960):

> anyone, anywhere, can now initiate cardiac resuscitative procedures. All that is needed are two hands. Supportive drug treatment and other measures may be given. The necessity for a thoracotomy is eliminated. The real value of the method lies in the fact that it can be used wherever the emergency arises, whether this is in or out of the hospital.

This simple technique allowed every death to be challenged by an effort at resuscitation. It was seized upon by the American Red Cross, the Royal Humane Society, and similar philanthropic organizations as a method that could easily be learned by the lay public. How could one argue with the worthiness of a technique that saved lives? Ironically, it also led to a reformulation of CPR as a professional technique. Although the lay public was now taught CPR with more dedication than before, the compelling purpose was to get the patient to the hospital, where physicians would take over.

It was initially believed that cardiac intensive care and improvements in resuscitation techniques would markedly reduce mortality from myocardial disease and cardiac arrest. Promising results were reported from the prompt diagnosis and treatment of previously undetected cardiac arrhythmias. Soon, the idea of intensive care was expanded from a room in which there was a concentration of nurses, physicians, and monitoring equipment, to a method of treating serious disease. The literature of the 1960s conveys the image of intensive care as a therapeutic modality. This initial enthusiasm was tempered by several factors.

5.2. Unexpected Difficulties

The tendency to place all seriously ill patients in specialized ICUs created several unexpected issues. First, ICUs had limited capacity, and there was significant competition for beds. What criteria should be used for decision-making at the intake stage? Second, a raft of problems arose when patients who were placed on life-support systems neither recovered nor died but simply languished. When could patients be removed from intensive care without risking accusations of malpractice or worse? Third, intensive care was perceived as the most modern and the "best"

*The so-called "technological imperative."

medicine. It carried new prestige and increased status, and led to a *de facto* division of hospital care into two tiers: intensive and nonintensive. How would hospitals function with a two-tier system of medical care? What were the implications of removing a patient from the ICU and transferring that individual to an "ordinary" ward? What to do with patients for whom intensive care had proved futile?

5.3. The "Right to Die" Movement

To complicate the picture, the lay press began to enunciate two contradictory apprehensions: first, a fear of that resuscitation would be carried out uncritically, purely in response to a technological imperative; and second, a fear that CPR would be arbitrarily denied. It was understood that the obligation to resuscitate would be absolute were health, youth, and "quality of mind" reinstated with cardiac output. As it became apparent to the public that resuscitation did not uniformly achieve these goals, disillusionment was translated into a desire for control of the time and manner of one's death. This grew into a movement for the "right" to die. The second apprehension never took root to the same extent.

5.4. Transplantation

The last consideration to affect the management of patients who failed to recover in the ICU was the burgeoning interest in transplantion. By the late 1960s, transplantation was no longer considered experimental. Potential recipients outnumbered available donors. While kidneys could be obtained from cadavers, other organs, especially the heart, could not. There was a felt need to define a category of patient from whom transplantable organs could be removed without damage to the organ, and without affecting the prognosis of the patient.

5.5. The Need to Redefine Death

These issues were met by a host of responses. One of the most appealing in its directness was the redefinition, reformulation, and reconceptualization of the meanings of death. If it were possible to declare death legitimately before a patient were removed from life-support systems, the competition for intensive care beds could be eased, organ transplantation would be facilitated, and fears of inappropriate prolongation of life could be assuaged. Two prerequisites had to be fulfilled before the reformulation of death could proceed: first, it would be necessary to discover a precedent for weakening the obligation to resuscitate and the obligation to prolong life, thereby reversing the trend of the past two centuries; and second, it would be necessary to define death by criteria that did not depend primarily on the cardiorespiratory function that life-support systems artificially preserved. New signs of death were sought.

5.6. Ordinary and Extraordinary Means

The stage had been set in 1957, when Pope Pius XII conceded that in cases of prolonged coma, the soul may have already left the body; that "extraordinary means" need not be employed to prolong life when recovery was hopeless; and that physicians were empowered to determine the time of death (Pius XII, 1957). This allocution confirmed the authority of the physician—at least in the Catholic world—to determine when patients could be treated as if they were dead for religious and legal purposes. The criteria to be used were not specified: it was understood that they would be grounded in medical science.

5.7. From Coma Dépassé to the Ad Hoc Committee

The second development occurred in 1959, when French neuroscientists provided the first detailed description of a condition they termed *coma dépassé* (Korein, 1978; Mollaret and Goulon, 1959): irreversible loss of consciousness in the face of electroencephalographic (EEG) silence. Postmortem examination of a group of patients showed profound structural damage and autolysis of the brain. Although this condition had been recognized in the past, it had not been studied well, nor had it been studied in the context of redefining death. Could this condition offer the key to declarations of death on grounds independent of continuing—if artificially sustained—cardiorespiratory function?

In 1967, the Harvard Ad Hoc Committee was created to consider this question (Beecher, 1968). The history from that point onward is well documented (Korein, 1978; Black, 1978; Veatch, 1981; Jonas, 1982; Walters, 1982; Veatch, 1982; Kaufman and Lynn, 1986). In adults, brain-based criteria for death became well established (Capron and Kass, 1972; Black, 1978) and, at last count, had been adopted with various modifications as statutory law in 37 states (Guidelines for the Determination of Death, 1981; Kaufman and Lynn, 1986). The problem of brain death in children was deferred. Technical standards for irrecoverability were not considered reliable in the pediatric age range.

Religious leaders in the United States were not adverse to accepting brain death as a new concept of death. Catholic thought was shaped by the allocution of Pope Pius XII. Protestant denominations on the whole were content to rely on medical expertise to use whatever criteria for death that seemed appropriate. Orthodox Jewish groups, however, could not accept brain-death criteria in their entirety because they conflicted with specific Talmudic statutes defining death and the treatment of the moribund (Preuss, 1978; Soleveichik, 1978; Tendler, 1978; Bleich, 1986; Rosner, 1986). It is interesting to note that an attempt to legislate the mandatory use of brain-death criteria in California was successfully opposed in 1985 by a coalition of surprisingly varied religious groups (Professor David Saperstein, Georgetown University Law Center, personal communication).

6. THE MEANING OF DEATH

For reasons that have already been noted, the proposal of brain based criteria for death led to a general reappraisal of the meaning of death. This was an unusual subject for physicians and scientists, and even for most modern philosophers to consider. Theology, on the other hand, had always speculated about eschatology and the experience of death, so much so that until relatively recent times, any attempt to speak of death in nontheological terms would have been considered highly controversial and would have attracted only limited interest. Yet both the Ad Hoc Committee and the President's Commission made a special point of continuing their deliberations to the secular realm. Why was this an issue?

6.1. Secular and Religious Interpretations of Death

It has been suggested that death in the secular sense alludes to "total and irreversible extinction of consciousness and sensation, including discontinuation of actual survival of the individual personality," whereas the religious notion "postulates actual survival of the individual personality and continuation of *post mortem* consciousness and sensation" (Walton, 1979). Thus, postmortem survival of consciousness is said to be the salient difference: I disagree.

What made some philosophies secular was not simply that they denied the survival of individual personality, but that they repudiated postmortem accountability for one's actions (Charon, 1963; Wolfson, 1965; Walton, 1979; Carrick, 1985).* Secular views of death also disagree about the involvement of preternatural forces in the afterlife and the significance of death to beliefs about cosmogony and human ontogeny.†

Secular thought does not depend on external authority for moral behavior; its view of life can be centered on man; and its ideas of cosmogony do not depend on the intervention of a prime mover preceding man, a predetermined purpose, or a non-natural explanation. Man's dominion is not subjugated to higher powers. If sacred and profane distinctions exist, they are explained rationally.

The secular view of death is satisfied to focus on individual experience up until, through, and including the moment of death. It need not be concerned with what happens afterwards. It requires neither speculation about the afterlife nor preternatural explanations about life or death in order to achieve theoretical completeness.

By contrast, religion is concerned with the definition and legitimization of moral precepts and the motivation of moral behavior by recourse to and by dependence upon actual external (suprahuman) authority.‡ The overall purpose of life is described in relation to god(s) or other objects of worship. Religions attributed the creation of the universe and the imposition of man's dominion upon earth to nonrandom, purposeful events, emanating from a suprahuman power, and dividing the world into the sacred and the profane. Thus, the religious view portrays death as a part of the continuum of human experience invested with moral significance.

Religious thought invariably includes beliefs about humankind that presume the powers of the human species to be both limited by death and comprehended within, but not coextensive with, the dominion (or dominions) of (an)other, and therefore more powerful force (or forces),** whose continuing existence is unaffected by the death of individual creatures.***

The distinctions between religious and secular interpretations of death are strikingly reflected

---

*Two ancient examples of secular approaches to death are Stoicism and Epicureanism. The Stoics believed that the individual soul is destroyed in death. In Epicureanism:

1. The soul was felt to be corporeal, dissolving, like the body, into atoms after death;
2. Because a soul without a body had no consciousness, an individual resurrected would have no recollection of his former life;
3. The disembodied soul, incapable of experiencing need, was equally incapable of experiencing pleasure—it had no wants and no desires (Wolfson, 1965).

Both the Talmud and the Church fathers worked to disprove these arguments: the Talmud because of a repugnance to the moral turpitude that overcame, in the view of rabbinical authorities, societies that abandoned a belief in the afterlife; and the Church fathers "not to explain why they believed in this twofold doctrine (of immortality and resurrection), but rather to show, on the basis of . . . philosophic testimonials and analogies, that it was not logically absurd (to hold this belief)" (Wolfson, 1965). Indeed, this is why Epicureanism was strongly rejected by Talmudic Judaism and patristic Christianity (Wolfson, 1965).

†Walton, I think, admits as much: "each of these views is related to a broad philosophical theory of *life* or *man* that does not stand or fall in any obvious way on any well-circumscribed set of observations concerning death."

‡Firth has an "ideal observer" theory of ethical authority, which hypothesizes what an ideal observer would do were it to exist. By not requiring, and implicitly denying, the *actual* existence of this observer, Firth avoids the pitfall of proposing an ethical system dependent upon an unidentified godlike entity.

**This use of dominion corresponds to the Hebrew *RST*. Cf. Segel (1977).

***It is possible for religions to find the afterlife irrelevant. This seems to have been a prominent motif in preMaccabean Judaism (prior to the 2nd century B.C.E.). Nonetheless, the doctrine of eventual accountability for one's actions is dominant in all religions, even if there is ambivalence between rewarding virtue by the quality of one's earthly existence and prolongevism, and rewarding virtue in the afterlife. This dilemma is highlighted, for example, in the Book of Job.

in differences between religious and philosophical interpretations of the soul.* In modern society, these differences are also reflected in ideas about the mind.

6.2. The Soul

It is not always possible to separate perceptions of reality from allegorical imagery in ideas about death. The soul, for example, may be depicted as an actual entity or as a metaphysical quality. It may be portrayed as life-making or life-giving. It may be thought to represent the essence of God in man. While the soul is sometimes construed as mortal (the existence of the soul ends with death of the body), this construction has usually fallen outside the stream of Western religious orthodoxy.†

Most religions, for example, teach that some distinct soul-like entity (however it may be known) exists within the body and contributes to it certain discrete characteristics associated with the presence of life. The fetus is at some point ensouled, at which point human life begins. Death, the end of terrestrial life as we know it, is marked by a disensoulment. The soul separates from the body and goes its own way.

What is the relationship between death and the separation of the body and the soul? Are they causally, even reciprocally related? Can both be caused by another force or event? Is the soul liberated with cessation of heartbeat? Is the soul a physical entity whose movement can be facilitated or impeded? If the soul is perceived as a physical entity, is there a specific organ it inhabits, so that the destruction of that organ is tantamount to losing the soul? Is resuscitation quite literally the recalling of a soul through a window in time, a period of "latent life" during which it hovers around the body, no longer present but not quite gone?

For the moment, let us focus only on the putative relationship between death and the soul. If it is believed that death occurs only after the soul has quit the body, the criteria for death are defined by the ways in which one can be sure that the soul has departed (e.g., it was once quite seriously suggested that the body could be weighed, and death could be proven by demonstrating that the corpse was lighter than the living body).

Some peculiar problems arise if one believes that a soul-less body can endure or "survive." Traditions that really believe that disensouled bodies can survive in a state of "apparent life" consider these bodies abhorrent, like vampires or zombies, and have no qualms about destroying them. They are not protected by the usual ethical principles that proscribe bodily harm to another human being, nor do they induce such ordinary human emotions as pity.‡

How, then, do we know that something is alive, or animate, rather than dead, or inanimate? If it has a soul, it is animate, and presumably alive. But how do we know it has a soul? Historically, religion, philosophy, and science have claimed the ability to distinguish through revelation or observation between classes of entities that are animate and those that are inanimate. The

---

*Orthodoxy surrounding beliefs about death has been very important historically, so much so that it often separated sects that could be tolerated as legitimate variations of institutionalized religious life from heresies that came to be repudiated (Segal, 1977).

†Significant departures from orthodoxy have taken two forms: views of death that are religiously oriented, but do not conform to orthodox belief; and beliefs about death that are independent of religion or even oppose religious thought (Piltcher, 1940; Aries, 1982; Anderson, 1986).

‡Defective souls have been invoked to explain many phenomena. In German concentration camps, for example, there was a special category of inmate called "Moslem" by the other inmates. this individual was closer to death, but in a different way from others. The Moslem had lost the will to live: some said the soul. It took great effort on the part of the spiritual leader of the camps to prevent these people from being treated as if they were dead before they were. The same type of phenomenon has been experienced by people in shipwrecks, epidemics, and other natural disasters.

question of whether a given representative of this class is alive or dead turns on the presence of some minimal function or spontaneous activity. The most frequently cited sign of life is movement, but there are others as well. Just as apparent death is not death, apparent life is not always life. A soul-less body is only apparently alive, and may be treated as a corpse, as if it were dead, even though it is capable of spontaneous motion—ordinarily one of the incontrovertible signs of life.

The concept of movement as a sign of life is called *quickening,* a word in Old English derived from congeners of the Latin *vivus* and the Greek *bios,* meaning "life" or "alive."* Quickening in contemporary speech is a technical term that refers to the first movements of the fetus *in utero*. It has been used liturgically to allude to the Divine ability to instill life into corpses: to *quicken* the dead.

Any entity that belongs to the class of living things is therefore presumed to be alive when it quickens, and so long as it quickens. The soul is presumed to be present in any member of the class as long as it quickens, because a soul is held to be characteristic of the class as a whole.

Historically, with the exception of certain instances of diabolical or preternatural possession, any human being capable of movement was considered ensouled and alive. The notion of movement extended to movement of the heart and lungs, which is one reason why the cessation of heartbeat and respiration have continued to maintain pre-eminence as criteria for death. Lack of movement was equated with apparent death. But the translation from apparent death to "real death" depended on one additional step historically couched first in spiritual terms as the irrecoverable departure of the soul, and later in technical terms as the failure of resuscitation. The irrecoverable departure of the soul meant that something essential (i.e., of the essence of the organism) and irreplaceable had been lost. But evidence of disensoulment was not usually sought until after movement had ceased. The failure of resuscitation was taken to mean simply that the absence of movement was irreversible.

Most belief systems have not dwelt on whether the loss of the soul is marked by or caused by a physiological event. They stress contemporaneity rather than causality: i.e, when the heart stops and when respirations cease such that a mirror held to the nostrils will not fog, then (and only then) may one assume that the soul has departed, and only then may one regard the body as a corpse rather than a living being. A period of "latent life" after death generally serves as a buffer for the uncertainty of death, especially when it is believed that the soul survives and may return to reinhabit the body or to haunt the surroundings of its own volition or in response to prayers, charms, or spells.

Most religiously derived soul-oriented belief systems, unlike other models of death, find some degree of uncertainty reasonably syntonic and do not require absolute certainty regarding the moment or the mechanism of death so long as the declaration of death or the rituals that follow are not obviously premature or in error. To the extent that a belief system regards liberation of the soul from the material body as preferable, the criteria for death become quite relaxed and relatively unconcerned with precise timing (the issue of premature burial is, as we have seen, altogether different). By contrast, belief systems that deny the continued existence of the soul after death are more likely to stretch the time accorded to life or, for reasons to be considered next, to seek control over the time and the manner of one's death.†

---

*The antonym is *still,* as in still-born, i.e., born without movement and therefore dead (Oxford English Dictionary, 1971).

†A great deal depends on whether death is considered good, bad, or indifferent. To the extent that one believes in an afterlife, death is the portal by which to attain it. If the afterlife is contemplated with pleasure, death holds little fear. If the afterlife is anticipated with dread, death becomes terrifying. If one believes that life is good, its prolongation becomes desirable. If one believes that the afterlife is preferable, the span of life becomes less relevant. If one believes that suffering predisposes to a better afterlife, suffering is wel-

In secular philosophy, the soul may be considered the essence of man, in whose absence a person may be treated as if he were dead, but in most religions, the presence of a sacred soul is equated with life, and its absence *is* death. Thus, the secular philosophical soul and the religious soul are not strictly analogous. The difference between them proves central to the understanding differences in the management of death.

6.3. The Soul and the Mind

Aristotle, in differentiating between human life and the lives of other living creatures, formulated a hierarchical organization that ranged from the lowest vegetative to the highest animal form. Man, however, he saw as qualitatively different, and Aristotle, as well as others, ascribed this difference to an attribute of mind or reason, a "human essence," a part of the soul.* So did many others. Plato for example, defined the soul as separate from the body, an independent entity. Whether one speaks of soul, in the classical philosophical sense, or whether one speaks of the more modern term, "mind," the belief that this entity maintains an existence independent of the body, but not necessarily material, is called the substantive view.† This dualist position attributes various experiences to the mind or the soul: It wills, it thinks, it feels. In addition to being separate from the body and substantial, it was typically construed as immortal. In this form, the dualist view has proved adaptable to most versions of Christianity, through which it has exerted a tremendous influence on Western ideas. It has also led to significant overlaps between the religious and the philosophical notions of the soul, particularly with respect to the worth of the soul as compared with the body.

It is important to note that the substantive view of the soul, for all its historical influence, no longer occupies the mainstream of philosophy. Hume was the first to reject substantialism by arguing that he could find no empirical or experiential evidence for an independent spiritual substance. Nonetheless, dualism has survived in other guises. For example, the concepts of "humanhood" or "personhood" as they are commonly used in medical ethics seem to express at least two important dualist ideas: first, that intellectual and experiential functions are what make a person; second, that these functions can be separated analytically from the body. These points are illustrated most convincingly in Veatch's discussions of personhood and irreversible brain damage (1981), and even, to a lesser extent, in the 1968 report of the Harvard Ad Hoc Committee.

The role of the secular soul (or the mind) may be subjected to the same analysis as the role of the religious soul. Loss of the religious soul can be equated with death, but what is the significance of absence of, or damage to, the secular soul? If it were the case that the "human" characteristics of an upright biped animal could be attributed to the uniqueness of its soul in a secular philosophical sense, and if this quality were in turn distinct from the body, what would be the status of a body from which this quality had been lost? Would it be human, and alive, though defective? Would it no longer be human, though still alive? Or would it no longer be considered alive in any operant sense because the human body, without this quality, may be treated as if it were dead, whether or not it is? If the philosophical system were to acknowledge a different set of moral obligations to entities that are human and those that are not, or to things

---

comed. But if, in the Epicurean manner, the successor to life is thought to be nothingness, suffering has no purpose. Thus, the fate of the soul is intimately associated with limits of propriety in the management of death.

*The concept of human essense has been used to refer both to a personal attribute and to an attribute of the human species as a whole. The distinction is unimportant in this discussion, however, and will not be further developed except as noted.

†The mind and the soul are obviously not the same. Within the limits of this discussion, the operative distinctions are so small that I will use the terms interchangeably when referring to the secular realm.

that are alive and to those that are not, or even to entities that once were "fully" human (perhaps because they had the power of reason) and now have lost that quality, then a basis for "levels" of death, so carefully avoided by the President's Commission, would be established.

The major difference between a soul in the religious sense and the soul or "human essence" in any of its secular forms is that the soul may be ascribed a separate existence beyond the body that houses it, whereas the "human essence" need be neither private to one specific individual nor even independent of the organism. The meaning of death in terms of disensoulment has been described. The meaning of death in terms of "human essence," for want of a less cumbersome phrase, is far more ambiguous. Does death occur at the moment that the "human essence" has departed or afterward? Is this essence truly metaphysical or can it be localized to an organ? If it is a quality of mind, and if mind is a function of the brain, does destruction of the brain mean that the "human essence" has departed? If the higher functions of the mind can be further localized to the cortex, should the destruction of the cortex be seen as a loss of the "human essence"?

Strictly speaking, it is difficult to argue that loss of humanhood really *is* death, either in the way that the religious equate disensoulment with death or in the way that a physiologist would equate irreversible cessation of heartbeat, respiration, and other vital functions with death. What some philosophers might argue, however, is that the loss of human experience that ensues when humanhood is lost depreciates life to the extent that one might as well be dead. This is the basis for treating someone "as if" he were dead, whether or not, physiologically, he is. The value system assumes that continued physiological or material existence in the absence of the unique set of qualities that contributes to or constitutes "humanhood" is not worth having. For this reason, it has been argued, obligations change when the "human essence" is lost, and it may become permissible to treat the individual as if he were dead.

The views of a tradition that rejects brain death in any except the strictest sense of the first meaning illustrates this point. The objection to brain-death criteria in strict interpretations of Talmudic law is based on the belief that death of the brain does not suspend the obligations due to a living human being until respirations have ceased (Rosner, 1986). Any effort that might hasten death is prohibited, even in the case of one who is obviously dying and considered moribund (Babylonian Talmud, Semahot, viii.1).* A transgression of this rule is considered murder (Bleich, 1986). Because decapitation is considered incompatible with life, death of the brainstem resulting in the loss of spontaneous respiratory drive is accepted as death by Tendler (1978), but not necessarily by others (Soleveichik, 1978; Rosner, 1986). Cortical brain death with preservation of spontaneous respiratory drive but diminution or loss of personhood in Veatch's sense of the term is not considered death in the Talmudic tradition. Indeed, this tradition takes exception to any formulation of the human condition that admits of a possible change in the obligation to preserve life before spontaneous respirations have ceased.

Thus, the state of the brain does not *ipso facto* influence whether someone may be treated as if he were dead, and certainly has no bearing on whether he is considered moribund *(goses)*. *Pari passu,* Jewish law rejects both the Platonic doctrine that prefers the soul to the body and the claim

---

*Although the Talmud recognizes that an individual may be moribund *(goses)*, a state in which there is no obligation to initiate new treatments, if, by any act of omission or commission, death is hastened, the act that led to the foreshortening of life is categorized as murder. The technical definition of *goses* stipulates that an individual will die within three days. The inability to make this prediction with certainty limits the use of this concept in the treatment of the terminally ill. It is for these reasons that the Babylonian Talmud goes to great pains to prohibit the treatment of someone as if he were dead (Semahot I):

Rule I. A dying man is regarded as a living entity in respect of all matters in the world. . . .
Rule IV. We may not close the eyes of a dying man. Whoever touches and moves him is a murderer. For R. Meir used to say: He can be compared to a lamp which is dripping, should a man touch it he extinguishes it. Similarly whoever closes the eyes of a dying man is considered as if he had taken his life. . . . .
Rule VI. We do not summon the people or recount his good deeds. . . . (begin his eulogy)

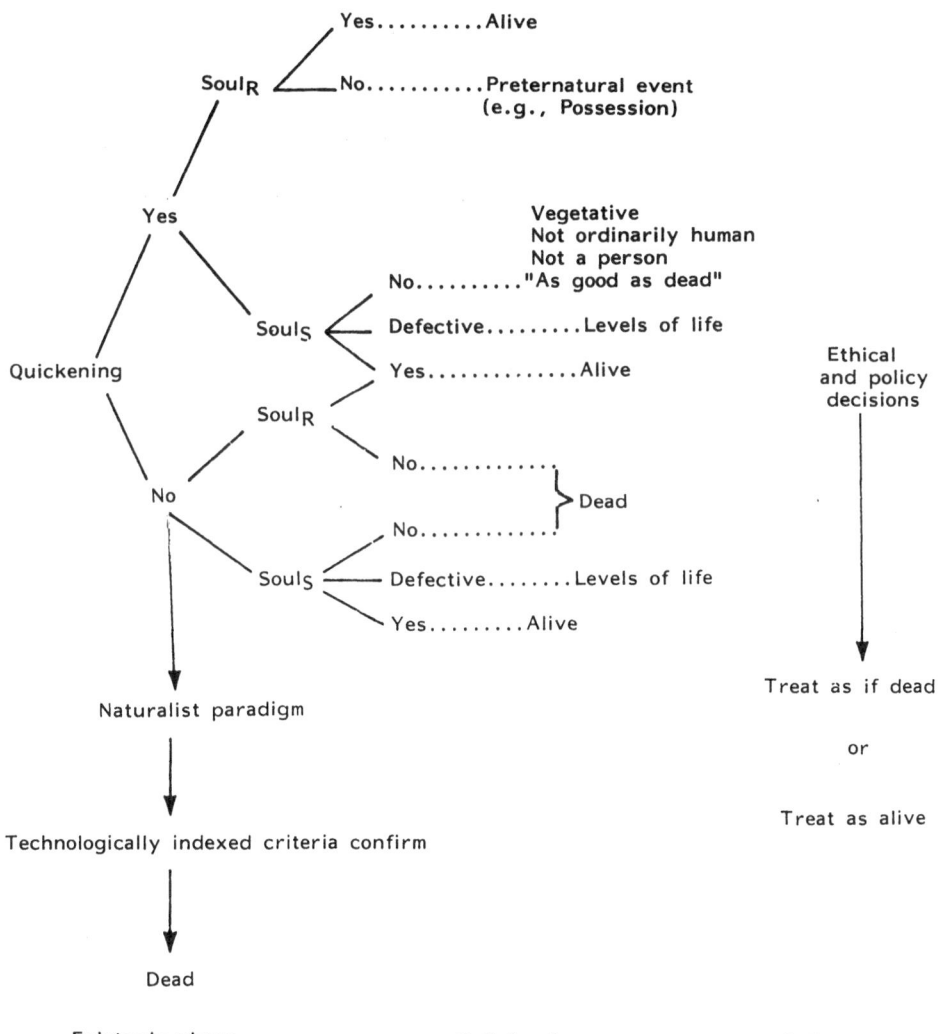

FIGURE 1. The conceptual sequence of managing death. There are three phases: the epistemic phase, during which evidence of movement is sought; the belief phase, during which the evidence is analyzed within the context of the operant belief system (i.e., naturalist versus non-naturalist, religious versus secular); and the ethical and policy phase, during which the results of the previous deliberations are analyzed in order to determine whether someone may be treated as if he were dead, and the appropriate responses are undertaken.

Epistemic (left) are confronted first: Is there evidence of quickening? If so, the individual is assumed to be alive unless, under very particular circumstances, there is reason to suspect that the human soul has been lost (zombie) or replaced (alien possession) or, even more speculatively, that the soul in the secular sense is defective. A defective soul may suggest some type of lesser, nonhuman life (see text). If there is no evidence of quickening, two paths are open. In the naturalist model, scientific signs of death are sought and confirmed. In the non-naturalist paradigm, the state of the soul is investigated. If the soul is present, life is present. If the soul is absent in the secular sense, the individual, having lost his personhood, is "as good as dead." If the soul is absent in the religious sense, life is absent. If the soul in the secular sense is defective and there is no quickening, there would be great reluctance to treat the individual as if he were alive. The third phase confronts ethical, legal, and policy issues. Soul$_S$, secular soul; Soul$_R$, religious soul.

that a human body without a functioning brain is any less human, any less of a person in the modern sense, than a human body with a fully functioning brain.

Those who have sought to explain death in purely physiological terms have considered naturalistic explanations of death—the "scientific" or "medical models"—to be free of adulteration by any supernatural notions of the soul or the spirit. These models, pursued, as we have seen, from the time of Bacon onward, evolved parallel to, and possibly as an outgrowth of, basic principles of rational empiricism: things that could not be measured or proved ought not to be invoked as explanations for natural phenomena. The soul could neither be demonstrated nor measured; for this reason, rational explanations for life and death could not revolve around the soul. This principle was seminal to the divergence of philosophy and natural science, whose estrangement increased as empiricism became the accepted intellectual paradigm for scientific exegesis.*

Thus, the physiological model for death began with the assumption that presence of quickening was necessary and sufficient to demonstrate the presence of life.† The absence of quickening in an animate organism constituted death. How to prove that there was no movement? This was the question that could be answered scientifically, and the answer evolved, without much paradigmatic change, from Bichat's experiments on guillotined bodies to our current tests for spontaneous respiration and cerebral function in brain-dead patients.

Nonetheless, it is important to realize that decisions about when to treat someone as dead involve scientific, ethical, and philosophical reasoning. A synthesis of the conceptual phases leading to the declaration of death is proposed in Fig. 1.

7. THE MEANING OF BRAIN DEATH

Thus far, the discussion has focused on the meaning of death and the role of concepts like the soul. In this section, the focus shifts to the significance of brain death specifically.

There are two ways of explaining what brain death means. The first looks at the brain as a vital organ. When brain death criteria are satisfied, the brain no longer functions, and, therefore, the person is dead. Since death of the brain is incompatible with life, death of the brain, proven by various tests, is an indicator of death in the same way that a flat EEG and absent respirations are indicators of death. The diagnosis of death is open to re-examination when new new or better criteria for brain function are devised. This is a technical issue that has been dealt with fully in the scientific literature on brain death and need not be reviewed here.

The second explanation sees in the brain the central organ for humanhood. The criteria for brain death are meant to prove that that the brain is not functioning, whereupon an individual is "as good as dead." Regardless of the condition of the rest of the body, the absence of a functioning brain suffices to treat someone as if they were dead, either because of what the brain represents or contains in the way of humanhood, or because the brain is the seat of something like the "spark of life" or even the soul whose continued association with the body is impossible once the seat has been irreversibly damaged. This view of death is intertwined with a number of evaluative assumptions that are rarely enunciated.

---

*Empiricism supplanted teleology and scholasticism. See Funkenstein, 1986.

†One question that has historically involved both science and philosophy is what kind of movement constitutes life, and how it is that molecules of protein and amino acids, whose inherent movement on a subatomic level is not considered life, can become quickened when they combine in certain ways. This question has not been answered to anyone's satisfaction. Most explanations revert to tenets of faith: all allude to a "vital element" in differentiating animate from inanimate objects. Whether this entity will be called "soul," "vital spark," or simply "X," where it comes from and what it is depend on the secular or religious paradigm invoked.

An example may serve to clarify the distinction. Plum and Posner (1980) divide consciousness into two parts: one includes arousal, a phasic attentional component of orientation, and wakefulness, a tonic activational component; the other includes intellectual and affective *content*, including emotion and cognition. In the first use of brain death, neither part functions. In the second model, one might postulate a hierarchy of importance even within consciousness. Someone who is awake but unarousable and devoid of intellectual and emotional content might be treated as if he were dead; by contrast, someone with obvious preservation of content at the expense of wakefulness of arousability might not. To be arousable for moments at a time but perfectly *compos mentis* is preferable to being awake but empty.

7.1. Brain Death and the Evaluative Assumption

The evaluative paradigm formulates death in terms of the loss of certain capacities that are postulated, *a priori*, to represent the essence of humanhood. The irreversible loss of these capacities is said to be, first, incompatible with participation in society as we know it, and second, characteristic of death in the sense that when people are dead, they do not display these functions. For example, Veatch (1981) described death as "the irreversible loss of the capacity for bodily integration," and he distinguishes between internal, or physiological, homeostatic or integrative mechanisms and external integrative mechanisms that allow conscious interaction with the environment. I have called this model "evaluative" because it depends ultimately on the subjective evaluation of what characteristics of living beings—here conscious interaction with the environment—are valued most highly.

Two assumptions are fundamental to the validity of this model: first, that the essence of humanhood can be expressed completely in terms of certain capacities or abilities; and second, that the meaning of death can be expressed completely in terms of their loss, and that the absence of these capacities either is the same as death or at least legitimately allows one to treat individuals as if they were dead. Although the first claim is the one most frequently advanced, it is the second that more accurately portrays what this model really does: it grants a sanction or dispensation to act in ways that would be otherwise considered ethically objectionable.

What seems to count most in Veatch's model is the loss of external integration (Veatch, 1976, 1982). He is not alone in this judgment. If internal integration were lost but external integration preserved, humanhood would not suffer. The link between external integration and the brain leads to a brain-based definition of death through the following train of logic: The function of external integration (consciousness*) is associated with the brain; loss of this function is characteristic of damage to the brain; this function is so greatly valued that its loss is either defined as or becomes tantamount to death of the individual; death of the brain is therefore taken to signify death of the individual. "It is not the collection of physical tissues called the brain but rather their functions—consciousness; motor control; sensory feeling; ability to reason; control over bodily functions . . . —which are given essential significance" (Veatch, 1982).

It is crucial to understand the assumptions on which this model relies. If one were to either deny that (1) this function, "packaged" as "external integration," constituted the essence of what we loosely call humanhood, or (2) its loss constituted the definition of death, granted dispensation to declare death, or sanctioned the treatment of individuals as if they were dead, the model would be invalidated. The model would be equally invalid if it could be shown that the brain were not the locus of this function.

A more radical expression of the evaluative model defines death as purely as "the irreversible loss of the capacity for social integration." Absence of consciousness and loss of the ability to

---

*There is more to it than just consciousness, but consciousness will serve as an abbreviation for the purposes of this discussion.

engage in social interaction become sufficient conditions to satisfy the definition. The capacity for "body integration" becomes irrelevant. This interpretation underlies the assertion that neocortical death should suffice to declare death (Veatch, 1976, 1982).

7.2.   Is the Evaluative Model Dualist?

The evaluative model has taken pains to distinguish itself from other figurative interpretations of death that are frankly dualist by virtue of distinguishing a metaphysical vital essence from a material body. Is it, nonetheless, dualist? The evaluative model justifies brain death by postulating two parts to the human existence, one part somatic and the other a metaphysical capacity. The metaphysical part is what counts. If internal integration were lost but the "package" of functions that Veatch and others describe in terms of consciousness and social interaction were preserved, humanhood would not be lost, and death would not have occurred. If the body and the physical brain perished but consciousness and social interaction continued, the so-called "disembodied brain," the evaluative criteria of death would not be satisfied.* Yet if these functions were lost, death has either occurred by definition or may be declared by dispensation, irrespective of the condition of the body. From this it appears that neither the brain nor the body, but only functions of the mind leading to consciousness and social interaction, convey the essence of life and humanhood.

The argument I am about to make pertains most strongly to neocortical definitions of death, but some points apply to whole brain definitions as well. This view of death either diminishes or eliminates the importance of the body in ascribing value to existence. The functions of consciousness and social interaction—in short, of the mind—are emphasized, appreciated, and otherwise endowed with primacy. These functions are thought to be located, on the basis of compelling scientific data, in the brain. If the brain were to be destroyed but these functions retained, resumed, replaced, or otherwise recovered, there is nothing in this view of death to explain why the individual under discussion should not be considered alive and human. Thus, the capacities whose absence is conceived as death are metaphysical and do not depend on the physical condition of the brain.†

Insofar as they rest on the value of life without the mind and admit that the mind and the body are separable, evaluative theories are dualist. Life is defined as the loss of a metaphysical quality that is preferred to the corporeal entity that it endows with humanhood. The body without this quality has insufficient worth to be (1) alive or (2) treated as if it were alive.

It may be argued that the evaluative model refers to the person and not to the body. It is the person that has died and the body that can be treated as if it were dead, once the capacity for mind has been lost. This argument is equally dualist in that it treats the body as an empty shell once a metaphysical element has been lost. The same argument has been used to sanction the removal of vital organs from anencephalic infants. Since the brain is absent, and no overt functions of mind are anticipated, there is no person, and the body can be treated as if it were dead.

One would have to presume that if the body were absent but the mind functioned normally, one would be obliged to create a somatic presence as the bionic soma—for the mind. This obligation would be conditioned by the activity of the mind.‡

---

*There is an entire literature on the subject of disembodied brains to which the interested reader is referred.

†Jonas (1982) remarks briefly that the primacy of the mind and the devaluation of the body in the report of the Harvard Ad Hoc Committee has gnostic overtones. This is an insightful observation that deserves further study.

‡This is not simply a theoretical consideration. One of my most painful personal recollections is of participating in a so-called awake resuscitation. A young man developed electromechanical dissociation of the myocardium. The heart would not capture externally supplied electrical impulses to develop a spontaneous

7.3. Must Brain-Based Criteria Be Dualist?

The brain-based definitions, particularly the neocortically based definitions, have never been satisfied to regard the brain as just another organ whose function is vital to life in the same way that the heart or the liver or the kidney is vital to life. The contribution of these organs is mechanical. Although their destruction leads to death, there is every reason to suppose that they will be fully replaceable within the forseeable future, either through transplantation or by artificial means. Two special qualities inhere to the brain, however; in Veatch's terms (1982), only one, "internal integration" can be replaced mechanically. This is precisely what life-support devices achieve. By contrast, the quality of external integration cannot be replaced mechanically, thereby justifying mind-based criteria for death.

Thus, the only irreplaceable function is this quality of mind. The quality of mind is distinct. The body and the brain may be integrated; the brain and the mind are not. The emphasis on the brain is based solely on its relationship to consciousness, communication, and the other functions esteemed as characteristic of humanhood. Were these functions to be translocatable to another organ, the brain would lose its primacy as an organ base for evaluative definitions of death. Were other capacities or functions to be appointed above consciousness and external integration, to use Veatch's term (1982), in figuratively conceptualizing humanhood, the locus of those functions would most likely replace the brain's.

Dualistic views of body and soul allowed for three conceptual relationships: body and soul together in terrestrial life; body and soul separated, but soul hovering around the body in a form of latent or vestigial life; and body decaying but soul immortal in the afterlife. There are obvious parallels between body–soul dualism and mind–body dualism. There are strong indications that society thinks in this way.* When mind and body function together, an individual is whole; when the body functions but the mind is deranged or damaged, an individual requires special protection because the instinctual moral and charitable responses in society cannot be depended on; when the mind is lost, it is very difficult to avoid treating an individual as if he were dead. It is easier to formulate this analogy with respect to the mind than the brain; it is the sense of an individual's mind and personality rather than the focal neurological functions of the brain that seem to make the difference.

7.4. The Problem of Relative Worth: Is the Mind Qualitatively Different from the Body?

There may yet be another way to look at the relationship between death and the qualities of mind. In contemporary culture, the mind has been endowed with primacy for purposes of defining death. Given sufficient injury to the body, a rational individual with a normal mind might well decide that life is as worthless as it would if the qualities of mind had been dissolved. It might take greater injury to the body than to the mind to affect the worth of life, but this is a quantitative

---

rhythm. So long as cardiac compression was provided, pulse and blood pressure were maintained and the patient was awake and speaking. The moment compression ceased, he lapsed into unconsciousness.

In most cases of cardiac arrest, patients are unconscious when found, and failure to achieve spontaneous or externally paced cardiac output after a suitable interval is easily interpreted as death. The body has died and the mind has died. In this case, however, the mind persisted even as the body had suffered irreversible loss of its homeostatic mechanisms. The decision to stop external cardiac compression was tantamount in the minds of the resuscitation team to burying someone alive. So long as he was conscious, he could not be treated as dead.

*A summary of the behaviorist view of mind and body is given by Fodor (1980).

rather than a qualitative difference. This line of reasoning suggests that the mind is a part of the body that holds greater worth, but not qualitatively different worth, than other parts.

That this analysis does not hold up is demonstrated by social conventions about competency and the limits of permissible behavior on the part of others. In the case of grievous bodily injury, an individual is allowed to determine what means of treatment he will undergo, as long as he is adjudged mentally competent; the proper functioning of the mind rationalizes decisions that affect the treatment of the body. In the case of damage to the mind, the capacity of an individual to make rational decisions is thrown into question. If I lost my eyes, I may feel as if I were as good as dead. My body image might change. I may even wish I were dead. But if I were to ask others to treat me as if I were dead, that would test the limits of acceptable behavior. By contrast, if I had left instructions that I be treated as if I were dead after an injury that destroyed my neocortex, that would be regarded as a reasonable request in present-day American culture.

Thus, the contention, on grounds of brain-based criteria for death, that brain death is the same as death must restrict the meaning of death to the irreversible and irreplaceable loss of somatic function controlled by the brain; otherwise, it must revert to a frankly dualist view of life that defines death as the loss of mind *irrespective* of the condition of the body and of the mind.

7.5. Implications for Neocortically Based Criteria for Death

Whereas whole-brain death is incompatible with life as we know it, neocortical death is incompatible with life as we desire it. Whole-brain death need not rely on mind-based justifications. Neocortical brain death cannot do otherwise. Whole-brain death need not be dualist, although many discussions of whole-brain death share a dualist orientation. Neocortical brain death is inescapably dualist, as well as intrinsically evaluative. The subjective nature of the dualist doctrine, its metaphysical qualities, and its hidden value-laden assumptions are of concern in establishing health-care policy.

8.   TREATING "AS IF DEAD"

Recent articles on CPR have reaffirmed the premise that the only valid proof of death in the face of apparent death is a failure of resuscitation (Bedell *et al.*, 1983; Bedell and Delbanco, 1984). But there have been many changes in the technical standards for resuscitation, and these developments have had inevitable consequences for testing the irreversibility of signs of death.

Death is irreversible by definition in the natural world. In the sense that no condition in medicine is ever diagnosed except by inference from signs, death is never diagnosed directly. To prove death means to show that the signs of death are irreversible. Some signs of death—decay, decomposition—are incontrovertible. Other signs of death are more relative in that their apparent irreversibility is a function of effort and technological sophistication: Cessation of respiration or heartbeat need not be irreversible unless the cause of cardiac standstill or respiratory arrest cannot be remedied. Thus, decapitation is irreversible, and the cardiorespiratory arrest that follows is equally irreversible. Some events are technologically indexed in that their consequences may be irreversible in some contexts but not in others: Kidney failure may be irreversible, but the condition it precipitates can be controlled with dialysis. Thus, reversibility of signs is, in part, a judgment linked to technological advances.

There are some difficult gray zones. If the entire brain is destroyed without physical separation from the body, the diagnosis of death is inferred from the combination of irreversible cardiorespiratory arrest (despite the fact that corporeal perfusion and gas exchange can be mechanically produced) and the irremediable destruction of the brain. The signs used to demonstrate irremediable destruction of the brain have evolved to the point that the use of the ventilator and pressor drugs can be thought of as prolonged resuscitation attempts. Failure of resuscitation is demonstrated by (1) failure of cerebral function, and (2) failure of spontaneous resumption of heartbeat and breath.

When the diagnosis of death is based on cadaveric decay, or decapitation, we accept the warrant* of these signs at face value. Obviously irreversible, they suffice to permit the treatment of an individual as if he were dead without further proof: they are equivalent to death. In the presence of "lesser signs," the warrant is less certain, and we would require that the signs be verified. What makes pulselessness a lesser sign is that, under most circumstances, we would be unwilling to treat a person as if he were dead purely on the basis of this sign; after all, it might be purely temporary or reversible. A failed attempt at CPR validates the "lesser sign" or pulselessness. In a triage situation, we might accept the lesser sign as sufficient warrant. It is not the criteria that have changed; it is the ethical decision that is based on the criteria. In a triage situation, the lesser signs might suffice to treat someone as if he were dead because of other competing needs. To treat someone as if dead implies that the moral obligation to verify that he is dead has been weakened or suspended. A weaker warrant becomes morally tolerable.

Clearly, a person need not be dead to be treated as if dead. Juliet was treated as if dead; death was diagnosed and the moral obligations of those around her changed from those referable to a living person to those referable to either the memory of that person or to its corpse. A person in this category may not yet be a corpse in any technical sense, but society will have begun to regard him as one. Treating someone as if dead in order that he might die is permissible only when the intent of having that person die is morally permissible on other grounds.† Thus, a person sustaining cardiopulmonary arrest is not treated as if dead unless a previous decision not to resuscitate has been taken.

The importance of the mind should not change the epistemic criteria for death. It is easy for empathic professionals to be swayed into the "as if" mode of reasoning. In actuality, they are expressing a desire to have the patient die, founded on a particular formulation of altruism: better the absence of suffering and the absence of life than the presence of suffering. Although this may accurately reflect the desires of some patients, it is incorrect to ascribe this mode of thought to all individuals, all patients, all cultures, and all faiths uncritically and should not be construed as a basis for health care policy on a larger scale.

9. SUMMARY AND CONCLUSIONS

Over the past 20 years, society has become more libertarian with respect to treating people as if they were dead. Several factors may be responsible for this development. First, the fear of premature interment or misdiagnosis of death is no longer acute. It is generally presumed that physicians are competent to declare death even if the precise moment is best determined in retrospect (Henry, 1980). While the *National Enquirer* continues to publish thrilling descriptions of dead bodies returning unexpectedly to life, and the medical literature contains scattered reports of patients who resumed respiration and heartbeat on the way to the morgue after failed resuscitation

---

*By warrant, I mean the justification for a belief that acts as a basis to assert that the belief is true.
†We seem to differentiate between (and prioritize) cardiac, respiratory, and neurological function in deciding the appropriateness of artificial life support. There is rarely any objection to maintaining respiration in the face of normal cardiac and cortical function: witness polio victims in the iron lung. There has been, until recently, hesitation to commit to longterm cardiac support, but the artificial heart and cardiac transplantation have diminished this reluctance. There remains a profound reluctance, however, to support either cardiac or respiratory function in the face of demonstrated destruction of the entire brain, and this reluctance is only slightly lessened when isolated brainstem function is preserved.

(Hartikainen *et al.*, 1982), a preoccupation with such examples would border on the eccentric. Second, with some well-defined exceptions, an awareness of the immanence of death no longer affects society as profoundly as it did in centuries past. Finally, and some might argue in consequence, the fear of death has been diluted, perhaps even replaced, by the fear of dying.

Today, the fear most commonly expressed is no longer that signs of residual life will be missed or ignored, but rather that they will be contrived and that the dying process will be prolonged at the expense of the person's comfort. The modern secular cosmology has difficulty justifying this course of events. Death has no obvious inherent purpose. The acceptability of both the empathic and the instrumental premises of the Harvard Ad Hoc Committee are beholden to this perspective.

The technical aspects of brain death in adults are no longer at issue. The level of certainty, the warrant required for brain-based criteria in children, will always be greater than in adults; this is an both a technical judgment (the brain has a higher potential for recovery in children) and an ethical posture.

Decisions on a policy level must confront and understand the phenomenon of warrant and the decision to treat people as if they were dead. It is the ethical and philosophical aspects of the decision that must be scrutinized. There is little question that whole-brain-based criteria can be gotten to satisfy virtually all standards of acceptability; evaluative assumptions that lead to partial brain-based criteria, however, are not universally acceptable and are open to abuse.

Many difficulties involving the management of patients at the end of life could be avoided by repeatedly posing one question in its starkest terms: Are we seeking to make a diagnosis of death, to determine whether someone has already died, or are we pursuing a fundamentally philosophical query—that is, whether it is permissible to treat the individual before us as dead?

ACKNOWLEDGMENTS. I wish to acknowledge the assistance of Jonathan and Jae Roosevelt and of Dr. Linda R. Dagi, who reviewed and criticized successive versions of this paper. Dr. Richard M. Swengel, Dr. William J. Meyer, Professor Lawrence McCullough, and Professor Stuart Spicker offered many helpful suggestions. The University Program in Health, Sciences and Technology at Case Western Reserve University provided, through the Zverina Lectureship, a forum for the discussion of an earlier version of part of this essay. The Secretary and Officers of the Royal Humane Society of Great Britain gave me access to invaluable archival documents. The History of Medicine Division of the Uniformed Services University of the Health Sciences provided facilities for research. The librarians of the Walter Reed Army Medical Center, the History of Medicine Section of the National Library of Medicine, and in particular, C. Pellegrino of the rare book collection at the Dahlgren Library of Georgetown University Medical Center, indulged my repeated requests for material with efficiency, humor, and encouragement.

REFERENCES

Adams, D., 1799, *An Inaugural Dissertaion on the Principle of Animation Read and Defended at a Public Examination held by the Medical Professor before the Hon. John Wheelock, L.L.D. President and the Governors of Dartmouth College for the Degree of Bachelor in Medicine, July 18, 1799*, Moses Davis, Hanover.

Ad Hoc Committee on Brain Death, 1987, The Children's Hospital, Boston, Determination of brain death, *J. Pediat.* **110:**15–19.

Anderson, R. S., 1986, *Theology, Death and Dying*, Basil Blackwell, London.

Aries, P., 1982, *The Hour of Our Death* (H. Weaver, transl.), Vintage, New York.

Bacon, F., 1638, *The Historie of life and Death. With Observations Naturall and Experimentall for the Prolonging of Life*, Humphrey Mosley, London.

Bedell, S. E., and Delbanco, T. L., 1984, Choices about cardiopulmonary resuscitation in the hospital. When do physicians talk with patients?, *N. Engl. J. Med.* **310:**1089–1093.

Bedell, S. E., Delbanco, T. L., Cook, S. F., *et al.*, 1983, Survival after cardiopulmonary resuscitation in the hospital, *N. Engl. J. Med.* **309**:569–575.

Beecher, H. K., 1968, A definition of irreversible coma, *JAMA* **205**:337–340.

Bernat, J. L., Culver, C. M., and Gert, B., 1982, On the definition and criterion of death, in: *Value Conflicts in Health Care Delivery* (B. Gruzalski and C. Nelson, eds.), pp. 155–170, Ballinger, Cambridge, Massachusetts.

Bichat, X., 1809, *Physiological Researches upon Life and Death* (T. Watkins, transl.), Smith and Maxwell, Philadelphia.

Black, P. McL., 1978, Brain death, I, *N. Engl. J. Med.* **299**:338–344; II. **299**:393–401.

Black, P. McL., and Zervas, N. T., 1984, Declaration of brain death in neurosurgical and neurological practice, *Neurosurgery* **15**:170–174.

Bleich, D., 1986, Establishing criteria of death, in: *Jewish Bioethics* (F. Rosner and D. Bleich, eds.), pp. 277–294, Hebrew Publishing Company, New York.

Bosworth, N., 1814, *The Accidents of Human Life; Within Their Preservation and Their Removal and Their Consequences*, Samuel Wood, New York.

Burns, N. T., 1972, *Christian Mortalism from Tyndale to Milton*, Harvard University Press, Cambridge, Massachusetts.

Capron, A. M., and Kass, L. R., 1972, A statuatory definition of the standards for determining human death: An appraisal and a proposal, *Univ. Pa. Law Rev.* **121**(1):87–88; 102–118.

Carrick, P., 1985, *Medical Ethics in Antiquity*, D. Reidel, Dortrecht.

Choron, J., 1963, *Death and Western Thought*, Collier, New York.

Coulter, D. L., 1987, Neurological uncertainty in newborn intensive care, *N. Engl. J. Med.* **316**:840–844.

Dagi, T. F., 1986, The obligation to resuscitate, *Bull. Am. Coll. Surg.* **71**:4–10.

Dagi, T. F., 1987, Revival, resuscitation and resurrection: The rights of passage, in: *Proceedings of the Eighteenth Trans-Disciplinary Symposium on Philosophy and Medicine* (S. Spicker and H. T. Engelhardt, Jr., eds.), D. Reidel, Dortrecht.

Dagi, T. F., 1988, Exhortations to resuscitate in eighteenth century Europe: Civic duty in poetry and prose, in: *Proceedings of the Second International Symposium on the History of Anesthesia*, Royal Society of Medicine, London.

Ducachet, H. W., 1822, On the signs of death, and the manner of distinguishing real from apparent death, *Am. Med. Rec.* **5**:39–53.

Fodor, J. A., 1980, The mind–body problem, *Sci. Am.* **240**(1):114–123.

Ford, F. L., 1961, The world of the enlightenment, in: *Chapters in Western Civilization* (J. Rothschild, D. Sidorsky, W. Wishy, eds.), pp. 530–580, Columbia University Press, New York.

Frazer, J. G., 1933, *The Fear of the Dead in Primitive Religion*, Vol. I, Macmillan, London.

Funkenstein, A., 1986, *Theology and the Scientific Imagination from the Middle Ages to the Seventeenth Century*, Princeton University Press, Princeton, New Jersey.

Gay, P., 1966, *The Enlightenment. An Interpretation. The Rise of Modern Paganism*, Norton, New York.

Gordon, B. L., 1959, *Medieval and Renaissance Medicine*, Philosophical Library, New York.

Gould, G. M., and Pyle, W. L., 1956, *Anomalies and Curiosities of Medicine*, Bell, New York.

Gruman, G. R., 1977, *A History of Ideas about the Prolongation of Life*, Arno, New York.

Guidelines for the Determination of Death, 1981, Report of the Medical Consultants on the Diagnosis of Death to the President's Commission for the Study of Ethical Problems in Medicine and Biomedical and Behavioral Research, Special Communication, 1981, *JAMA* **246**:2184–2186.

Hartikainen, M., Cozanitis, D. A., and Heikkila, J., 1982, Resurrection, *South. Med. J.* **75**:1301.

Hawes, W., 1782, An address to the public, appendix I, in: *An Address to the King and Parliament of Great Britain on the Important Subject of Preserving the Lives of its Inhabitants, by means of which, with the Sanction and Assistance of the Legislature, would be rendered Simple, Clear, and Efficacious to the People at Large*, J. Dodsley, Pall-Mall, T. Cadell, Strand, C. Dilly, Poultry, Dennis and Son, Bridge Street, pp. 22–24.

Hawes, W., 1780, *An Address to the Public*, "printed privately for W. Hawes, London, and bound with an account of the late Dr. Goldsmith's illness, so far as it related to the exhibition of Dr. James' powder."

Henry, J. B., and Smith, F. A., 1980, Estimation of the Postmortem Interval by Chemical Means, *Am. J. Forensic Med. Pathol.* **1**:341–347.

Jonas, H., 1958, *The Gnostic Religion*, Beacon, Boston.

Jonas, H., 1969, Philosophical reflections on experimenting with human subjects, *Daedalus* **98**(2):219–247.

Jonas, H., 1982, Against the stream: Comments on the definition and redefinition of death, in: *Contemporary Issues in Bioethics* (T. L. Beauchamp and L. Walters, eds.), 2nd ed., pp. 288–293, Wadsworth, Belmont, California.

Kaufman, H. H., and Lynn, J., 1986, Brain death, *Neurosurgery* **19**:850 856.

Korein, J., 1978, The problem of brain death, in: *Brain Death: Interrelated Medical and Social Issues* (J. Korein, ed.), pp. 19–38, New York Academy of Sciences, New York.

Kouwenhoven, W. B., Jude, J. R., and Knickerbocker, G. G., 1960, Closed-chest cardiac massage, *JAMA* **173**:1064–1067.

Kristeller, P. O., 1961, The moral thought of Renaissance Humanism, in: *Chapters in Contemporary Civilization,* 3rd ed. (J. Rothschild, D. Sidorsky, and B. Wishy, eds.), pp. 289–235, Columbia University Press, New York.

Mollaret, P., and Gouloun, M., 1959, Le coma dépassé, *Rev. Neurol.* **101**:3–15.

Pinkus, R. L., 1984, Families, brain death, and traditional medical excellence, *J. Neurosurg.* **60**:1192–1194.

Pius XII, 1957, *Acta Apostolocae Sedia* **45**:1027–1033.

Plum, F., and Posner, J. B., 1980, *Diagnosis of Stupor and Coma,* 3rd ed., F. A. Davis, Philadelphia

Preuss, J., 1978, *Biblical and Talmudic Medicine* (F. Rosner, transl.), Sanhedrin, New York.

Rosner, F., 1986, *Modern Medicine and Jewish Ethics,* Ktav, Yeshiva University Press, New York.

Say, B., 1799, *An Annual Oration Pronounced before the Humane Society of Philadelphia on the Objects and Benefits of Said Institution, 28th Day of February, 1799,* William Young, Philadelphia.

Segel, A. F., 1977, *Two Powers in Heaven. Early Rabbinic Reports About Christianity and Gnosticism,* E. J. Brill, Leiden.

Snart, J., 1824, *An Historical Enquiry Concerning Apparent Death and Premature Interment,* Sherwood, Neely and Jones, London.

Soleveichik, A., 1978, Jewish Law and time of death, *JAMA* **240**:109.

Tendler, M. D., 1978, Cessation of brain function: Ethical implications in terminal care and organ transplants, *Ann. NY Acad. Sci.* **315**:394–397.

The President's Commission for the Study of Ethical Problems in Medicine and Biomedical and Behavior Research, 1981, *Defining Death: Medical, Legal, and Ethical Issues in the Determination of Death,* U. S. Government Printing Office, Washington, D. C. (abbreviated the President's Commission on Bioethics).

Veatch, R. M., 1976, *Death, Dying, and the Biological Revolution: Our Last Quest for Responsibility,* Yale University Press, New Haven, Connecticut.

Veatch, R. M., 1981, *A Theory of Medical Ethics,* Basic Books, New York.

Veatch, R. M., 1982, Defining death anew: Technical and ethical problems, in: *Contemporary Issues in Bioethics* (T. L. Beauchamp and L. Walters, eds.), 2nd ed., pp. 278–288, Wadsworth, Belmont, California.

Walker, B., 1983, *Gnosticism. Its History and Influence,* Aquarian Press, Wellingborough, Northamptonshire.

Walters, L., 1982, The definition and determination of death, in: *Contemporary Issues in Bioethics* (T. L. Beauchamp and L. Walters, eds.), 2nd ed., pp. 274–278, Wadsworth, Belmont, California.

Walton, D. N., 1979, *On Defining Death. An Analytical Study of the Concept of Death in Philosophy and Medical Ethics,* McGill-Queens University Press, Montreal.

Whiter, W., 1819, *A Dissertation on the Disorder of Death* Booth and Ball, privately printed for the author, Norwich.

Winslow, J. B., 1740, *Quaestio Medico-chirurgica . . . an Mortis Incertae Signa Minus Incerta a Chirurgis, Quam ab Aliis Experimentis,* Quillan, Parisiis.

Winslow, J. B., 1742, *Dissertation sur l'incertitude des signes de la mort et de l'abus des enterrements et embaumements précipités* (J.-J. Bruhier d'Ablaincourt, transl.), Paris.

Winslow, J. B., 1746, *The Uncertainty of the Signs of Death; and the Danger of Precipitate Interments and Dissections . . . With Proper Directions, both for Preventing Such Accidents, and Repairing the Misfortunes Brought on the Constitution by Them. To the Whole is Added, a curious Account of the Funeral Solemnities of Many Ancient and Modern Nations, Exhibiting the Precautions they made use of to Ascertain the Certainty of Death* (J.-J. Bruhier d'Ablaincourt, transl.), M. Cooper, London.

Wolfson, H. A., 1965, Immortality and resurrection in the philosophy of the Church Fathers, in: *Immortality and Resurrection* (K. Stendahl, ed.), pp. 54–96, Macmillan, New York.

2

A Jewish Approach to Ethical Issues in Brain Death and Organ Transplantation

Rabbi Moshe Tendler

1. INTRODUCTION

Western civilization is firmly rooted in biblical ethics. The Judeo-biblical heritage of Christianity is still the major, primary source of moral and ethical standards by which we measure man and society. A review of these standards can serve to guide the medical practitioner, as well as society at large, through the complexities of the donor–recipient interactions when transplant surgery is considered.

2. BIBLICAL FOUNDATION

2.1. Man Instructed to Master the Physical World

> From all the trees of the Garden of Eden you may eat. But of the Tree of Knowledge of good and evil, you should not eat therefrom. (*Gen.* **1**:16–17)

Man may eat of all. But there is a limitation. Not everything that man can do, may he do. In verse **1**:28, man was given mastery of the biotic world: "God blessed Adam and Eve and commanded them to be fruitful and multiply, fill my earth and master it." But no permission was granted to master fellow man. The inviolate nature of human life was reiterated when the earth was reborn after the flood. Noah was granted dominion over "all living animals . . . like the vegetation of the earth which you may eat . . . but your blood even for your own lives I will demand, from every man I will demand the life of fellow man" (*Genesis* **9**:3–5).

Not only is fellow man's life inviolate, but suicide or self-mutilation and injury are also forbidden. Whose life is it anyway? Not yours! Your life given to you to enjoy and protect. It can be taken away only by the "Giver of All Life."

RABBI MOSHE TENDLER • Yeshiva University, New York, New York 10033.

2.2.   The Duty to Heal

Three biblical instructions concern the duty to heal:

1. *Exod.* (21:19) "and he shall heal." This verse is understood to be a licensure or permission for man to meddle in the affairs of God, who is the Supreme Healer. It implies that God works through natural laws, including those that govern the health of mortals. The development of modern medical science—a prime example of man's exercise of his right of "mastery"— is a proper arena for human endeavor. It is not confrontational with God the Healer, who expects man to seek medical help as the first stage in the healing protocol. The last stage is still reserved for God.

2. *Lev.* (19:17) "You are forbidden to stand idly by when your friend is in danger." We are commanded to intercede even at personal financial expense or at some acceptable level of personal risk. High risk or self-sacrifice is not permitted even to save a life. The bottom-line figure does not warrant the loss of one life to save another. Since suicide is not man's option, his own life is as valuable as any other.

3. *Deut.* (22:1) "You cannot hide your eyes from the last ox or sheep of your brother; you must return them to your brother." If we are commanded to return lost objects, how much more concerned must we be to return someone's lost health!

This emphasis on duty and obligation rather than on rights and privileges shifts the focus temporarily from the confrontational to the problematic. It is the dilemma of what is best for the patient when risks and benefits are compared. However, triage concerns due to the finite resources available compel a decision to allocate these resources in accord with some priority scale. At this point, conflict and confrontation enter the evaluation process.

In this process, some projects and some patients will be denied a share of these limited resources. Projects will conflict with each other for higher-priority ratings. Medical care budgetary allotments will impinge on the budgetary requests from proponents of better housing, transportation, and security services. Our resolve to provide maximum benefits to all our citizenry may be a goal to be achieved rather than an actual protocol to be administered. A multitiered system of medical care based on the patient's ability to pay is inevitable, at least for the present. What must be avoided, lest the ethical fabric of our society be rent asunder, is the criterion of "social worth" in patient selection. "Cost-effective" medicine, concepts of "human capital," and age limits for access to expensive medical technology are synonyms for "social worth." They are but thinly disguised eugenic doctrines applied to the economy of our democratic society.

3.   BRAIN DEAD AND BRAIN ABSENT: AN ISSUE OF HUMANHOOD

3.1.   Brain Dead

From earliest biblical days, breathing determined the living state. "And He blew into his nostrils the living soul" (*Gen.* 2:7) established independent respiration as the *sine qua non* of the living state. However, cardiac or respiratory arrest can often be reversed. Even when death of the brain cell controlling respiration occurs, a respirator can inflate the lungs. Brain death, or the total cessation of all brain function including the brainstem, has therefore become a widely accepted indicator of death. The ability to keep organs viable after the organism has died by the use of drugs and machines also allows for the transplantation of vital organs such as heart and liver.

But neurological death has not been understood by much of the laity. Confusion introduced by the inaccurate use of the brain death diagnosis, as in the Karen Quinlan case, coupled with increased publicity about the advances in transplantation surgery and the shortages of donor organs, has placed a cloud of suspicion on the medical profession. The accepted practice of using separate teams to declare the patient brain dead and to do the transplantation surgery is but one response to this climate of suspicion. A further response is needed. The routine use of angiogram or blood-flow studies to ascertain that the base of the brain is not being perfused would surely allay the suspicion of many that "almost" brain dead is good enough for the transplant surgeons.

There are unique problems in determining pediatric brain death (Report of Special Task Force, 1987; Volpe, 1987). Unlike the adult, a pediatric patient under the age of 2 can survive many months in the "brain dead" state. Blood-flow studies are critical in determining that brain death has occurred (Alvarez *et al.*, 1988). The limitations of available equipment to detect blood flow in the small vessels of the neonate may require a minimum age before brain death can be declared—possibly no younger than 14 days (Coulter, 1987).

3.2. Brain Absent

3.2.1. Anatomical

Brain absent is a new designation, developed to describe the anencephalic fetus. This fetus is anatomically deficient in most of the brain above the brainstem or medulla. But this child can breathe independently for the short life span allotted it by the creator of all life. During this brief hold on life, its life is inviolate and cannot be terminated in order to use its organs for others whose tenuous hold on life can be strengthened by such transplanted organs. Brain absent is a euphony to make the unthinkable—infanticide—acceptable. The anencephalic is a critically ill neonate, not an organ farm. When life begins to ebb, it is quite proper to place the child on a respirator. When it is declared brain dead by repetitive apnea testing and blood-flow study (Belsh *et al.*, 1986; Goodman *et al.*, 1985), the organs can be made available for transplantation to other infants with life-threatening deficiencies.

3.2.2. Physiological

The brain-absent designation is being extended to the adult population. The permanent vegetative state (PVS) patient is being treated as if he were brian dead due to the absence of a functioning cerebrum. This physiological "absence of the brain" has permitted both physician and Christian clergy to approve withdrawal of all life support, including hydration and nutrition. This is tantamount to active euthanasia, unless indeed the brain-absent state is equated with the brain-dead condition. Surely this equation cannot be justified on scientific merit. It is a value judgment on the basis of social worth or utility—a most disturbing demonstration of the "slippery slope" in ethics. The justification for this equation is the concern for "human dignity," hence "death with dignity" as a basic human right. The absence of human intelligence or of minimal self-awareness is viewed as loss of humanity and therefore loss of all rights of the patient and exemption of society from all duties and obligations to this patient. There is no historical basis for such a discounting of the infinite worth of the human created in God's image. The concern for human dignity is best expressed by a refusal to move the boundary line between living and dead to a new location based on social and economic considerations.

REFERENCES

Alvarez, L. A., Moshe, S. L., Belman, A. L., Maytal, J. Resnick, T. J., and Keilson, M., 1988, EEG and brain death determination in children, *Neurology (NY)* **38**:227–230.

Belsh, J. M., Blatt, R., and Schiffman, P. L., 1986, Apnea testing in brain death, *Arch. Intern. Med.* **146**:2385–2388.

Coulter, D. L., 1987, Neurological uncertainty in newborn intensive care, *N. Engl. J. Med.* **316:**840–844.

Goodman, J. M., Heck, L. L., and Moore, B. D., 1985, Confirmation of brain death with portable isotope angiography: A review of 204 consecutive cases, *Neurosurgery* **16:**492–297.

Report of Special Task Force, 1987, Guidelines for the determination of brain death in children, *Pediatrics* **80:**298–300.

Volpe, J. J., 1987, Brain death determination in the newborn, *Pediatrics* **80:**293–297.

3

Catholic Considerations of Brain Death and Organ Retrieval

John J. Paris

1. INTRODUCTION

The Vatican's *Declaration on Euthanasia* (1980) highlights the fact that technological advances not only increase the capacity of medicine to cure and prolong life but bring with them complex and trying issues of the appropriateness of those treatments to specific cases. The moral dilemma now has become not how to apply the treatments, but whether to do so. When the decision is made to withhold or withdraw treatment, it is sometimes met with unreflective charges of euthanasia, suicide, or murder.

The confusion on this topic is frequently compounded by a failure to distinguish among patients who are "dead," "brain-dead," "in a chronic vegetative state," "comotose," and "terminally ill but conscious." To that list we must now add, as Capron's article (1987) makes clear, the distinction between the brain dead and those born without a brain but who are otherwise living and breathing: the anencephalic. In each of these instances, it may be appropriate to stop treatment; in some cases, it is a moral imperative. That is, one ought not expend scarce medical resources ventilating a corpse.

How then do we know the person is dead? The traditional answer was simple: The heart or the breathing has stopped. If there is no pulse or respiration, the patient is dead. In the postbiblical language of the theologians: "The soul has left the body." What remains is thus no longer a person but a corpse.

Today, advanced cardiopulmonary techniques take us beyond the traditional understanding of death. With these techniques, it is possible to generate breathing and heartbeat even after both have stopped. In many instances, the person then resumes a normal life. For others those functions are restored, the patient never regains the capacity for spontaneous breathing or, worse, is unable to sustain integration of bodily functions, consciousness, or human experiences. Such artificially maintained bodies—the Karen Ann Quinlans, Melanie Bacchiochis, and Paul Bro-

John J. Paris • Department of Ethics, College of the Holy Cross, Worcester, Massachusetts 01610; Department of Community Medicine, Tufts Medical School, Boston, Massachusetts 02111.

phys—present a new category, or, more specifically, new categories, of persons for whom the traditional means of determining death is neither clear nor fully satisfactory.

To bring clarity, consistency, and principled guidance to a determination of whether such bodies are alive or dead, the President's Commission for the Study of Ethical Problems in Medicine and Biomedical and Behavioral Research conducted a 2-year study on defining death (1981). Its final report on the medical, legal, and ethical aspects of death, was issued in July 1981 along with a proposal for a uniform statute on the determination of death, i.e., the Uniform Determination of Death Act (UDDA) (see Section 2.3). That proposal has now been adopted by some 16 states as part of a uniformly agreed upon understanding of when death occurs. Some 20 other states and the supreme courts in some six other jurisdictions have adopted various formulations of that determination of death.

It is important to be clear on what those determination of death statutes involve, how they have evolved, and the need for them. It is equally important to understand the objections to such legislation, to analyze and evaluate them, and to devise a coherent public policy position on the issue. That policy must be medically sound, ethically appropriate, and theologically acceptable.

2. BRAIN DEATH

2.1. The Definition of Brain Death

Thirty years ago, the definition of death was uniformly agreed upon and easy to assess: When the heart and breathing stopped, the patient was dead. Two technological developments have challenged that understanding: the advent of artificial life-support systems and the possibility of organ transplants. The first allows the revival of patients whose hearts or breathing have stopped. A patient who had not suffered more than a few minutes of oxygen deprivation would resume a normal life. Alternatively, in a patient who underwent prolonged oxygen deprivation (15–20 min), heart action might be restarted and breathing maintained by a respirator, but the destruction of the brain cells would mean that the patient would be unable to maintain either of those functions on his own.

Neurological examinations are able to assess the extent of brain cell destruction and to distinguish patients who have suffered neocortical damage from those who have lost all brain functions, including that of the brainstem. The first are in a persistent vegetative state. The overwhelming majority of these patients never regain mental functions of any type. Others may recover from the sleeplike coma after days to weeks and then have periods of wakefulness during which their eyes are open and move. There may even be rare instances of recovery of consciousness months or—as in the case of Sgt. David Mack—almost 2 years after the initial trauma. All these patients, including those such as Karen Ann Quinlan, who have suffered overwhelming destruction of the higher brain centers, continue to have functions of, and circulation to, the brain. These patients are clearly alive.

By contrast, brian-dead patients have no flow to the brain. Clinical examinations indicate no evidence of any brain functions. The pupils do not respond to light, nor is there any eye movement. Spontaneous respiration ceases because of the permanent destruction of the vital respiratory centers in the lower brainstem, and the patient is entirely dependent on mechanical respiratory support. Since cardiac functioning is not dependent on neural regulation from the brain, the heartbeat can continue indefinitely in a respirator-supported brain-dead patient, although heart stoppage usually occurs within a few days. There are, however, published cases of confirmed brain-dead children maintained for a month or more; Parisi et al. (1982) report on a case of a 49-year-old New York man who survived 74 days in a brain-dead condition before the court-ordered removal of his respirator "terminated" his life.

2.2. Requirements for Transplantation

With the ability to "sustain" patients through ventilator assistance came the realization that, with such technology, organs of brain-dead patients cold be kept "fresh" for transplant purposes. But in order to harvest the organs, the person must be dead. Physicians and society then faced two critical questions: When is the individual dead? And is it legitimate to ventilate the cadaver to preserve the organs? Moralists quickly agreed to an affirmative answer to the second query. The first proved more problematic.

2.3. The Law and Brain Death

That issue was sharply focused with the advent of cardiac transplant surgery. As is true with many medicomoral topics, it was the courts that first confronted the problem publicly. In the celebrated case of *Tucker v. Lower* (1972), a Virginia court had to determine whether the physicians who removed a brain-dead Bruce Tucker from a respirator and then transplanted his heart into a patient who was dying of cardiac failure were guilty of a wrongful death. The judge instructed the jury in a new definition of death: "In determining the time of death you may consider the following elements . . . among them the time of complete and irreversible loss of all function of the brain." The jury took less than an hour to return a verdict of not guilty.

To clarify the issue for physicians and families and to obviate the costly, burdensome, and often traumatic trial of court battles, various states, beginning with Kansas in 1970, enacted brain-death statutes. Some 36 states and the District of Columbia have followed suit.

To provide for greater uniformity on this subject and avoid the strange situation of the same "body" being "alive" in one state and "dead" in the next, and the still more paradoxical situation of a "body" being alive or dead in the same state, depending on as extrinsic a factor as a signed anatomical gift card, the President's Commission for the Study of Ethical Problems in Medicine was charged by the Congress with developing a uniform determination of death statute. In its 1½-year study, the Commission heard testimony from a wide variety of medical, legal, ethical, and religious viewpoints. Among the positions considered was Jean-Jacques Winslow's eighteenth-century text, *The Uncertainty of the Signs of Death and the Danger of Precipitate Interments,* in which the author argued that putrefaction was the only sure sign of death.

From the outset, the Commission was determined to take extreme caution in formulating public policy in this area. Proposed changes in the existing laws would be designed to produce a minimal shift in the definition as well as a maximal acceptance among laymen, scientists, and clinicians. To that end, the Commission took a conservative posture in its hearings, in its findings, and in its final report. It evaluated, but did not accept, the philosophical understandings of death as the loss of personality or personal identity. It likewise studied and rejected the proposal that "death" be defined as the permanent loss of higher brain functions. In its understanding, those who, like Karen Ann Quinlan, Paul Brophy, or Nancy Jobes, who were in a persistent vegetative state, are not dead.

The commission adopted as its position the widely accepted whole brain-death standard, i.e., death is established when "all functions of the brain including the brain stem have permanently and irreversibly ceased." Thus, even if life continues in individual cells or organs, without the complex integration of the entire system, a person cannot properly be regarded as alive. It proposed the following UDDA: "An individual who has sustained either (1) irreversible cessation of circulatory and respiratory functions, or (2) irreversible cessation of all functions of the entire brain, including brain stem, is dead. A determination of death must be made in accordance with accepted medical standards." With so careful and conservative a formulation—one that had already been adopted with slight variation in 26 states, 20 state supreme courts, and 13 nations, and that had the approval of the American Medical Association, the American Bar Association, the National Conference of Commissioners on Uniform State Laws, and the American Academy of Neurology—it would appear that the remaining jurisdictions would quickly adopt the model statute.

3. OPPOSITION TO THE CONCEPT OF BRAIN DEATH

Nevertheless, opposition soon arose from several quarters. Various right-to-life groups and the Rev. Edward Bryce, chairman of the United States Bishops' Committee for Pro-Life Activities, released position papers denouncing the proposed statute as "unnecessary, dangerous and a stepping stone to euthanasia." Father Bryce's statements, which constitute a replay of the old arguments of the National Conference of Catholic Bishops against living-will legislation, have no application to brain-death statutes. They do reflect, though, the hysteria that exists among some of the right-to-life groups with regard to any attempt to deal with the subject of death and dying.

For example, the Minnesota Citizens Concerned for Life, a 25,000-member organization, testified at a legislative hearing that "it opposes not only brain-death legislation but any imposed definition of death." Such an action, contends Mary Winter, president of People Concerned for the Unborn Child, a powerful Pittsburgh-based antiabortion group, "would be the first step to the 'dehumanization' of the critically ill and to euthanasia." "Once you get that established," she continued, "you're on your way to a Holocaust."

People Concerned's memorandum attacking the UDDA shows the thinking behind their position. It begins by "exposing" support for the legislation by "euthanasia-prone" groups and then articulates their true worry: "As prolifers, we hold what science has proven: that human life begins at fertilization. A definition of death which refers to brain function is anti-life because in the early stages of human development there is no brain. . . . A Statute equating brain function with life would further legally dehumanize the unborn." While the antiabortion stance is admirable, the statement fails to distinguish those with future potential for brain function from those who have exhausted that capacity.

In failing to make crucial distinctions, they follow the leading spokesmen for the positions, Dr. Paul Byrne, an Omaha neonatologist, and the Rev. Paul Quay, a Chicago Jesuit who writes on medical issues. Dr. Byrne and Father Quay, together with the late Sean O'Reilly, authored a well-known article, "Brain Death—an Opposing Viewpoint" in *The Journal of the American Medical Association* (1979), in which they maintain that destruction of the brain, not merely cessation of function, is required for death. Lest there be any doubt as to their standard for irreversible function, the authors provide examples of evidence of death: "If someone's head has been completely crushed by a truck or vaporized by a nuclear blast, or if his brain has been dissolved by a massive injection of sulfuric acid."

What, one might ask, would lead to such a demanding standard? Father Quay's testimony before the President's Commission demonstrates a fear that physicians would be willing "to kill someone who is still alive" in order to obtain transplant organs. His standard of nuclear vaporization or "the total physical disintegration of the individual organs and tissues" not only precludes that grisly possibility but guarantees no harvesting whatsoever. It also recalls Winslow's questionable criterion for certitude: putrefaction.

Dr. Byrne and Father Quay are not content to state their position. They claim that a brain-function criterion "stands in flat contradiction to the religious beliefs of Christians, Jews, Moslems, Hindus and many others." A thorough search of the literature finds no Catholic moral theologian, no Protestant ethicist, and but one Orthodox Jewish spokesman supporting their contention. Rabbi J. David Bleich of Yeshiva University opposes brain-death standards on the grounds that independent cardiac activity still occurs.

Rabbi Bleich (1977), in fact, is the source of the Byrne-Quay dysfunction/destruction thesis.

He articulated it at a 1977 conference on Biomedical Ethics in the Perspective of Jewish Teaching, when he stated "Dysfunction of the brain should not be confused with destruction of the brain. Only *destruction* of the brain can be entertained as a possible definition of death." Rabbi Moses Tendler (Rabbi Bleich's colleague at Yeshiva University), Rabbi Seymour Siegal, and Dr. Isaac Franck took issue with his interpretation of the tradition. They support the validity of total brain-death criteria for the determination of death.

None of this evidence dissuades the prolife forces from continued opposition to the legislation. The prolife groups merely repeat the familiar refrain that legislation is unnecessary and dangerous and on the road to euthanasia. The unfortunate aspect of that mantra is that it influences, if not determines, the political statements of many Catholic bishops. The bishops, in turn, influence and control the policy position of many legislators.

Speaking to that issue, State Senator Louis Bertonazzi of Massachusetts noted the fact that, "the mere presence of an auxiliary bishop of Boston speaking in opposition to the brain-death bill on 'moral grounds' has resulted in a fairly even split among members despite the fact that proponents outnumbered opponents." This, he observed, is not because of reasoned arguments advanced by the opponents but because of their well-known ability to punish or reward legislators. The fear of that punishment will become mobilized, Senator Bertonazzi warns, if brain-death proposals become enmeshed with emotional cries against premature organ transplants or "pulling the plug."

That is precisely what happened in Minnesota, where the Minnesota Citizens Concerned for Life held information meetings to demonstrate the evils of brain-death legislation. Their star witness was Dr. Paul Byrne, who awed a dozen of the legislators with the story of a "brain-dead" patient rescued from a transplant surgeon's knife by a last-minute movement of his Adam's apple. Dr. Byrne further dramatized the issue for the assembled lawmakers by describing the reality of "brain-dead" patients: "The heart is beating, there's blood pressure, they put out urine, they sweat, they're warm, they look like a human being and someone decides they're dead." After his presentation, no one in the Minnesota legislature wanted to decide that such a patient was dead. Not a single member wanted to sponsor the UDDA—this for a bill that in one form or another had already been enacted into law in 31 states.

Similar influence was demonstrated by the Missouri Catholic Conference, when it opposed "any statutory definition of death." After describing brain death as "an esoteric creation of neurologists and neurosurgeons who are seeking to speed up the declaration of death for transplant purposes," the Missouri Catholic bishops presented several objections to a brain-death statute:

1. There is no need for a statutory definition of death. No physician has ever been prosecuted for using brain criteria, and no Missouri case prohibits physicians from doing so.
2. There is strong disagreement among the medical profession about the acceptance of that standard.
3. There are foreseeable adverse consequences to patient, family rights, physician rights, and the welfare of society from such a statute.

On its face, points 1 and 2 are incompatible. If there is strong disagreement among physicians on the acceptance of a brain-death standard, to employ it as a criterion for death without legislative or judicial authorization would be cavalier, if not foolhardy. The Missouri Conference also acknowledges that there are physicians who, while accepting the criterion as valid, believe it is illegal to use it under the present circumstances. Consequently, they keep "dead" patients on respirators.

On that topic, there is no longer any doubt as to what the medically accepted standards are. "The Guidelines for the Determination of Death" (1981), a landmark document that reflected a summary of currently accepted medical practices, was published in *The Journal of the American Medical Association*. It is signed by the nation's leading authorities in neurology, neurosurgery, critical care, and legal medicine. In the words of the accompanying editorial, it represents "a consensus that is truly a remarkable achievement, [one] of which the medical profession can be proud." That document endorses the UDDA.

The charge of impure motives on the part of neurologists and neurosurgeons likewise falters under examination. Dr. Shelley Chou, a neurosurgeon writing in *The Lancet* (1981), reports that at the University of Minnesota Hospital there are "about 20 brain-death cases per year and less than 50 percent of them become organ donors." Reporting on a similar study done over a 5-year period at Queen Elizabeth Hospital in Birmingham, England, Tomlin *et al.* (1981) note that only 15 of the 66 patients diagnosed as brain dead became organ donors. Similar figures are found in the President's Commission Report (1981), where we learn that "only six of 36 subjects declared dead by neurological criteria in the commission's survey were organ donors."

The third cluster of concerns of the Missouri Catholic Conference is the least defensible. It objects that a legal definition of death would prevent the family of a brain-dead individual from continuing life-support treatment if they so desired, would assist hospitals in refusing to care for "dead bodies," would aid insurance companies and the government in stopping payment for such care, and would inhibit the freedom of the individual physician from practicing medicine according to his or her own best judgment. Do the members of the conference really believe that the determination of death should be subject to the designs of families, the idiosyncratic judgments of physicians, or the desires of third-party payers? The wishes, hopes, or fantasies of the family or physician will not change the reality of death, nor should they influence its diagnosis.

In addition to the various Catholic conferences, the Catholic Hospital Association has given its attention to the subject. In a thoughtful and well-documented booklet entitled *Determination of Death,* the Reverend Albert S. Moraczewski and J. Stuart Showalter (1982) explore the theological, medical, ethical, and legal implications of brain death. They conclude their analysis with the statement, "We pose no legal or moral objection to UDDA." Yet, they continue, "one cannot thereby simply assert that legislation of such criteria is justified." to be justified, they claim, there must be evidence that the absence of legislation results in injustice to patients, families, or physicians, evidence that they maintain has not yet been established.

They hold that the way to achieve public acceptance of the brain-death criteria is not by legislation—the usual way in which society codifies its social values—but by education.

4. EXAMPLES OF PROBLEMS ATTRIBUTABLE TO LACK OF STATUTES

It is difficult to obtain public acceptance of a standard that is repeatedly attacked by some Catholic bishops as being morally suspect and potentially dangerous. It is yet more difficult to get physicians to follow the Moraczewski–Showalter exhortation that they should rely on their medical judgment rather than fret over legal liabilities. In our litigious society, physicians and lawyers are understandably unwilling to go forward under the threat of civil or criminal liability. A tragic example of that reality was the case of Melanie Bacchiochi, a 23-year-old Connecticut woman who was maintained in a brain-dead condition for 43 days until a court finally authorized the physician to follow the appropriate medical response to her condition.

Still other reported travesties of justice were provoked by a lack of brain-death legislation. For example, the wife of a brain-dead New York policeman, who had been ambushed and shot in the head, was asked by Queens County District Attorney John Santucci not to disconnect the respirator lest that action jeopardize a potential first-degree murder conviction. The wife, a Catholic, replied that she would never remove the respirator under such circumstances, saying, "It would be against my religion."

Similar fears were expressed by the Nassau County District Attorney's Office in the case of Richard Berger, a 19-year-old who was wheeled into the emergency room of the Smithtown

General Hospital, Long Island, New York, with a robber's bullet in his brain. Comatose as the result of massive brain damage, the patient had no reflex responses. His pupils were dilated and fixed, and there was no response to light or intense pain. His electroencephalogram (EEG) was flat. He was unable to breathe without a respirator. The boy's father had but one question: "Is he dead?" The physician replied, "He is brain dead." The father pressed further. Was his son legally dead? The physician's response is instructive: "Medically he is dead. Legally . . . I don't know. I am not a lawyer."

That confusion set up 6 days of agony for Berger's parents as physicians, lawyers, district attorneys, and transplant coordinators tried to sift through the competing claims, hopes, and expectations for the boy. The physicians, though convinced Richard was dead, would not pronounce him so unless the parents either sought a court order declaring him dead or decided to donate his organs. In the latter case, the doctors and the hospital would be legally protected by the state's Uniform Anatomical Gift Act, which authorized the removal of organs from brain dead individuals.

The physicians explained the issues to the family and the complications resulting from the fact that in New York there was no definition of death statute. The district attorney compounded the family woes by alerting them to the fact that the assailant probably would argue that the parents, not he, had caused their son's death. Although no court had ever accepted such a defense, that would not prevent things "from getting very, very ugly at the trial."

Yet a further burden for the parents as they viewed their son breathing on the respirator day after day was the hope that though brain dead, he might somehow miraculously come out of the coma. That hope was finally dashed on the sixth day, when Richard suffered cardiac arrest. The parents were confronted with the decision of immediately permitting the removal of his organs or facing the prospect of both his death and the destruction of his organs. At that point, for reasons that had nothing to do with the law, they determined that the miracle of life would go to the waiting recipient rather than to their son. They authorized the transplant.

5. RECENT DEVELOPMENTS AND CURRENT STATUS

If there were but a few brain-death cases, and if they all ended within a day or two, the misuse of the medical personnel and resources might be a tolerable price to pay. But as a survey done by the President's Commission indicates, there are 204 such cases per month in major medical centers. And as Parisi *et al.* (1982) show, not all such patients succumb quickly to cardiac failure. In addition, we know that brain-dead children have substantial "survival rates." When these data are evaluated, it is apparent that the misallocation of resources, the financial costs, and the emotional strain of continued "treatment" become vastly disproportionate to any putative benefits.

During the past few years, there have been shifts in the stand taken by some prolife activists and Catholic conferences on the UDDA. Such well-known prolife spokesmen as Dr. Joseph Stanton, attorney Dennis Horan, and Dr. C. Everett Koop have supported determination of death statutes. In the words of Surgeon General Koop, "I think the Uniform Act addresses the critical issues of brain-stem death and therefore should be a piece of legislation which prolife groups could sincerely and honestly support."

It was that realization and the growing awareness that the idea of brain death "has become widely accepted in the medical profession" that led the Wisconsin Catholic Conference to withdraw its longstanding opposition to a uniform determination of death act. With the Wisconsin bishops no longer actively lobbying against the bill, the UDDA passed.

Yet more striking was the change in Pennsylvania, where the Catholic conference announced that it now supports the President's Commission proposal. In a position paper explaining its shift, the Pennsylvania bishops provide a point-by-point refutation of the frequently repeated charge that such legislation is unnecessary, dangerous, and the first step to euthanasia. They argue that technological changes make it imperative that we update our understanding of death. They then declare that it is far better to enact clarifying legislation than to leave the determination to the vagaries of court opinion and the burden of unnecessary litigation. They argue that if, as is possible, someone proposes a radical departure from the intent of this law in favor of euthanasia, that is the time to enter battle.

The Pennsylvania Catholic bishops have provided a model of how church involvement in the public policy process should proceed. Rather than merely join the chorus shouting "euthanasia" every time an issue involving death is raised, they have followed Archbishop John Roach's admonition that when the church enters the political arena, it must do so on the basis of reasoned argumentation. To provide this, the Pennsylvania bishops subjected the traditional charges against the legislation to critical analysis, found them inadequate, and revised their position.

That the shift in Catholic opposition to brain-death legislation is now nearly complete is found in the recent statement of the Pontifical Academy of Science (1985), the Vatican's official scientific advisory body, that:

> A person is dead when he has irreversibly lost all capacity to integrate and coordinate the physical and mental functions of the body. Death occurs when:
> (a) the spontaneous cardiac and respiratory functions have definitively ceased, or
> (b) if an irreversible cessation of every brain function is verified.

With that official pronouncement, it is hoped that the criticisms and political lobbying against the UDDA by prolife activists and their allies in the Catholic hierarchy will end. If that should occur, such states as Minnesota, Massachusetts, and New York, where the UDDA legislation has been stymied by the lobbying of the Catholic bishops, ought to be able to enact appropriate brain-death legislation.

Once a brain death statute has been enacted, the traditional Catholic teaching on transplants of cadaver organs, a teaching summarized in Pope Pius XII's (1956) statement, applies:

> A person may will to dispose of his body and to destine it to ends that are useful, morally irreproachable and even noble, among them the desire to aid the sick and suffering. One may make a decision of this nature with respect to his own body with full realization of the reverence which is due it. . . . This decision should not be condemned but positively justified.

That teaching was reinforced by the Pontifical Academy of Science's observation that cadaver "transplants deserve the support of the medical profession, of the law and of people in general." As they added, "the donation of organs should, in all circumstances, respect the last will of the donor, or the consent of the family, if present."

REFERENCES

Barber, J., Becker, D., Behrman, R., Bennet, D. R., and Beresford, R., 1981, Guidelines for the determination of death, *JAMA* **246**:2184–2186.

Barclay, N. R., 1981, Editorial: Guidelines for the determination of death, *JAMA* **246**:2194.

Bertonazzi, L. P., 1981, Brain death: A political process, *Conn. Med.* **45**:452–455.

Bleich, J. D., Neurological criteria of death and time of death statutes, in: *Jewish Bioethics* (F. Rosner, J. D. Bleich, eds.), pp. 303–316, Hebrew Publishing Co., New York.

Byrne, P. A., O'Reilly, S., and Quay, P. M., 1979, Brain death: An opposing viewpoint, *JAMA* **242**:1985–1990.

Capron, A. M., 1987, Anencephalic donors: Separate the dead from the dying, *Hastings Ctr. Rep.* **17**(1):5–8.

Chou, S., 1981, Brain death, *Lancet* **214**:282–283.

Moraczewski, A. S., and Showalter, J. S., 1982, *Determination of Death,* Catholic Health Association, St. Louis.

Parisi, J. E., Kim, R. C., Collins, G. H., and Hilfinger, M. F., 1982, Brain death with prolonged somatic survival, *N. Engl. J. Med.* **306:**14–16.

Pius XII, 1956, Allocution to a group of eye specialists, quoted in Ashley, B. M., and O'Rourke, K. D., 1978 *Health Care Ethics: A Theological Analysis,* Catholic Health Association, St. Louis.

Pontifical Academy of Science, 1985, Ethical, medical and legal questions on the artificial prolongation of life, *L'Osservatore Romano,* **11:**10.

Tomlin, P. J., Martin, J. W., and Honigsberger, L., 1981, Brain death: Retrospective surveys, *Lancet* **214:**282–283.

Tucker v. Lower, 1972, No. 831, Richmond, Va L. and Eq. Ct., May 23, 1972.

Vatican Congregation for the Doctrine of Faith, *Declaration on Euthanasia,* 1980, United States Catholic Conference, Washington, D.C.

4

PROTESTANT PERSPECTIVES ON ORGAN DONATION

JAMES F. CHILDRESS

1. INTRODUCTION

My assigned task is to examine Protestant perspectives on organ retrieval, particularly organ donation, with some attention to brain death. Because of the diverse traditions and denominations that are labeled Protestant, I cannot hope to be comprehensive. Instead, I will offer some rough generalizations about perspectives that can legitimately be considered Protestant, while raising more general issues as well.

Why attend to religious perspectives at all, when our aim is to develop public policies in a pluralistic society? A first reason is historical: Many of the laws, policies, and practices regarding bodies and their parts have been influenced by religious traditions. To understand and reconsider these laws, policies, and practices, we need to identify and examine the beliefs and values that may have originally supported them.

A second reason is that religious traditions still shape the ethical values of many people, influencing many people's beliefs and practices regarding the body, as well as the donation of organs. A third, and closely related, reason is that policy-makers must anticipate the responses of religious communities when they attempt to determine which policies will be politically feasible as well as ethically acceptable and ethically preferable. For example, vigorous opposition from religious organizations may defeat a policy.

2. RELIGIOUS ATTITUDES TOWARD THE BODY AND ITS PARTS

William May (1985) developed a typology that expresses "several basic religious attitudes and their implications for recovering body parts." This typology provides a context for differentiating various Jewish and Christian beliefs and practices. The first type of religious perspective is idealistic, monistic, and optimistic. It recognizes the reality of the spiritual realm but denies the reality of the body, sickness, and death. A modern version is Christian Science.

JAMES F. CHILDRESS • Departments of Religious Studies and Medical Education, University of Virginia, Charlottesville, Virginia 22903.

The second type is dualistic and pessimistic. Recognizing the reality of both the body and the spirit, it views the body as evil and the spirit as good. As represented in the ancient Manichaeans, it divides the world into rival powers, light and darkness, spirit and flesh, good and evil. Although rarely explicitly defended in official theological statements, it often appears in popular religious discourse.

The third type, as represented by the Gnostics, is also dualistic but it views the body as incidental, rather than unreal or evil. Salvation is gained through knowledge, and the body is not essential to human identity and fulfillment.

By contrast, the fourth type, which appears in the mainstream of Judaism and Christianity, views the body as real, as good, and as essential to human life and personhood. May (1985) states:

> As opposed to the Christian Scientists or other idealists, the [Judeo-Christian] tradition says that the body is *real* rather than unreal; as opposed to the Manichaeans, it affirms the body to be *good* rather than evil, worthy of preserving. Both affirmations converge to justify medical intervention. But, as opposed to the Gnostics, the Judeo-Christian tradition affirms a profound link and identity of the spirit with its somatic existence. Thus it would not be so ready as the Gnostic to justify invasion of the body, living or dead, without explicit consent.

Furthermore, May argues, the Judeo-Christian tradition "sympathizes with [natural] aversions to tampering with a living body or corpse," while it also develops symbols and rituals for disciplining those aversions.

Because of variations among and within Judaism, Catholicism, and Protestantism, it is difficult to speak of the Judeo-Christian tradition unless that phrase refers to one shared source (the Hebrew Bible/Old Testament) and some common though very general themes. Following are some themes that are widespread among these traditions and are prominent in Protestant denominations, which usually appeal to Scripture as their fundamental authority.

3.   CREATION IN THE IMAGE OF GOD

God created the world, including human beings, as good. Human beings themselves were created "in the image of God." "Then God said, 'Let us make man in our image, after our likeness; and let them have dominion. . . .' So God created man in his own image, in the image of God he created him; male and female he created them" (Gen. 1:26f; cf. 5:1 and 9:6). While the image of God *(imago dei)* has been variously interpreted as reason, free will, or spiritual capacities, some theologians have objected to the concentration on intellectual and spiritual aspects of humanity to the neglect of the external body. Some have even argued that the image of God is the body, while others have argued that it is a combination of the spiritual and the physical in a psychophysical unity.

The modern debate about the image of God has focused on what is distinctive about persons, particularly their use of reason, exercise of will, and decision-making. In short, the *imago dei* has often been seen as a theological basis for the principle of respect for persons. Even though there are some important historical and conceptual connections between Protestantism and liberalism, it would be a mistake to construe the image of God as equivalent to autonomy in the modern liberal tradition. Respect for persons is one way to state the implications of the theological doctrine of the *imago dei*, but for most Protestant theologians the *imago dei* implies respect for embodied persons, not simply their wills. The main tendency in Protestant theology is to view the person as an animated body, or as an embodied spirit, even though at times Protestant beliefs and practices have represented more Hellenistic convictions about the separation of soul and body. In any event, the *imago dei* does not imply unlimited self-determination (autonomy) because what human beings may will and choose is limited by God's creation and will (heteronomy or theonomy).

In practice, it is often difficult to determine which actions are required by the principle of respect for persons, as an expression of the *imago dei*. Nevertheless, several implications of the *imago dei* are important for discussions of the body and the transfer of body parts. The passage in Genesis connects creation in the image of God with God's authorization of human "dominion" over the rest of creation. Human beings are in but are distinguished from the rest of nature. Some commentators have interpreted the image of God in relation to the royal ideology of the ancient Near East: Human beings are God's representatives in parts of his kingdom. Their dominion should not be viewed as domination but as stewardship, trusteeship, or deputyship, and their rule should be like God's and never exploitative. As stewards and trustees, human beings do not have unlimited power. The earth and all that is in it, including living and dead human beings, belong to God; they are God's property. And God has set limits on what human beings may do with and to their own bodies and those of others, living and dead. For example, Gen. 9:6 connects the prohibition of taking human life with creation in God's image. And this prohibition has also been applied to suicide, particularly through such analogies as property relationships, e.g., life is a gift or a loan from God, and personal or role relationships, e.g., human beings are God's children, servants, or sentinels (Battin, 1982).

Respect for the human cadaver is also significantly connected to human creation in the image of God. Indeed, the body of the dead is symbolic of human persons and their dignity. As May (1985) argues, this respect recognizes and supports (within limits) the aversion to tampering with the body, whether living or dead. However, in contrast to the Jewish tradition, Protestants generally have no major problems with autopsies. The traditional belief in the resurrection of the body does not constrain organ or tissue removal, because that belief affirms God's power and does not imply that "the expected resurrection of the body will be a reconstituting of bone, flesh and blood" (Nelson, 1984).

Obviously, different interpretations of the doctrine of the *imago dei* have different implications for the conception of death. In general, Protestant thinkers, ranging from Joseph Fletcher to Paul Ramsey, have recognized the appropriateness of determining death by the use of brain criteria. Most Protestants have adopted the whole-brain death conception rather than the higher-brain conception. However, as Robert Veatch (1986a) has noted, Protestant theologians are divided over the "question of whether an irreversibly unconscious person with lower-brain function including intact respiration should be considered dead. Some who answer yes argue that, in Christianity, the human being represents an essential unity of body and soul (mental function being a modern analogue for the soul). They hold that when consciousness is irreversibly lost, what remains is only the mortal remains of the person. More conservative critics argue that an individual should be considered alive as long as capacities remain for bodily integration, even if consciousness is no longer possible."

The traditional Protestant view of human sinfulness, i.e., that human beings are created in the image of God, but they are also fallen, sinful creatures, has played a role in some Protestants' emphasis on the need for procedures and barriers to prevent the removal of organs under inappropriate circumstances. For example, Ramsey (1970) argued that it is important, on the practical level, to separate the role of pronouncing death from the role of organ transplantation in order to avoid a conflict of interest; thus, the potential recipient's physician should not determine when the donor is dead. Similarly, Ramsey argued, on the theoretical or intellectual level, society should not update the criteria for determining death primarily in order to increase the supply of organs. There are sufficient reasons to update these criteria in care of dying patients themselves, without reference to benefits to others.

For most Protestant theology, the New Testament norm of *agape* (neighbor love) is the main norm of ethics. Viewed as a summary of the law and the prophets, and expressed in the parable of the Good Samaritan, neighbor love is freely giving to benefit the neighbor. It would be possible to interpret neighbor love as obligating the donation of one's own organs after death or the organs of a dead relative. Even though Protestantism tends to permit, and even to praise, donations of cadaver organs, it has rarely recognized an obligation to do so. Connecting several Protestant themes, the Rev. Foster McCurley, a Lutheran, has insisted that "organ donations can be an important way of continuing in partnership with our Creator in the life process—responsible and benevolent stewardship of our bodies." He continues, "alleviating suffering, serving others in wellness and in death, is part of the self-sacrifice and crossbearing of Christians" (Geiser, 1985). It is not clear, however, why such donations are only praiseworthy rather than obligatory, since they are low in cost and high in benefit. Such gifts could even be seen as obligatory within the context of secular beneficence.

In summary, Protestant theologians, drawing from their biblical interpretation, hold that human beings are created in the image of God and thus derive their dignity and worth from this creation; they are animated bodies or embodied selves, not a composite, and their bodies are real, good, and essential to their identity; God has given humans dominion over nature, including their own bodies and parts of bodies. This dominion is best conceived as stewardship, trusteeship, or administration, because human power and authority are limited by God's will. There are certain obligations toward the body, including the cadaver, as a symbol of the image of God. The image of God does not imply unlimited autonomy of the individual or of family members because God sets limits and points a direction of neighbor love. Even though human beings are created in God's image, they are fallen, sinful creatures, and institutions are thus needed to limit and control the effects of sin, as well as to provide opportunities for neighbor love. These are very general theological–ethical perspectives, and a bridgework is required to connect them to particular judgments about actions and policies.

4.   DONATION AS THE PREFERRED MODE OF TRANSFER OF ORGANS AND TISSUES

There are several possible modes of transfer of body parts: gifts (explicit and implicit), abandonment, sales, and expropriation. The gift relationship marks the current system of organ donation in the United States. It is largely a matter of explicit gifts, including both living donors (e.g., of kidneys, blood, and bone marrow) and cadaver organs (e.g., kidneys, hearts, and livers). But several states also have presumed consent statutes for corneas; the sale of blood plasma persists; and some tissues, such as spleens removed during surgery, may be transferred through abandonment.

Protestants tend to put a high premium on explicit gifts and donations (as in the Uniform Anatomical Gift Act) without necessarily excluding implicit gifts (as in presumed or tacit consent). In addition, for most Protestants, transfer (or acquisition) by abandonment, sales, or expropriation would not always be wrong, depending on the body parts or tissues in question, but there are special concerns about them. For example, arguments against commercialization include the dangers of exploitation and coercion of vendors, risks to vendors, risks to buyers, and threats to the society, particularly its attitudes toward and practices regarding the body. In general, Protestants argue, the gift relationship is preferable, where gifts are donated to others, including strangers, in accord with the norm of neighbor love. For instance, Ramsey (1970) does not argue that presumed consent—what we might call presumed or tacit gifts—is ethically unacceptable, but that a policy of explicit gifts is ethically preferable because it expresses and supports an altruistic community.

It is important to be clear about our language—the term "donor" is applied indiscriminately to the decision-maker and to the source of the organs, even if the decedent never could or never did make a decision to donate. We should reserve the term "donor" for the decision-maker. Even the term "donor family" may be misleading. It is important not to obscure the import of our policies and practices by misusing such terms as "donor" and "donation" because of their positive connotations. Focusing on cadavers, we can say that the decedent is the source. The decedent may also be the donor if he or she made a decision to donate before dying. Often, however, the family will be the donor. In principle, the Uniform Anatomical Gift Act is individualistic; it assigns primacy to the individual. In practice, the family's role in donation has been crucial.

There are various types of generosity, whether expressed by the decedent or by the family. In organ donation, generosity may be expressed in ways other than through the initiation of the gift. For example, the decedent may have feared the consequences of signing a donor card—opinion polls (Gallup Organization, 1985) indicate that potential donors fear that their deaths may be allowed or hastened in order to benefit others if they have signed a donor card—whereas the family may be so distraught about its tragedy that it fails to consider donation. An affirmative response to an inquiry displays generosity as much as initiation of donation. Even in a system of presumed consent or donation, which would be opposed for various reasons, generosity may be expressed in the refusal to opt out.

Various opinion polls indicate a decline in expressed willingness to sign donor cards because of distrust of the system, as reflected in the fear that patients with signed donor cards may be declared dead prematurely in order to provide organs for others. Such fears are especially prominent among groups that view themselves as marginal to the society. It may not be possible to alter this attitude of distrust through educational efforts, but information about certain and consistent criteria for determining brain death could help.

In general, respondents indicate a greater willingness to donate a family member's organs because they are in control. For example, according to a Gallup poll (1985), 45% indicated that they were very or somewhat likely to donate their own organs, while 85% indicated that they were very or somewhat likely to donate the organs of a dead family member. Such attitudes provide a major reason for the recent state and federal legislation mandating that hospitals routinely inquire about the family's willingness to donate when a relative has died under circumstances in which the organs could be salvaged for transplantation.

5. PEDIATRIC ORGANS: SPECIAL PROBLEMS

Two preliminary points are in order as we turn to the serious problem of obtaining pediatric organs. First, the child cannot serve as a donor, because he or she cannot make an advance gift; the child is only the source of organs, which are donated by others. However, in some cases children may indicate their wishes to their families. Second, a Gallup poll (1985) indicated that 65% of the population is very or somewhat likely to donate their own child's organs. Thus, people are more likely to donate their child's organs than their own, but less likely to donate their child's organs than the organs of another family member.

The Task Force on Organ Transplantation (1986) heard testimony from a woman whose young child suffered brain death following the rupture of a cerebral aneurysm. The mother indicated that she had not considered organ donation until a procurement coordinator discussed it with her. She attributed her positive response to the way she was provided this opportunity to donate her daughter's organs and to the consolation it appeared to offer:

> I can honestly admit that out of my personal tragedy something beautiful has blossomed, a living memorial to my daughter. And, I truly believe that this was made possible because I was contacted by someone who epitomized my concept of what compassion is all about.

Special ethical problems have emerged in the pediatric area because of the possibility of using aborted or delivered anencephalics. Since anencephalics can survive only briefly—their death is inevitable and imminent—their parents often want to donate the organs in order to benefit other children. The need for pediatric organs is great; approximately 400–500 kidneys and hearts and 500–1000 livers are needed each year (Capron, 1987; Fletcher *et al.*, 1986). Each year the organs of approximately 1,800–3,500 anencephalics could probably be salvaged to benefit children in need. However, parental donations of anencephalic organs cannot be accepted within the current legal framework, consisting of the Uniform Anatomical Gift Act and whole-brain death criteria. If the conditions of that framework are met, the organs of the anencephalic will probably not be satisfactory for transplantation. A fundamental question is whether the legal framework should be altered in order to facilitate the donation and transplantation of anencephalic organs. Any of the major alterations that would be necessary and sufficient is fraught with serious difficulties, largely because of the demands of clarity, certainty, and consistency in organ procurement.

On the one hand, it would be possible to create an exception for anencephalics in the requirement of whole-brain death for the removal of organs. but anencephalics can breathe spontaneously, and it is conceptually difficult to distinguish them from patients who are irreversibly comatose. Using the language of "brain absent" in contrast to "brain dead" does not resolve the problem. Creating an exception in the whole-brain death requirement would endanger other patients who do not now qualify as acceptable sources of organs.

On the other hand, it would be possible to create an exception in the Uniform Anatomical Gift Act by allowing anencephalics to be killed in the process of removing their hearts and livers. This alteration would be a serious breach in important societal rules against killing human beings to benefit others.

Alexander Capron (1987) rightly argues that adopting either of these possible policies in order to obtain additional pediatric organs would threaten organ donation in the United States by introducing further unclarity, uncertainty and inconsistency in a system that already generates some distrust. Another possibility would not be as problematic for the system of organ procurement. John Fletcher *et al.* (1986) focus on the management of dying anencephalics as sources (not donors) of organs. With parental consent, physicians could gradually cool the body to protect the organs from ischemia. This practice, which is already used for some adult sources of organs, would probably hasten the anencephalic's death. It would not be tantamount to killing, for it could be brought under the rule of double effect, employed widely in Roman Catholic thought but also accepted in much Protestant thought (e.g., Ramsey, 1970). Even though this is a complicated medical and ethical maneuver, which also raises other important questions, e.g., about the management of pregnancy after a diagnosis of anencephaly, it is appropriate as a way to avoid tampering with other rules (the standard of whole brain death and the prohibition of killing) while also trying to help infants in need of organ transplants. The system of organ procurement, which depends on public generosity, is very fragile, and tampering with some rules that are important for clarity, certainty, and consistency may further threaten public trust.

6.   MORAL CONNECTIONS BETWEEN ORGAN PROCUREMENT AND DISTRIBUTION

There are several important connections between organ procurement and organ distribution. Obviously, an increase in the supply of organs would reduce scarcity and problems of patient selection. But one important moral connection works the other way: It is essential that potential donors perceive the system of distribution of donated organs as fair. Otherwise, their suspicion and distrust, which are already fundamental reasons for their reluctance to donate organs, will perpetuate scarcity.

Cases of designated recipients include virtually all living donations of kidneys and some donations of cadaver organs. For example, in a dramatic and poignant case, a teenager in California had a premonition of his death and indicated that he wanted his heart given to his girlfriend, who needed a heart transplant; he died unexpectedly, and his family donated his heart according to his wishes. More recently, when a teenager was killed in an accident, his family donated his heart to his grandfather. However much we may be moved by, and may even praise, such donations, we have to be concerned about some practices of designated or specified donees.

In the first place, there are the particularistic appeals by the President and others for donations of organs for an identified child in need. Such particularistic appeals are often defended on the grounds that they will lead to an overall increase in donations, but critics note that such increases, even if apparent, are at most only temporary. In addition, because parents have unequal access to the media and to public figures, such particularistic appeals are often criticised as unfair. It is more important to design a system of organ procurement that will tap the latent, responsive generosity of the public in order to secure gifts of organs for unidentified strangers.

In the second place, apart from such particularistic appeals and donations to particular recipients, some donors want to attach strings to their gifts, for example, by restricting them to certain races or to certain groups. Even though it is difficult to decline any gift of organs because of the need for them, gifts with certain strings attached should be declined, as the Uniform Anatomical Gift Act permits. In the long run, acceptance of those gifts would probably subvert the system of impersonal altruism; it would probably lead to counterdonations and increase suspicions of the system's lack of trustworthiness.

In general, apart from organs donated for specific donees, or with certain strings attached, donated organs belong to the community. According to the federal Task Force on Organ Transplantation (1986), donated organs should be viewed as scarce public resources to be used for the welfare of the community. Thus, organ procurement and transplant teams receive donated organs as trustees and stewards for the community, and they should distribute donated organs according to public criteria that have been developed with public input and are just.

Many, although not all, Protestant theologians and ethicists argue that agape or neighbor love is most congruent with an egalitarian conception of justice that distributes the scarce good of health care according to need (Outka, 1974). Although Protestants may appeal to independent secular grounds in support of egalitarian patterns of distribution, they often invoke specifically theological arguments (Veatch, 1986b). For example, Ramsey (1970) contends that scarce life-saving medical resources should be distributed according to need, rather than merit or other standards of social worth, because God's care is indiscriminate. When needs are roughly equal and resources are inadequate to meet all of them, Ramsey continues, a lottery or queuing may approximate God's indiscriminate care because it provides rough equality of opportunity.

Most conceptions of justice permit rationing under conditions of scarcity, while ruling out criteria of selection that reflect such morally irrelevant characteristics as race or sex. There is general agreement that the primary criteria should be medical: medical need and probability of success (Task Force on Transplantation, 1986). However, there is debate about whether these medical criteria should be defined broadly or narrowly, about how to specify them, about the relevance of such factors as age and the number of previous transplants, and about whether need or probability of success should have priority in cases of conflict. In view of such uncertainties, the task force recommended a public process that could determine the parameters of just allocation, particularly by making sure that medical criteria are not corrupted by covert judgments of social worth. It also recommended that time on the waiting list be decisive when medical factors are roughly equal. Furthermore, it argued that ability to pay should be irrelevant to access to donated organs, largely because it is unfair for the society to ask rich and poor people alike to donate organs if poor people cannot gain access to donated organs when they need them. As part of the argument against the commercialization of the transfer of organs, the Task Force on Transplantation (1986) recommended that the federal government as a last resort provide funds to ensure that ability to pay will be irrelevant.

Even when Protestant perspectives, especially regarding *agape*, push in the direction of equal access in health care, the debates just identified will still be significant. A final example will illustrate this point. Agape is considered universalistic; this implies that all human beings should be treated equally because they are created in the image of God and are the objects of God's love. Such a conception of agape might appear to imply that donated organs should be distributed to patients in need regardless of accidents of geography or national origin. It might appear to require that nonresident aliens be granted unrestricted access to cadaver organs retrieved in the United States. However, even a universalistic conception of agape may be qualified in practice, and it may, for example, recognize the legitimacy of giving priority to near-neighbors over distant neighbors when it is impossible to meet the needs of everyone. It may also recognize a standard of sharing, such as tithing. Thus, it is not clear what policy recommendations about nonresident aliens would follow from these general Protestant perspectives. The major debate centers on whether (1) to allow nonresident aliens access to a certain percentage of U.S. cadaver organs, e.g., a maximum of 5 or 10%, but to treat those admitted to the waiting list equally according to need, probability of success, and time on the waiting list or (2) to put nonresident aliens on the bottom of the waiting list or on a separate waiting list, so that they would not be eligible for donated organs unless no U.S. citizens or residents could benefit from those organs. Confronting its most divisive issue, the Task Force on Transplantation (1986) recommended policy (1) for renal organs, proposing that nonresident aliens comprise no more than 10% of the total number of kidney transplant recipients at any transplant center until the Organ Procurement and Transplantation Network, now developed by United Network for Organ Sharing, could review the issue. It recommended policy (2) for extrarenal organs.

Which policy would follow from Protestant perspectives? It is not easy to move directly from general Protestant (or other religious) perspectives to recommendations about policies. Even though such general perspectives as the *imago dei* and agape may set limits and point directions, adherents to such perspectives will often have considerable latitude in defining appropriate policies, frequently invoking secular moral norms as well.

REFERENCES

Battin, M. P., 1982, *Ethical Issues in Suicide,* Prentice-Hall, Englewood Cliffs, New Jersey.

Capron, A. M., 1987, Anencephalic donors: Separate the dead from the dying, *Hastings Ctr. Rep.* **17**:5–9.

Childress, J. F., 1985, Love and justice in Christian bioethics, in: *Theology and Bioethics* (E. E. Shelp, ed.), pp. 225–243, Reidel, Dordrecht, Holland.

Childress, J. F., 1986, The Implications of Major Western Religious Traditions for Policies Regarding Human Biological Materials, Office of Technology Assessment, Contract No. 633–2425.0 (May 13, 1986).

Childress, J. F., 1987, Some moral connections between organ procurement and organ distribution, *J. Contemp. Health Law Policy* **3**:85–110.

Fletcher, J. C., Robertson, J. R., and Harrison, M. R., 1986, Primates and anencephalics as sources for pediatric organ transplants, *Fetal Ther.* **1**:150–164.

Gallup Organization, 1985, The U. S. Public's Attitudes Toward Organ Transplants/Organ Donation, conducted for Golin/Harris Communications, on behalf of the American Council on Transplantation, Jan. 1985.

Geiser, F., 1985, Sharing body and blood is familiar to Christians, *Lutheran* April 17:5–7.

May, W. F., 1985, Religious justifications for donating body parts, *Hastings Center Report* **15**:38–42.

Nelson, J. R., 1984, Protestant Christian perspectives, *Report of the Massachusetts Task Force on Organ Transplantation,* presented to the Commissioner of Public Health and Secretary of Human Services, Oct. 1984, pp. 97–99.

Outka, G., 1974, Social justice and equal access to health care, *J. Relig. Ethics* **2**:11–32.

Ramsey, P., 1970, *The Patient as Person,* Yale University Press, New Haven, Connecticut.

Task Force on Transplantation, 1986, *Organ Transplantation: Issues and Recommendations,* U.S. Department of Health and Human Services, Washington.

Veatch, R. M., 1986*a*, Death, determination of, *Dictionary of Christian Ethics,* 2nd ed. (J. F. Childress and J. Macquarrie, eds.), pp. 144–146, Westminster Press, Philadelphia.

Veatch, R. M., 1986*b*, *The Foundations of Justice,* Oxford University Press, New York.

5

THE LEGAL STATUS OF BRAIN-BASED DETERMINATIONS OF DEATH

ALEXANDER MORGAN CAPRON

1. INTRODUCTION

The simple answer to the question posed in this volume—What is the legal status of brain death?—is that determinations of death based on the complete and irreversible cessation of all functions of the entire brain are legally sanctioned by statute or judicial decision in 47 jurisdictions in the United States. Furthermore, there is no reason to think that they would be found invalid in any of the remaining four. Thus, were one addressing his subject solely from the view of the practicing lawyer, the answer to a client's question "What is the legal status of brain death?," would be easy and noncontroversial. Why, then, does interest in this topic persist? There are several reasons. Prime among these is the confusion in nomenclature that has led to a conceptual or philosophical confusion, which is to be discussed below.

I intend to advance the thesis that the subject of determining death is no longer a matter of dispute in medical or legal circles. In support of this position, I address three arguments: first, that the problems with terminology have led to a misperception that what is involved is a "redefinition" of human death, when all that is actually involved is a reformulation of the standards for measuring death; second, that the medical profession has articulated reliable, appropriate, and generally accepted criteria and tests to implement the reformulated standards; and third, that we can expect the states that have not yet done so to enact the Uniform Determination of Death Act (UDDA) or its equivalent in the coming years (although, needless to say, my view is that the UDDA and *not* some "equivalent" statute should be the one adopted).

2. THE CONFUSION OVER *BRAIN DEATH*

The first problem is illustrated by the title of this book, which speaks of *brain death*. That terminology has been widely used. Indeed, it has probably been familiar to the general public

ALEXANDER MORGAN CAPRON • The Law Center and the School of Medicine, University of Southern California, Los Angeles, California 90089–0071.

since the first human-to-human cardiac transplant in December 1967. How, the public wondered, could a live heart be taken from the chest of a dead man? The answer came back from medicine: This is possible because the man was "brain dead," which is not inconsistent with having a functioning heart.*

The term *brain death* causes problems in several ways; this chapter addresses three, which I call (1) the seat-of consciousness confusion, (2) the means-as-ends mistake, and (3) the separate phenomenon muddle. All reflect a reductionist approach to the understanding of life and death.

2.1. The Seat-of-Consciousness Confusion

The first confusion is understandable because in many ways our concept of a person is associated primarily with conscious functioning and social interaction. Once the brain no longer functions, these qualities are lost and the person seems to be gone. But these qualities may disappear before the brain ceases functioning, and so in terms of life and death of a human organism, it is misleading to look to only certain—albeit very important—attributes of the brain. The disappearance of social, rational, and interactive qualities can result from a total loss of higher brain functioning, such as with a persistently vegetative patient, or from profound impairment of brain functions, such as with a patient who is very severely retarded or has advanced dementia of the Alzheimer type.

Yet it seems clear to me that whatever state the latter persons are in—from deep coma to stupor to the general social inaccessibility that characterizes advanced Alzheimer patients—that state is not death. Many people would not want their lives extended by medical intervention were they to be in such conditions, and medical groups, judges, and commentators have concluded that ethical duties are not necessarily violated when life-sustaining treatment is withheld from patients who are irreversibly comatose or near inevitable death (President's Commission for the Study of Ethical Problems in Medicine and Biomedical and Behavioral Research, 1983; *Barber v. Superior Court,* 1983; American Medical Association, 1986). But, whether made by the patient in advance, or by the health care team and the patient's surrogates at the time, a decision is still involved, not simply the application of an alleged definition that would label "dead" persons who spontaneously respire, metabolize, excrete, and even go through sleep–awake cycles.

Thus, the first problem with the term *brain death* is that it invites us to think in terms of only certain functions of the brain and then to regard persons lacking in the higher functions as dead or, what is worse, "as good as dead," which is a judgment on the quality of their lives but which risks becoming a conclusion about the fact of their death.

2.2 The Means-as-Ends Mistake

The second way a problem arises from the terminology is an extension of the first, namely, the mistaking of a means of determining death with death itself. Although this point may seem obvious, I think it is worthwhile to rehearse it briefly here. The use of artificial support for respiration, together with drugs and other surgical and medical interventions, such as electrical stimulation of the heart (either on an emergency basis or through the use of an implanted pacemaker), can sustain the lives of patients who would otherwise die. The conceptual problems occur because sometimes the use of such interventions does not restore a patient to normal functioning.

---

*The public may also have wondered how this heart could be transferred into a person who was alive even though this heart had been removed. The answer was that a person does not need a heart to survive because, at least for awhile, oxygenation and circulation of the blood can be carried out by a machine.

In those circumstances, the question arises as to whether the result is a living patient supported by artificial means or a dead body in which the signs of life are being artificially created.

To answer that question, physicians developed tests that bypass the artificially generated "life signs" of respiration and circulation and instead measure brain functions. When such functions are absent, physicians may state that the patient is "brain dead." That is shorthand for saying that the patient's death has been determined neurologically, but it suggests that somehow the physicians have found that the brain—rather than the patient—is dead.

Yet the very notion that an organ is "dead" is erroneous. Organisms die; organs cease functioning. Ironically, this point should have been manifest from the very provocation for the issue itself, namely, that some patients lack either a functioning heart or lungs, or both, and yet remain alive. It is the integrated functioning of the organism that is at issue, not the ability of particular organs to function. Although the irreversible cessation of any of the primary organs—heart, lungs, and brian—has traditionally been associated with the death of the organism, the ability of contemporary physicians to provide artificial means of respiration and circulation means that death no longer inevitably attaches to the failure of the heart or lungs. Instead, the question becomes: Has the integrated functioning of the organism ceased?

In certain cases, when artificial support is provided, integrated functioning remains because the substitution of the machines for the heart and lungs has been successful in maintaining the circulation of oxygenated blood to the rest of the body, including the brain. The problem arises when the nature of the injury or the duration of anoxia is such that the brain has been irreversibly damaged and is incapable of playing its role as coordinator of the body's homeostasis. This role involves the upper and mid-brain as well as the brainstem. Although the upper brain is usually thought of largely in terms of such neocortical functions as reasoning and consciousness, it also plays a role in other basic bodily activities that are primarily controlled and modulated through the brainstem.

The task for medicine, then, was to find ways of determining when all the functions of the brain, including those of the brainstem, had ceased so that a determination could be made that the body's ability for integrated functioning had been irretrievably lost. This task is one that medicine has admirably fulfilled, as will be seen.

2.3. The Separate Phenomenon Muddle

What I have said thus far has, I hope, established that a good deal of confusion centers around *brain death*, despite the actual clarity about the congruence of the circulatory–respiratory and the brain-based criteria for determining that death has occurred. This is what I meant when I stated at the outset that the task was one of reformulating the means for determining that death had occurred, not for "redefining" life and death. The state being measured has remained the same—it is a single phenomenon. The ability to sustain respiration and circulation made it necessary to have a means of ascertaining the occurrence of the same phenomenon when its traditional signs—absence of spontaneous circulation and respiration—could no longer be employed. By steering clear of the term *brain death*, we avoid what I term the separate phenomenon muddle.

A recent illustration of this problem comes from a headline in *American Medical News* (Aug. 15, 1986), "Brain-Dead Pregnant Woman Ordered Kept Alive." The suggestion that there are different categories of death, that in effect some bodies are "more dead" than others, is particularly a problem when organs are to be transplanted. Yet, as the President's Commission noted, although public consciousness of this subject may have been stimulated by the need for reliable means of determining death in persons who are candidates for organ donation, organ donation is not actually a prospect in the overwhelming majority of cases in which brain-based determinations are made (President's Commission, 1981). Moreover, the brain-death muddle is particularly confusing to the public, since in most instances declarations of death continue to be based on the absence of circulation and respiration. It is only for that fraction—perhaps 10–20%—who die while undergoing intensive treatment, including artificial support of circulation and respiration, for whom new means of diagnosing death had to be developed.

3. THE MEDICAL CONSENSUS ON TESTS AND CRITERIA

This discussion only touches on the topic of the medical consensus that has emerged around the relevant tests and criteria, as so many other chapters in this book examine the topic in detail. The move to reformulate the criteria for diagnosing death is usually traced to the work of several French neurophysiologists, who in 1959 published the results of the research that they had conducted with respirator-supported patients whom they found to be in a condition "beyond coma" (Mollaret and Goulon, 1959). Postmortem examination of these patients, who lacked reflexes and electrophysiological activity, indicated extensive destruction of the brain. Stimulated by these findings and by the growth of organ transplantation and the general problems in having a firm basis for diagnosing respirator-supported patients, the Ad Hoc Committee of the Harvard Medical School to Examine the Definitions of Death (1968) produced the first formal statement in the United States on criteria for the use of neurological measures to diagnose what the committee unfortunately called *irreversible coma*.

The committee described the following characteristics of a permanently nonfunctioning brain: (1) unreceptivity and unresponsivity, (2) no movements or breathing, (3) no reflexes, and, as a confirmatory measure, a flat electroencephalogram (EEG) showing that there is no discernible electrical activity in the cerebral cortex. In the Harvard formulation, all the tests were to be repeated at least 24 hr later without showing any change, and the physician had to rule out drug intoxication and hypothermia (below 90°F). The initial Harvard criteria did not single out special tests for pediatric patients. Subsequently, experience showed that extra care is necessary in such cases to make sure that the loss of function is indeed irreversible, just as it is necessary in cases in which drug intoxication might have occurred leading to a reversible loss of functions (President's Commission, 1981).

In the nearly two decades since the Harvard criteria were first published, there has been extensive confirmation of the concept of diagnosing death through neurological measures, as well as a continuous refinement of those measures. Certain of the intervening findings have indicated the incompleteness of the Harvard criteria, e.g., those criteria failed to recognize that spinal cord reflexes actually persist or return after the brain has permanently ceased functioning. Likewise, subsequent neurological studies emphasized the need for more adequate tests of brainstem reflexes, especially apnea, and some neurologists preferred tests that measured the absence of intracranial blood flow directly, e.g., by radioisotope cerebral angiography by bolus or static imaging or by four-vessel intracranial contrast angiography.

Guidelines of the Medical Consultants

Although different medical centers developed somewhat different criteria, generally reflecting differing assessments of the technical skill and instrumentation available to the physicians, a consensus emerged that the *sine qua non* of diagnosis is careful clinical assessment that includes identifying a cause of the damage to the brain sufficient to explain the clinical findings.

By the time the President's Commission that I directed began its examination of this subject in 1980, it was obvious that neither the concept of determining death by neurological measures nor the methods to be used were a matter of great dispute among knowledgeable physicians, especially the leading neurologists and neurosurgeons who had written on the subject. Therefore, in furtherance of our statutory mandate on this subject, the Commission determined that rather than attempt to formulate our own criteria, we would instead try to bring together the leading physicians from a variety of fields to formulate a set of guidelines for the determination of death that would be widely accepted. Several of the contributors to this book, including its editor, Dr. Howard Kaufman, participated in the process of preparing these guidelines, which were eventually published in the *Journal of the American Medical Association,* where they were hailed by the editor as a "landmark" (Medical Consultants, 1981; Barclay, 1981).

As the President's Commission (1981) stated in its report, for ethical reasons having to do with the certainty that must attach to any life-and-death action, the aim of any tests in this field is

> to reduce mistaken diagnoses that a patient is still alive, without incurring risks of erroneous diagnoses that a patient lacks all brain functioning when such functions actually remain or could recur. This is achieved by establishing first that all brain functions have ceased and then ascertaining that the cessation is irreversible.

The Commission employed the technique of convening a group of medical consultants to emphasize the notion that the formulation of criteria is a medical task and ought to be undertaken, and periodically reviewed and updated, by knowledgeable physicians based both on their clinical experience and on studies that show the adequacy of the criteria being used in light of new medical developments and findings.

In setting forth their criteria, the Medical Consultants to the President's Commission (1981) stated that criteria for determining death should accomplish the following five goals:

> (1) eliminate errors in classifying a living individual as dead; (2) allow as few errors as possible in classifying a dead body as alive; (3) allow a determination to be made without unreasonable delay; (4) be adaptable to a variety of clinical situations; and (5) be explicit and accessible to verification.

In my judgment, the warm acceptance that greeted the consultants' *Guidelines* indicates how very well they meet these objectives. Of special note is the parallel construction of the document, which states the criteria establishing "cessation" and "irreversibility" for both circulatory–respiratory and brain functions.

4. LEGAL RESPONSES TO THE NEW CRITERIA

The development of the medical tests and criteria for determination of death is a relevant topic in a discussion of the legal status of death. First, the existence of a consensus on the tests and criteria is important according to the terms set by the law. For example, the UDDA requires that "A determination of death must be made in accordance with accepted medical standards." Thus, the existence of such accepted standards is a predicate for the implementation of the statute.

Second, the Commission's assignment of the criteria-drafting role to a group of medical consultants underlines the distinct function that a public body plays separately from the process of formulating medical criteria. Biomedical scientists and clinicians can explain certain phenomena and show the consequences of certain actions, but in the end it is up to society—through its law-giving organs—to attach significance to the phenomena and consequences (Capron and Kass, 1972). This is what occurred in the development of statutory and decisional law on the "definition" of death, as through the formulation of the UDDA and its adoption in 24 jurisdictions (see Table I).

4.1. Remaining Philosophical Debate

Despite the legal and medical acceptance of the UDDA, philosophical debate has persisted on several points. Nonetheless, the legislatures and courts have not adopted either of the principal

TABLE I.   Current Law on the Definition of Death[a]

Type of law[b]	Statutory/judicial citation (alphabetically by jurisdiction)[c]
N	Ala. Code §§22-31-1 to 22-31-4 (1987), [1979] (permits use of other, unspecified medically accepted standards; must have second confirmation of death when determination is based on cessation of brain function or when part of body is to be used in transplantation; limits liability for civil/criminal actions)
N	Alaska Stat. §09.65 120 (1987), [1984] (similar to UDDA; explicitly permits pronouncement of death before removal of artificial supports)
(N)	Arizona (State v. Fierro, 124 Ariz. 182, 603 P.2d 74 (1979); homicide law)
UDDA	Ark. Stat. Ann. §§82-537 to 82-538 (1985), [1985]
UDDA	Cal. Health and Safety Code §§7180 to 7183 (1988), [1982] (includes sections on independent confirmation of brain-based determinations and of organ donors, and on patient records)
UDDA	Colo. Rev. Stat. §12-36-136 (1987), [1981]
N	Conn. Gen. Stat. Ann. §19a-278(b)&(c) (1987), [1979] (part of UAGA)
UDDA	Del. Code tit. 24, §1760 (1986), [1986]
UDDA	D.C. Code Ann. §6-2401 (1987), [1982]
N	Fla. Stat. Ann. §382.085 (1987), [1980] (determination must be made by two physicians—one a neurologist, neurosurgeon, internist, pediatrician, surgeon, or anesthesiologist; limits liability)
N	Ga. Code Ann. §31-10-16 (1987), [1982] (limits legal liability; allows other, unspecified medically recognized criteria)
N	Hawaii Rev. Stat. §327C-1 (1985), [1982, am. 1983, 1984 & 1985] (modified 1979 C-K statute; limits brain-based determinations to organ donation cases; requires biennial review of medical and legal developments)
UDDA	Idaho Code §54-1819 (1987), [1981] (defines accepted medical standards to be usual and customary procedures of the community)
B	Illinois Ann. Stat. ch. 110½ §302(b) (1987), [1975] (part of UAGA)
UDDA	Indiana Ann. Code §1-1-4-3 (1987), [1986]
C-K	Iowa Code Ann. §702.8 (1987), [1976]
UDDA	Kan. Stat. Ann. §§77.204 to 77.206 (1987), [1984]
N	Ken. Rev. Stat. §446.400 (1986), [1986]
C-K	La. Rev. Stat. Ann. §9:111 (1987), [1976]
UDDA	Me. Rev. Stat. Ann. tit. 22, §§2811 to 2813 (1987), [1983]
UDDA	Md. Ann. Code §§5-201 to 5-202 (1987), [1982]
(N)	Massachusetts (see Commonwealth v. Golston, 373 Mass. 249, 252, 366 N.E.2d 744, 747 (1977), cert. denied, 434 U.S. 1039 (1978); homicide law)
C-K	Mich. Comp. Laws Ann. §§333.1021 to 333.1024 (1987), [1979] (requires pronouncement of death before terminating artificial support; applies to trials of all civil and criminal cases)
UDDA	Miss. Code Ann. §41-36-1 to 41-36-3 (1987), [1981]
N	Mo. Ann. Stat. §194.005 (1988), [1982]
UDDA	Mont. Code Ann. §50-22-101 (1987), [1983]
(N)	Nebraska (see State v. Meints, 212 Neb. 410, 414, 322 N.W.2d 809, 812 (1982); homicide law)
UDDA	Nev. Rev. Stat. §451.007 (1986), [1985]
UDDA	N.H. Rev. Stat. Ann. §§141-D:1 to 141-D:2 (1987), [1986].
(UDDA)	New Jersey (Strachan v. John F. Kennedy Memorial Hosp., 109 N.J. 523, 538 A.2d 346, 351 (1988)
K	N.M. Stat. Ann. §12-2-4 (1978), [1973]
(C-K)	New York (see People v. Eulo, 63 N.Y.2d 341, 346, 482 N.Y.S.2d 436, 438 (1984))
N	N.C. Gen. Stat. §90-323 (1987), [1979]

TABLE I. (*Continued*)

Type of law[b]	Statutory/judicial citation (alphabetically by jurisdiction)[c]
M	Ohio Rev. Code Ann. §2108.30 (1986), [*1982*] (mentions brain stem and artificial support)
UDDA	Okla. Stat. Ann. tit. 63, §§3121 to 3123 (1988), [*1986*]
UDDA	Or. Rev. Stat. §432.300 (1987), [*1987*]
UDDA	Pa. Stat. Ann. tit. 35, §§10201 to 10203 (1987), [*1982*]
UDDA	R.I. Gen. Laws §23-4-16 (1984), [*1982*, am. *1985*]
UDDA	S.C. Code 1976, §44-43-450 & §44-43-460 (1987), [*1984*]
UDDA	Tenn. Code Ann. §68-3-501 (1987), [*1982*]
C-K	Tex. Rev. Civ. Stat. Ann. art. 4447t (1988), [*1979*]
UDDA	Vt. Stat. Ann. tit. 18, §5218 (1987), [*1981*]
K	Va. Code §54-325.7 (1987), [*1973*, am. *1986*]
(UDDA)	Washington (*see In re* Bowman, 94 Wash.2d 407, 421, 617 P.2d 731, 738 (1982))
UBDA	W. Wa. Code §§16-10-1 to 16-10-3 (1987), [*1980*]
UDDA	Wis. Stat. Ann. §146.71 (1987), [*1981*]
UDDA	Wyo. Stat. §§35-19-101 to 35-19-103 (1986), [*1985*]

[a] As of August 1, 1988.
[b] B, ABA proposal (1975); C-K, Capron-Kass Proposal (1972); K, Kansas Model (1970); M, AMA Proposal (1979); N, Nonstandard statute; UBDA, Uniform Brain Death Act (1978); UDDA, Uniform Determination of Death Act (1980) (endorsed by the NCCUSL 8/80, AMA 10/80, President's Comm. 11/80 and ABA 2/81, and published in *President's Commission Defining Death*, July 1981).
[c] Roman date indicates latest statutory material; italicized date indicates enactment.

variations urged by such philosophers as Englehardt (1975, 1982) and Veatch (1975). A proposal particularly favored by the latter commentator, under the heading of "a statute for a confused society," is to permit freedom of choice regarding the standard for determining death that will apply to oneself or to others (such as a parent, spouse, or child) on whose behalf one speaks (Veatch, 1976). Yet even Professor Veatch is bothered by the "antinomian [and] anarchical" potential in letting "any individual no matter how malicious or foolish . . . specify any meaning of death which the rest of society would be obliged to honor." He would thus limit choice to those three "concepts of death" that he finds reasonable: respiratory–circulatory, whole brain, and higher brain. Yet from his own discussion, it seems apparent that the real thrust of Professor Veatch's concerns is with preserving choice about the "treatment of persons" in a way consistent with the wishes of the patient and of his or her relatives, concerns well addressed by the growing body of law on forgoing treatment (President's Commission, 1983) and by the actual language of the UDDA, which does not command that any particular actions follow on a pronouncement of death.

The freedom-of-choice death statute is advanced by Veatch as a way out of an alleged "social policy impasse" that is, as far as I can tell, solely a result of the position that he shares with Engelhardt and others that it should be possible to declare dead a person who lacks neocortical function, despite the persistence of brainstem capacity. The philosophical arguments here are complex; they revolve around arguments about either personal identity (Green and Wikler, 1980; Gert 1971) or personhood (Engelhardt, 1982). It does not surprise me that this philosophical debate has not much affected public policy, given its tenor, which is well illustrated by the following excerpt from a recent ethics article:

> [A] human organism that has been irrevocably stripped of personal being is no longer in any ethically interesting sense, alive. The former person's body is however alive and has a definite but distinct ethical status (Gillett, 1987).

But the law, in speaking of "persons," as in the abortion context, is plainly concerned with live human bodies, without differentiating those capable of continuity of personal identity or of a high level of "personal being." Whether a body is ready for burial, whether it is murder to stop it from breathing, and so forth, is not dependent on whether it has any "ethically interesting" qualities left, although how vigorously it should be treated may be dependent on such qualities. As another commentator stated, one should not solve the terribly difficult problems surrounding medical decisionmaking for very sick patients by attempting to define them away (Stanley, 1987).

It may well be objected that the failure of legislators to respond to the arguments of philosophers is hardly proof positive of the wisdom of the former and the folly of the latter. Yet on the present subject, I think the judgment of the lawmakers should be applauded, both for its good sense and for its accurate reflection of the wisdom of the community about who is alive and who is dead.

4.2. The Future of the Law

The momentum of history is clearly behind the UDDA, even if there is no rush toward adoption in the remaining states because there is little pressure from organized groups that might have an interest in seeing the law clarified. In New York, a decision has apparently been made by the governor's Life and the Law task force to avoid the political battlelines that might be drawn were a determination of death statute to be debated in the legislature; instead, a regulation establishing the same standards as the UDDA will be issued by the Health Department.*

The closest to a new direction in the determination of death law came in 1986 in California Senate Bill 2018 which, as originally proposed, would have amended the UDDA to establish that "an individual born with the condition of anencephaly is dead."† This proposal could be seen as embodying the first recognition of a "higher brain" standard for death declarations. The risk that such a law would open the door to subsequent enlargements of the category of dead patients to include others who lack higher brain functions, such as patients in a persistent vegetative state, seems quite real, as I have argued elsewhere (Capron, 1987). Yet the proponents of the statute deny that any grand theory underlies their proposal; it makes an exception for anencephalic infants because of the certainty that they will die, and only incidentally because they are decorticate. Indeed, Harrison (1986) argues that "the failure of the brain to develop is clearly different from injury to a functioning brain."

It would not be appropriate to rehearse all the arguments as to why it would inadvisable to amend the UDDA to declare anencephalics dead (Capron, 1987). Suffice it to say that the manifest desire to make use of the anencephalic to achieve an admirable end (extension of the life of babies who might benefit from experimental transplant procedures) only serves to emphasize the need for uniform and dispassionate decision-making about who is alive and who is dead. The various Baby Doe regulations and statutes, whatever their many problems, certainly serve as a warning that society—skeptical about the withdrawal of life-prolonging treatment from seriously ill newborns—is going to be justifiably resistant to any proposal that involves actively taking the life of such infants, even to achieve a good for other persons.

---

*This strange result is mirrored by the task force's recommendation that a statute be issued on the subject of Do Not Resuscitate (DNR) Orders; in most jurisdictions, DNR policy is established by hospitals pursuant to general rulings by the state health department, but not by a statute.

†The bill was subsequently modified merely to establish a commission to study the subject of pediatric organ transplants, including the possible use of anencephalic babies as a source of organs; no proposal was introduced in the current legislative session.

REFERENCES

Ad Hoc Committee of the Harvard Medical School to Examine the Definition of Death, 1968, A definition of irreversible coma, *JAMA* **205**:337–341.

American Medical Association, Council on Ethical and Judicial Affairs, 1986, *Current Opinions* (¶2.18), American Medical Association, Chicago, pp. 12–13.

Barber v. Superior Court, 1983, 147 Cal. App.3d 1006, 195 Cal Rptr. 484.

Barclay, W., 1981, Defining death, *JAMA* **246**:2194.

Capron, A., 1987, Anencephalic donors: Separate the Dead from the Dying, *Hastings Ctr. Rep.* **17**(1):5–9.

Capron, A., and Kass, L., 1972, A statutory definition of the standards for determining human death: An appraisal and a proposal, *U. Pa. Law Rev.,* **121**:87–118.

Engelhardt, H., 1975, Defining death: A philosophical problem for medicine and law, *Annu. Rev. Respir. Dis.* **112**:587–590.

Engelhardt, H., 1982, Medicine and the concept of person, in: *Contemporary Issues in Bioethics* (T. Beauchamp and L. Walters, eds.), pp. 94–101. Wadsworth, Belmont, California.

Gert, B., 1971, Personal identity and the body, *Dialogue* **10**:458–478.

Gillett, G., 1987, Fiddling and clarity, *J. Med. Ethics* **13**:23–28.

Green, M., and Wikler, D., 1980, Brain death and personal identity, *Philos. Pub. Aff.* **9**:105–133.

Harrison, M., 1986, Organ procurement for children: The anencephalic fetus as donor, *Lancet* **2**:1383–1385.

Medical Consultants on the Diagnosis of Death to the President's Commission for the Study of Ethical Problems in Medicine and Biomedical and Behavioral Research, 1981, Guidelines for the determination of death, *JAMA* **246**:2184–2186.

Mollaret, P., and Goulon, M., 1959, Le coma dépassé, *Rev. Neurol.* **101**:5–15.

President's Commission for the Study of Ethical Problems in Medicine and Biomedical and Behavioral Research, 1981, *Defining Death*, U. S. Government Printing Office, Washington, D. C.

President's Commission for the Study of Ethical Problems in Medicine and Biomedical and Behavioral Research, 1983, *Deciding to Forego Life-Sustaining Treatment*, U. S. Government Printing Office, Washington, D. C.

Stanley, J., 1987, More fiddling with the definition of death, *J. Med. Ethics* **13**:21–22.

Veatch, R., 1975, The whole-brain oriented concept of death: An out-moded philosophical formulation, *J. Thanatol.* **3**:13–30.

Veatch, R., 1976, *Death, Dying, and the Biological Revolution*, Yale University Press, New Haven, Connecticut.

6

BRAIN DEATH
Historical Perspectives and Current Concerns

JOANNE LYNN

1. HOW WE'VE COME TO WHERE WE ARE

Brain death is widely accepted as death by medical and legal professionals and by the public generally, even though having brain death occur substantially before cardiovascular death has become possible only during the past few decades. The first description of what was then termed *coma dépassé* appeared in 1959 (Mollaret and Goulon, 1959). Nearly 10 years later, a particularly persuasive article was published by a prestigious committee at Harvard Medical School that made widely acceptable the criteria for diagnosing death on the basis of neurological signs in the presence of continuing cardiorespiratory support (Ad Hoc Committee, 1968).

The Harvard criteria were quite influential in generating widespread acceptance of neurological criteria but also led to some difficulties. The use of the term *irreversible coma*, as used by the Harvard committee, has caused confusion between permanent loss of consciousness (as in the case of Karen Quinlan) and *whole brain* death. The criteria were also justified because no patient meeting them had ever had any recovery of neurological function, which is true. However, this contention created a sense that the criteria were predictive of death rather than diagnostic of the status of being dead. Also, the Harvard criteria were incorrect in stating that spinal reflexes were generally absent; later experience showed that spinal cord reflexes frequently persist and are actually increased by the loss of cortical suppression. Finally, the Harvard criteria encouraged the electroencephalogram as a confirmatory test, engendering a controversy that has sometimes delayed progress in this field.

Nevertheless, the Harvard criteria were accurate and widely adopted. Minor variations were published and debated over the next decade, as reviewed by Black (1978) and by Powner *et al.* (1977), although courts tended still to rely on the Harvard criteria. Most likely, some of the criteria proposed would have permitted erroneous declarations of death. For example, the criteria proposed by the Collaborative Study of Cerebral Death (1976) included a definition of apnea that required only the absence of spontaneous respiration, evidenced by no effort to override the ventilator in 15 min. This standard is readily met by some persons who are not even comatose.

JOANNE LYNN • ICU Research and Geriatrics, George Washington University Medical Center, Washington, D. C. 20037.

Failure to meet this criterion is certainly adequate to ascertain that a person is not dead, but meeting it is scant reassurance that a person is actually dead.

This shortcoming is not particularly egregious and is not likely to have led to serious error. In practice, the fact that a person is suspected of being brain dead is probably already an indication of a greater than 95% accuracy in the eventual diagnosis. All the tests used to make the definitive determination will be quite accurate in such a population, if accuracy is measured by dividing the number correctly determined by the total number tested. A better statistical test to ascertain the relevance and merit of the criteria proposed would be to measure the reliability of the diagnosis both before and after application of the proposed criterion. With this evaluation, apnea testing proposed in the Collaborative Study criteria would have been nearly useless; making the diagnosis very little more certain than it would have been on clinical grounds alone.

However, there never was a debate of this sort about this subject. Instead, there were multiple sets of criteria, most of which aimed to determine the same status—that of being dead— although at least two prominent sets (Conference of Royal Colleges, 1979; (Collaborative Study of Brain Death, 1976) claimed to determine only that the patient was certain not to recover any function and had passed the "point of no return." There were fierce defenders of the need to establish isoelectric encephalograms. There were equally fierce denigrators of the role of EEG, who might be promoters of clinical diagnosis alone, of four-vessel intracranial angiography, or of newer techniques such as isotope angiography or evoked potentials. In fact, the multiplicity of criteria and the unintelligibility to the layperson of the debates among advocates had become a major stumbling block to the adoption of legislation authorizing determination of death on the basis of neurological criteria.

The President's Commission

By 1980, a uniform statute had been developed and had gained the support of all the major professional groups and of the President's Commission for the Study of Ethical Problems in Medicine and Biomedical and Behavioral Research (1981). The Commission's director was Alexander Capron, who presents more of this history in Chapter 5. Capron had devoted considerable time and effort to the endeavor of developing a uniform statute and gaining for it widespread support; he found it disconcerting that the appearance of discord in medical circles was delaying acceptance. Therefore, he asked me to see whether a clear and broadly acceptable set of criteria might be published with the Commission's report on brain death, due to be published some 6 months later.

As a recently trained specialist in internal medicine, I knew something of determining brain death, but not much. Very shortly, I found that nearly everyone in the field had some deep-seated reason to dislike, distrust, or oppose at least some of the leaders in the field. I called nearly everyone who had published a set of criteria or a major clinical study of brain death. Nearly all said that they would be glad to be of help but that some other leaders in the field would never cooperate. Some felt that they had been mistreated in the Collaborative Study of Brain Death because others had published data prematurely, some felt abused by others with abrasive styles and perceived arrogance, and some just favored their own procedures and defended them vigorously. Only a few persons who were knowledgeable about the issues were also on speaking terms with most of the others, and these persons would be critical to the success of the Commission's efforts to generate guidelines.

With the blessings of stunning naïveté, I began formulating proposed criteria from those that were published and began sending them for comment to those I had contacted. With the imprimatur of the President's Commission and the eagerness of the experts to see that the government did not come out with something that was wrong-headed, we began to revise and circulate drafts. There were at least a dozen. The circle of advisors continued to grow, as each person contacted and asked to comment was also asked whether he knew of others who should be included. We also solicited the involvement of all authors of brain death research who could be located. Since who else was involved was generally unknown to the participants, I could request scientific substantiation from those who favored a particular resolution of an issue and then present the gathered scientific data to those with other views. This approach downplayed the history and the personalities and required everyone to adopt the rules of scientific evidence. In this way, we ended up with a fairly widely acceptable document, with only a few substantial controversial points that would need to be resolved by clinical judgment and professional authority. Six of those who had been most involved in the process and who had conflicting concerns were convened to discuss the issues for 1 day. The resulting document was accepted by 56 of the 58 experts who had advised the Commission during the process and was published with the report *Defining Death* (*President's Commission for the Study of Ethical Problems in Medicine and Biomedical and Behavioral Research*, 1981) and in the *Journal of the American Medical Association* later that year.

This has now become the standard statement of the criteria for determining death and has served its purpose well. In fact, it has been well enough accepted that it may be able to endure some criticisms, within the context of providing some guidance to those who would like to generate a similar document in regard to determining death in young children, a group excluded in the Commission Guidelines.

2. WHERE WE MIGHT HAVE GONE INSTEAD

Before confronting the specific problems in developing criteria for the determination of death under the current definition, it would be worthwhile to reflect briefly on the fact that the current societal resolution is not the only possible means of authorizing cessation of treatment and donation of organs from the bodies of persons with what the Uniform Determination of Death Act (UDDA), developed by the President's Commission (1981), calls "the irreversible cessation of all functions of the entire brain." The society had come upon a phenomenon that had not previously been encountered, or indeed even been possible. Human bodies were lying in hospital beds looking like patients and having all manner of treatment aimed at sustaining the functions of the body, but had already had complete and irreversible loss of the brain. Until the 1950s, such a situation could rarely exist, for loss of the brain meant loss of respiration, and artificial measures were not adequate to substitute for that loss. Until then, death of brain and heart was always virtually simultaneous. Artificial respiration precipitated the issues of defining appropriate care of a person who has permanently lost all brain function but could still have adequate function in all other vital systems.

This society has chosen to call such patients dead and to authorize treatment of the body as property. Two other sorts of resolutions would have been coherent and practical, and the fact that they continue to have adherents complicates discussions of brain death, even today. One alternative would have been to continue to rely on the permanent cessation of heartbeat as the indicator of death, while recognizing that for some persons who are not dead, treatment to sustain life is correctly withheld and that others who are not dead can be used as sources of organs for transplant.

The other major alternative would have been to accept that certain functions of the brain that support consciousness are essential to human life and that those persons who have permanently lost these functions are considered dead. Treatment to sustain other physiological functions would then not be warranted, and organ donation could be allowed, although some such persons would continue to breathe, mitigating against proceeding with burial or removal from caregiving settings.

This is not the place to play out the arguments for or against any of these three resolutions:

higher brain death, heart death, or whole-brain death (which has been adopted). Nevertheless, it is important to realize that there is not a conceptual argument that makes whole-brain death the only correct one. This societal resolution has relied upon the perceived clarity of medical criteria for neurological death (as opposed to the obvious uncertainties and delays with most forms of higher brain death) (Lynn, 1983), the pressures to achieve permission to save other lives with transplantation, and the political acceptability of incremental change. Not only do many people still intuitively feel themselves closer to an alternate view of the matter, but also changes in the applicable scientific or political milieu could alter the long-term acceptability of ''whole brain'' criteria of death.

3. UNFINISHED BUSINESS

Every social upheaval leaves some unfinished business, some rough edges. Some of these are eventually made unimportant and are forgotten, but some remain important and either are resolved or become the substrate for a future upheaval. Which, then, are the skeletons in the brain death closet?

I have selected five such issues to discuss here: (1) the theoretical reliability of the criteria for determining death, (2) the meaning of the term *functions*, (3) the discord over the time of death, (4) the reliability of the criteria in actual use, and (5) the reliability of the methods proposed to cope with ''complicating conditions.''

3.1. The Theoretical Reliability of the Criteria for Determining Death

How reliable are our criteria? This is the sort of question that often generates more hostility than illumination, but it is the most central question for this entire endeavor. For the Commission guidelines, no case has met the criteria and (1) gone on to evidence any recovery of neurologic function prior to cessation of cardiac function, (2) shown evidence of intracranial oxygen consumption or normal intracranial circulation, or (3) demonstrated discernible amounts of potentially viable intracranial neural tissue at autopsy. External criteria of the adequacy of any proposed criteria are crucial; otherwise, not only would there be no way to assess their reliability but they would be self-fulfilling as well. Once widely accepted, criteria for death lead to the decision to forgo treatment to sustain heart and lung functions, which would be lethal to a person erroneously classified but would constitute an undetected error. It is difficult to engender external criteria, however, and it seems that the only ''gold standards'' available are nonrecovery despite vigorous treatment, angiography, and autopsy findings (Black, 1978). All are clearly somewhat less than perfect, since they, too, could be in error.

Nevertheless, it is worthwhile to inquire as to how adequately we now know that the Commission guidelines criteria meet this sort of gold standard. There are two lines of evidence. According to one line, about 200 cases in the medical literature have been examined by these criteria (or a closely similar set) and by a ''gold standard'' test. The criteria have not failed in any such case. If one sets the odds to be correct 99% of the time, and if there are 200 such cases, the odds of there being a future case in which the criteria are in error are about 2.5% (Hanley and Lippman-Hand, 1983). By contrast, if there are 1000 such cases (which might be the case if those that are not published are included), the odds are about 0.5%.

In other words, statistics alone would not be comforting enough to endorse adopting a set of criteria that would be self-fulfilling and that could cause serious damage to a patient and to the general trust in the criteria if ever it were to be shown that the criteria could err. In patients beyond infancy, however, there is a corroborating line of evidence that substantially improves on these odds. Once the skull has matured, substantial brain injury from any cause leads to raised intracranial pressure. Injury severe enough to eradicate the testable functions of the brain will have caused increased intracranial pressure sufficient to cut off circulation for enough time to eliminate any real possibility that functioning brain will survive. This understanding of the pathophysiology of the sequence of injury encourages confidence that the criteria are correct, despite the relatively small numbers of cases that have tested the criteria against any gold standard. Nevertheless, it would certainly be worthwhile to collect and publish the experience of those few cases that continue to receive cardiorespiratory support until cardiac standstill or that undergo autopsy or other special examinations to ascertain irreversible cessation of all functions of the entire brain. The current statistical risk of error in regard to adults is unsettling and is probably readily reduced.

3.2. Meaning of Functions

The second of the "skeletons in the brain death closet" concerns the definition of the term *functions*. There is no short, clear definition of this term. Loss of all functions clearly does not mean the death of every cell. The traditional heart–lung criteria for determining death meant that there was no circulation or oxygenation and not that each and every heart and lung cell or group of cells was dead. Similarly, one must mean that the brain's functions are irreversibly stopped and not that every brain cell or group of cells is dead. But the functions of the brain are more complex, varied, and separable than are the functions of the heart and lungs. If one could somehow have a situation in which it was clear that a patient's entire brain was dead except for the few neurons necessary to have a pupillary response to light, would that alone count as a function, or would it be construed as being analogous to showing that a piece of myocardium can still contract when stimulated a few hours after death? Conveniently, all discernible functions have tended to stop simultaneously, probably in part due to the mechanism of assured widespread neural destruction with increased intracranial pressure. But there are known exceptions. Hypothalamic and pituitary function may be retained (Hall *et al.*, 1980; Schrader *et al.*, 1980; Outwater and Rockoff, 1984). Some hemodynamic responses to organ-donation procedures, responses ordinarily thought to be centrally mediated, have been reported (Wetzel *et al.*, 1985). In one case, visual-evoked potentials were reported in a patient who met all criteria in the Commission's Guidelines for the Determination of Death (Ferbert *et al.*, 1986).

There is no easy answer, but there will have to be some attention to delineating what will count as "feeble and ineffective electrical activity" (Fackler and Rogers, 1987) and what will count as the "functions of the entire brain" (i.e., UDDA, the President's Commission, 1981), the latter serving to define the patient as still being alive.

3.3. Discord over Time of Death

A third "skeleton" that has had the staying power to resist efforts to resolve it is the issue of what time to give as the time of death in the case of a person who died with brain death. At one level, this is a legal issue of no particular importance: Just let the legal system define it, and the rest of us should go along. In most cases this is true, since nothing important turns on whether the patient died on Tuesday or on Wednesday. However, our inability to establish a common practice in this regard reflects that there are very troubling aspects to every available choice and that any choice as to the time to list is, in effect, a statement as to which problems are to be discounted.

There are three potential times to list as the time of death, none of which actually corresponds to the time at which all brain functions ceased irreversibly:

• Earliest time: the first time at which all brain functions seem to have ceased, whether or not a full examination was undertaken

- Middle time: when all brain functions were known to have ceased, a situation later verified to be irreversible
- Last time: when irreversibility was determined and the death certificate could be signed.

The earliest is the closest to actual death, the least manipulable, the most subject to error from inadequate observations or from complicating conditions, such as barbiturate intoxication, and the most removed from the time when death can be ascertained. The middle is reliable but manipulable and does not correspond to any important change in the relationship of the patient or family to others (as do the first and last times, which correspond to the time of fatal injury and to the time when burial becomes appropriate). It also can be separated by many days from the time of cessation of functions and from the time that cessation was shown to be irreversible. The last time proposed is eminently manipulable but does correspond best to social behaviors, such as burial and organ donations. I do not presume to have the wisdom to settle this debate, but I do believe that how it is settled has more to say about the relative merits of maintaining social comfort with brain death and of controlling the manipulability of the determination than is commonly recognized.

3.4. Reliability of the Criteria in Actual Use

A fourth "skeleton" certain to come out of the closet at some point is the reliability of the Commission guidelines, or any other set, in the hands of those who actually apply them. Criteria may be entirely adequate, but inattentive application may well engender substantial error. In reporting data that encourage the use of radioisotope angiography, Goodman *et al.* (1985) note that clinical assessment of brain death was in error in 3 of 204 cases referred for radioisotope studies. While the examining physician would perhaps have taken a more careful or conservative approach if radioisotope scanning were not available, which might have eliminated this error rate, it is still true that an error rate in a self-fulfilling diagnostic test of 1.5% is enough to give one pause. Some have proposed restricting the use of brain-death criteria to certain specialties (e.g., neurology, neurosurgery, and anesthesia), but there is no evidence that these specialists would be more knowledgeable or careful than would others with substantial experience. Perhaps experience itself should be the qualification, but extensive experience might lead to complacency.

3.5. Complicating Conditions

The last of the skeletal ghosts of past and unsolved troubles that I will take up is the group of issues having to do with the reliability of the advice regarding complicating conditions. More than any other aspect of the Commission guidelines, this section relies on clinical judgment and not empirical evidence. This may prove an unacceptably uncertain footing. How extensive should the testing be for drug intoxication? What is the impact of therapeutic levels of drugs on the functioning of damaged brain? At what levels do hypothermia and shock become contaminants of good determinations, and at what levels are they merely the evidence of death? Most of the known cases of "recovery" after a "diagnosis" of brain death have involved drug intoxication, yet the consultants to the President's Commission were unable to agree about which drugs should be assessed in which settings.

4. WHERE WE SHOULD BE GOING

Obviously, I believe there is substantial unfinished business in regard to the determination of death. Major research endeavors to shore up the contentions now being made with scant empirical backup are needed. Even in adults, careful reporting of large numbers of persons whose physiology is maintained as long as possible, whose brains are studied carefully at autopsy, or who have had multiple confirmatory tests would be helpful. Animal and human studies of some of the complicating conditions would be expected to reduce the uncertainty over the modifications to be required in these circumstances. Serious public discussion of the time of death and the appropriate uses and care for dead bodies would also be useful.

But this volume concerns determinations of brain death in children. What special concerns arise? Mostly those discussed earlier—only even more seriously. The most serious of these concerns arises with the very young child, for whom we cannot postulate that increasing intracranial pressure necessarily ensures destruction of the entire brain, if widespread destruction is documented on other grounds. How many infants under 2 years of age have been declared brain dead on the basis of a "gold standard" test *and* on the basis of a proffered more limited and more transplant-encouraging test? It is hard to say, for most series do not split out the young children to report these issues. My best estimate is that no more than a few dozen are reported. Since young children's skulls may be too flexible to engender the pathophysiology of increased intracranial pressure (and probably other effects) that ensures progressive destruction of the brain, we are left to rely on the statistics. If there are 10 cases of brain death in which the proffered criteria are shown to conform to a "gold standard" test, and if one hopes to be correct 99% of the time, the odds that there will be cases showing that the proffered criteria are in error as compared with the gold standard can be no less than 46%. With 50 cases, the odds of error are reduced to 9%, and with 100 cases to 5%. At 1000 cases, the odds are 0.5% that there will be a case that demonstrates that the criteria proposed would call a person dead at a time that a "gold standard" would not. Only if there is better understanding of the pathophysiology can we claim to do better than these odds. And we must bear in mind that our "gold standard" tests are one shade short of being accurate, as they too are subject to interpretation and technical error.

Circulation studies for determining brain death have not been validated on infants, who probably have more resistance to anoxia than do adults. It is not known whether isotope angiography is sensitive enough to detect flow rates just barely high enough to sustain some brain tissue. It is not even clear how long four-vessel angiography must demonstrate no flow before brain death can be considered definite in infants.

What should we be doing in regard to declaring death on the basis of "irreversible cessation of the functions of the entire brain" in infants? I would conclude that the evidence is solid enough to continue to make this determination, but I would also conclude that we must be quite willing to forgo the determination whenever there is the least doubt, to do "gold standard" tests such as four-vessel angiography often, to collect and report corroborating and confusing cases assiduously, and to carry on the necessary discussions in the spirit of collaboration and concern that should mark scientific and medical enterprises at all times. Finally, we probably should not endorse any limited set of criteria, including isotope angiography or extended observation, at this time. Wide professional acclaim for any one set of criteria would preclude doing the sorts of testing of criteria that are needed if we are ever to stand on firmer ground. The two experts who refused to sign the Guidelines of the Advisors to the President's Commission did so because they believed that the empirical data base was inadequate and that the Commission's publishing authoritative criteria would preclude further research as to the adequacy of the criteria. Whether or not they were right about criteria for adults and older children, their criticism would certainly be true for criteria regarding infants.

REFERENCES

Ad Hoc Committee of the Harvard Medical School to Examine the Definition of Brain Death, 1968, A definition of irreversible coma, *JAMA* **205**:337.

Black, P. M., Brain death, 1978, *N. Engl. J. Med.* **299:**338–344, 393–401.

Collaborative Study of Brain Death 1976, An appraisal of the criteria of cerebral death: A summary statement, *JAMA* **237:**982–986.

Conference of Royal Colleges and Faculties of the United Kingdom, January, 1979, Memorandum on the Diagnosis of Death.

Fackler, J. C., and Rogers, M. C., 1987, Is brain death really cessation of all intracranial function?, *J. Pediatr.* **110:**84–86.

Ferbert, A., Buchner, H., Ringelstein, E. B., and Hacke, W., 1986, Isolated brain-stem death: Case report with demonstration of preserved visual evoked potentials (VEPs). *Electroencephalogr. Clin. Neurophysiol.* **65:**157–160.

Goodman, J. M., Heck, L. L., and Moore, B. D., 1985, Confirmation of brain death with portable isotope angiography: A review of 204 consecutive cases, *Neurosurgery* **16:**492–497.

Guidelines for the Determination of Death: Report of the medical consultants on the diagnosis of death to the President's Commission for the Study of Ethical Problems in Medicine and Biomedical and Behavioral Research, *JAMA* **246:**2184–2186.

Hall, G. M., Mashiter, K., Lumley, J., and Robson, J. G., 1980, Hypothalamic–pituitary function in the brain dead patient, *Lancet* **2:**1259.

Hanley, J. A., and Lippman-Hand, A., 1983, If nothing goes wrong, is everything all right? Interpreting zero numerators, *JAMA* **249:**1743–1745.

Lynn, J., 1983, The determination of death, *Ann. Intern. Med.* **99:**264–266.

Mollaret, P., and Goulon, M., 1959, Le coma dépassé, *Rev. Neurol.* **101:**3–15.

Outwater, K. M., and Rockoff, M. A., 1984, Diabetes insipidus accompanying brain death in children, *Neurology (NY)* **34:**1243–1246.

Powner, D. J., Snyder, J. V., and Grenvik, A., 1977, Brain death certification: A review, *Crit. Care Med.* **5:**230–233.

President's Commission for the Study of Ethical Problems in Medicine and Biomedical and Behavioral Research, 1981, *Defining Death,* U. S. Government Printing Office, Washington, D. C.

Schrader, H., Krogness, K., Aakvaag, A., Sortland, O., and Purvis, K., 1980, Changes of pituitary hormones in brain death, *Acta Neurochir.* **52:**239–248.

Wetzel, R. C., Setzer, N., Stiff, J. L., and Rogers, M. C., 1985, Hemodynamic responses in brain dead organ donor patients. *Anesth. Analg.* **64:**125–128.

II

CRITERIA FOR THE DECLARATION OF
BRAIN DEATH IN CHILDREN

7

BRAIN DEATH IN CHILDREN
Guidelines and Experience at the Massachusetts General Hospital

PETER McL. BLACK AND I. DAVID TODRES

1. INTRODUCTION

The determination of death by brain criteria in children remains an area in which official guidelines are vague but one in which practical needs have mandated the adoption of specific criteria. This chapter presents the guidelines that have been developed for children at the Massachusetts General Hospital (MGH), comments on their use over the past 2 years, and discusses several problems in their practical application.

2. THE BASIS FOR BRAIN DEATH DECLARATION

The Report of the Consultants to the President's Commission on Brain Death encouraged the development of specific institutional guidelines for the determination of death by brain criteria. At the MGH, specific guidelines were adopted by the General Executive Committee shortly after the Commission report (President's Commission for the Study of Ethical Problems in Medicine and Biomedical and Behavioral Research, 1981). These guidelines attempted to bring to the bedside general principles elaborated by the Commission, specifically addressing such problems as severe facial trauma, possible drug intoxication, and the determination of brain death in children.

Table I outlines the local rules adopted by the governing board of the hospital in 1982. They require clinical determination that brainstem reflexes are absent and that there is no cortical function. The Pco_2 level has to be at least 50 mm Hg on apnea testing. One electroencephalogram

PETER McL. BLACK • Neurosurgical Service, Brigham and Women's Hospital and the Children's Hospital; Department of Surgery, Harvard Medical School, Boston, Massachusetts 02115. I. DAVID TODRES • Pediatric Intensive Care Unit, Massachusetts General Hospital, Boston, Massachusetts 02114; Department of Pediatrics and Anesthesiology, Harvard Medical School, Boston, Massachusetts 02115.

TABLE I.   MGH Guidelines for Determination of Brain Death

I. Preface
The medical and legal communities have indicated that "locally accepted guidelines" are to be used for the diagnosis of brain death. The following are proposed guidelines that may be helpful in determining brain death. These guidelines do not replace the physician's judgment in individual cases, since brain death is a clinical diagnosis. These are not intended to encourage the use of resources in order to establish the diagnosis of brain death nor do they indicate the physician's role once the diagnosis has been made. They may, however, be referred to as reasonable, current, and generally acceptable criteria.

II. Technical criteria
With the exception of guideline II.B.2 (ancillary testing), all the following criteria should be met:
  A. Clinical
    1. Cerebral unresponsiveness: The patient should be deeply comatose with no evidence of withdrawal or posturing to painful stimuli. Spinal level movements such as the flexor toe response or isolated triple flexion do not preclude the diagnosis of brain death.
    2. Brainstem unresponsiveness
      a. Apnea test: The proper determination of severe medullary damage requires an apnea test. The patient should be removed from the respirator and CO_2 allowed to accumulate while the thorax is observed and palpated carefully for spontaneous respiration. At the end of a period of time estimated to bring the $Paco_2$ to above 50 mm Hg, (a Pco_2 rise of approximately 2.5 mm Hg/min can be expected in most patients), a blood-gas sample is drawn and the patient is reconnected to the ventilator. If the $Paco_2$ at the end of the test exceeds 50 mm Hg and the pH is below 7.35, apnea has been adequately demonstrated.
      During this test, vital functions are supported by the use of diffusion oxygenation. This may be accomplished by preoxygenation for 5 min with 100% O_2 and the use of a tracheal cannula supplying 8–12 min O_2 through the tracheal tube (not a T piece). An unacceptable change in pulse or blood pressure or the appearance of cyanosis requires termination of apnea testing.
      b. Absence of other brain functions
        i. Pupils: The pupils should be 4 mm in diameter or larger and nonreactive to bright diffuse light. They should not be oval in shape, as this demonstrates residual midbrain function.
        ii. Eye movements: There should be no spontaneous eye movement. Oculovestibular testing with 30 ml ice-water irrigation of each ear separately should produce no eye movement. The patient's head should be elevated 30° during testing and the external auditory canals cleared.
        iii. Other: There should be no corneal reflex, external facial movement, or bulbar function, such as gagging or coughing, with tracheal stimulation.
        iv. Spinal reflexes: The presence of deep tendon or other spinal-mediated reflexes does not preclude the diagnosis of brain death; however, decerebrate or decorticate posturing does.
  B. Laboratory testing
    1. Electroencephalogram: An EEG recording of at least 30-min duration should show no electrocerebral activity, i.e., the absence of nonartifactual activity greater than 2 μV in amplitude with electrode impedences of 100–3000 Ω and interelectrode distances of $\geq$10 cm. There should be no change with auditory, visual, or painful stimulation. ECG artifact should be visible. There is no need for the patient to be normothermic, and recordings with core body temperature above 90°F are acceptable. A recording showing no EEG activity should be read by a staff member before the determination of brain death and documented in the record.
    2. Ancillary testing: Radionuclide or contrast angiographic demonstration of absent cerebral blood flow is not necessary but can be used in special cases (see below). Evoked potential testing may be helpful in the diagnosis of brain death but is not diagnostic alone.

III. Period of observation and underlying illness
A period of observation of at least 24 hr without clinical neurological change is recommended and necessary if brain hypoxemia–ischemia has occurred. Toxicological screening for CNS-depressant drugs is recom-

TABLE I. (*Continued*)

mended in all cases in which such toxins may play a role. If the cause of coma is known with certainty and drug or metabolic causes have been excluded, then in extraordinary circumstances a period of observation of 6 hr with no change in clinical state is adequate.

IV. Special cases
    A. Children and neonates: The above criteria in general form can be applied to children and neonates under the following conditions and with the following exceptions:
        1. A diagnosis that the brain has ceased to function is precluded if there is a phenobarbital level of >10 μg/ml, a pentobarbital level of >2 μg/ml, a thiopental level of >5 μg/ml, or a valproate level of >40 μg/ml.
        2. Brain blood-flow technology is not sufficiently well established or understood to justify its use in determining that the brain of a child/infant has ceased to function.
        3. 24 hr must elapse between that time when the guideline criteria have been met and the determination of death has been made.
        4. The Infant Care Committee (an *ad hoc* committee of the Critical Care Committee) is to be consulted. If there is disagreement as to whether death has occurred, then the Optimum Care Committee (a subcommittee of the Critical Care Committee) should be asked to mediate the difference of opinion.
        5. Documentation that death has occurred is to be entered into the patient's record by the patient's physician or his/her designee. It must include a record of those examinations (and the times they were performed) which led to the determination that the brain had ceased functioning, and that, therefore, the patient was dead.
    B. The previous therapeutic use of high-dose barbiturates for raised intracranial pressure or seizures does not preclude the diagnosis of brain death if serum levels at the time of examination are very low (i.e., <1 <10 μg/ml). Brain death flow examination may be useful in circumstances where barbiturates are present.
    C. Inability to examine the brainstem. When circumstances do not permit the examination of the eyes or pupillary reaction and eye movements, the diagnosis of brain death may generally be made by demonstrating EEG inactivity and apnea. In questionable cases, cerebral blood flow studies are recommended.
    D. Hypothermia and hypotension. Except when extreme (below 90°F), hypothermia does not produce the clinical or EEG phenomena associated with brain death. The diagnosis of brain death should not be made if the systolic blood pressure is <90 mm Hg.

V. Consultation and recording
If the patient is under the care of a nonneurological physician, then a staff neurologist or neurosurgeon should concur in the diagnosis of brain death. A note to the effect that the patient is declared dead and the explicit criteria used for this determination should be written, dated and signed in the patient's chart. Physicians associated with the transplantation team or a potential organ recipient should not be involved in the determination of brain death.

(EEG) is recommended but not required. Blood-flow testing may be used, but it is not central to the diagnosis because of limited experience with it at the MGH. Drug levels must be minimal but not absent because of the range of error with the test and the very low likelihood that minimal levels would make the diagnosis inaccurate.

    These rules represent a practical attempt to adapt general principles to specific cases. They are not arrived at by extrapolation from a clinical series but by applying the best combined judgments of clinicians dealing with brain death to the day-to-day problems of medical practice. As such, they must be seen as provisional guidelines, constantly open to modification.

TABLE II.   Guidelines for the Determination of Brain Death in Children[a]

I. History
The critical initial assessment is the clinical history and examination. The most important factor is determination of the proximate cause of coma to ensure absence of remediable or reversible conditions. Most difficulties with the determination of death on the basis of neurological criteria have resulted from overlooking this basic fact. Especially important are detection of toxic and metabolic disorders, sedative-hypnotic drugs, paralytic agents, hypothermia, hypotension, and surgically remediable conditions. The physical examination is necessary to determine the failure of brain function.

II. Physical examination criteria
    A. Coma and apnea must coexist. The patient must exhibit complete loss of consciousness, vocalization, and volitional activity.
    B. Absence of brainstem function as defined by:
        1. Midposition or fully dilated pupils which do not respond to light. Drugs may influence and invalidate pupillary assessment.
        2. Absence of spontaneous eye movements and those induced by oculocephalic and caloric (oculovestibular) testing.
        3. Absence of movement of bulbar musculature including facial and oropharyngeal muscles. The corneal, gag, cough, sucking, and rooting reflexes are absent.
        4. Respiratory movements are absent with the patient off the respirator. Apnea testing using standardized methods can be performed but is done after other criteria are met.
    C. The patient must not be significantly hypothermic or hypotensive for age.
    D. Flaccid tone and absence of spontaneous or induced movements, excluding spinal cord events such as reflex withdrawal or spinal myoclonus, should exist.
    E. The examination should remain consistent with brain death throughout the observation and testing period.

III. Observation periods according to age
The recommended observation period depends on the age of the patient and the laboratory tests utilized.
    7 days to 2 months. The Task Force recommends two examinations and electroencephalograms (EEGs) separated by at least 48 hr.
    2 months to 1 year. The Task Force recommends two examinations and EEGs separated by at least 24 hr. A repeat examination and EEG are not necessary if a concomitant radionuclide angiographic (CRAG) study demonstrates no visualization of cerebral arteries.
    Over 1 year. When an irreversible cause exists, laboratory testing is not required and the Task Force recommends an observation period of at least 12 hr. There are conditions, particularly hypoxic–ischemic encephalopathy, in which it is difficult to assess the extent and reversibility of brain damage. This is particularly true if the first examination is performed soon after the acute event. Therefore, in this situation, the Task Force recommends a more prolonged period of at least 24 hr of observation. The observation period may be reduced if the EEG demonstrates electrocerebral silence or the CRAG does not visualize cerebral arteries.

IV. Laboratory testing
    Electroencephalography. Electroencephalography to document electrocerebral silence should, if performed, be done over a 30-min period using standardized techniques for brain death determinations. In small children it may not be possible to meet the standard requirement for 10-cm electrode separation. The interelectrode distance should be decreased proportional to the patient's head size. Drug concentrations should be insufficient to suppress EEG activity.
    Angiography. A cerebral radionuclide angiogram (CRAG) confirms cerebral death by demonstrating the lack of visualization of the cerebral circulation. A technically satisfactory CRAG that demonstrates arrest of carotid circulation at the base of the skull and absence of intracranial arterial circulation can be considered confirmatory of brain death, even though there may be some visualization of the intracranial venous sinuses. The value of this study in infants under 2 months is under investigation. Contrast angiography can document lack of effective blood flow to the brain.

TABLE II.   (*Continued*)

Techniques under investigation. The Task Force recognizes that other tests, including xenon computed tomography, digital subtraction angiography, visualization of cerebral arterial pulsations by real-time cranial ultrasound, Doppler determination of cerebral blood flow velocity, and evoked potentials are under investigation.

"Task Force for the Determination of Brain Death in Children, 1987.

3. GUIDELINES FOR CHILDREN

Several guidelines for brain death in children have been published, including those of The Children's Hospital, Boston (Ad Hoc Committee on Brain Death, 1987). Physicians concerned with the care of infants and children at our institution also believed that further modifications of adult guidelines were required to deal with brain death in children. Initially, these guidelines were modified by local criteria but subsequently the recommendations of the Task Force for the Determination of Brain Death in Children (1987) were accepted. These are presented in Table II and are applicable one week after the cerebral insult to all infants over 38 weeks of gestation.

4. PRACTICAL APPLICATION OF THE BRAIN-DEATH GUIDELINES

This section reviews the implementation of brain-death guidelines in our practice in the pediatric intensive care unit (ICU) at the MGH for 2 years from January 1985 through December 1986. The staff physicians who participate in the diagnosis of brain death were selected from the pediatric neurology service, neurosurgery service, and ICU. During this period, 894 children aged 2 weeks to 17 years were admitted. Fourteen (1.6%) were declared brain dead. The etiology of brain death is summarized in Table III.

TABLE III.   Brain Death in the Pediatric Intensive Care Unit

No. of cases	Etiology	Ages
1	Osteodystrophy with subglottic stenosis (anoxic encephalopathy)	22 mo
1	Meningomyelocele with Arnold–Chiari malformation (cardiac arrest → anoxic encephalopathy)	5 yr
1	Hanging	13 yr
1	SIDS	4 wk
2	Aspiration	4 yr
		12 yr
2	Intracranial hemorrhage (thrombocytopenic purpura)	15 yr
		17 yr
6	Head trauma	7 mo
		16 mo
		22 mo
		4.5 yr
		8 yr
		12 yr

The patients studied in our unit were diagnosed as brain dead 1–20 days following admission to the ICU (mean 5.2 days). Neonates were not included in this study because of current uncertainties regarding the validity of applying criteria established for older children and adults to neonates. Of particular concern is the establishment of brain death in the low-birth-weight infant, when clinical neurological evaluation and EEG interpretation are fraught with difficulties in interpretation.

Several conditions were routinely excluded prior to the diagnosis of brain death: hypotension (shock), temperature $< 34°C$, toxic drugs, and barbiturate level > 10 $\mu g/ml$. In four of our patients, high doses of barbiturates necessitated waiting a few additional days for the barbiturate levels to fall below therapeutic levels. In all cases, clinical examination revealed (1) cerebral unresponsiveness, and (2) brainstem unresponsiveness. Of particular importance in assessing brainstem unresponsiveness was the apnea test (Outwater and Rockoff, 1984; Rowland et al., 1984), which was always carried out by a physician experienced in this procedure.

The patient was ventilated to a Paco$_2$ level of 40 mm Hg and then preoxygenated for 5 min with 100% O$_2$. The respirator was then disconnected, but O$_2$ was insufflated through the endotracheal tube. Blood gases were monitored. If no respirations occurred when the Paco$_2$ level had reached 55 mm Hg, apnea had been demonstrated.

Ancillary tests included the EEG, which in some cases (9 of 15) was repeated at 24 hr, demonstrating "electrocerebral silence"; this was considered to indicate absent cortical function (American Encephalographic Society, 1986).

Blood-flow studies, either radionuclide scans or angiographic studies, were not performed on our patients. Earlier experience with blood-flow studies had at times confused the issue rather than clarified it. New advances in technique and experience would suggest that this ancillary test might be of value in selected cases, e.g., in those patients who received high doses of barbiturates to control raised intracranial pressure (Drake et al., 1986; Goodman et al., 1985; Schwartz et al., 1984).

In six patients, an intracranial measuring device was placed. In five cases, this consisted of a subarachnoid bolt, and in one an external ventricular drainage system. Five patients demonstrated markedly elevated pressures at the time of declaration of brain death.

Notations in the chart were consistent and explicit. An example of such notation reads as follows:

> Patient unresponsive. No response to noxious stimuli. No voluntary or involuntary movements.
> Pupils dilated and unresponsive to light. Ocular movements absent on doll's head (or calorics).
> Corneals and gag reflex absence. Apnea test performed—no spontaneous respirations with Paco$_2$
> > 55 mm Hg. EEG—no cortical activity.

Organ donation was carried out in five patients. In five others, the underlying physical condition of the patients, i.e., shock with severe organ ischemia and sepsis, excluded the patient from organ donation. In the remaining five patients, permission for organ harvesting was not granted.

5. SPECIAL ISSUES

This section presents the authors' opinions on two issues relevant to declaration of death by brain criteria in children. They are not to be construed as policy statements of the institution but rather as personal attitudes.

5.1. Should Family Consent Be Required for the Declaration of Brain Death?

The determination of death is a medical matter. Where there is firm legal or statutory recognition of brain death as a criterion for death, and where there is well-documented fulfillment of criteria, it is our opinion that declaring death by brain criteria should be managed in the same way as declaring death by heart criteria.

This statement is made despite the fact that there may be uncertainty in the family's mind about brain death as a criteria for death. Although in some cases there may be opposition to the concept, it is only in rare cases that we believe the diagnosis should not be carried through for this reason.

5.2. What about Patients Who Don't Fulfill Criteria at the Moment but Are Likely to Do So?

Patients who are in the "waiting period" for fulfillment of brain death criteria are not by definition brain dead; they cannot be declared dead. An important question to be resolved with patients' families is whether full support should be carried out: In some cases a "no code" order is appropriate, and at times a family will ask for support to be stopped. Decisions here should be made on the basis of surrogate decision-making as to what the patient would want.

A further problem occurs in fully maintained patients who become unstable. Cardiovascular instability may require volume replacement which counteracts an attempt to keep the patient dehydrated. In general, we have found that maintenance of cerebrovascular stability by crystalloid infusion is the best course of action.

ACKNOWLEDGMENTS. The authors would like to thank John Fugate, M.D. for his help in collection of data for this chapter and for his assistance in analyzing the cases.

REFERENCES

Ad Hoc Committee on Brain Death, The Children's Hospital, Boston, 1987, Determination of brain death, *J. Pediatr.* **10**:15–19.

American Encephalographic Society, 1986, Guidelines in EEG, *J. Clin. Neurophysiol.* **3**:131–168.

Drake, B., Ashwal, S., and Schneider, S., 1986, Determination of cerebral death in the pediatric intensive care unit, *Pediatrics* **78**:107–112.

Goodman, J. M., Heck, L. L., and Moore, B. D., 1985, Confirmation of brain death with portable isotope angiography: A review of 204 consecutive cases, *Neurosurgery* **16**:492–497.

Outwater, K. M., and Rockoff, M. A., 1984, Apnea testing to confirm brain death in children, *Crit. Care Med.* **12**:357–358.

President's Commission for the Study of Ethical Problems in Medicine and Biomedical and Behavioral Research, 1981, Guidelines for the determination of death, *JAMA* **246**:2184–2186.

Rowland, T. W., Donnelly, J. H., and Jackson, A. H., 1984, Apnea documentation for determination of brain death in children, *Pediatrics* **74**:505–508.

Schwartz, J. A., Baxter, J., and Brill, D. R., 1984, Diagnosis of brain death in children by radionuclide cerebral imaging, *Pediatrics* **73**:14–18.

Task Force for the Determination of Brain Death in Children, 1987, Guidelines for the determination of brain death in children, *Ann. Neurol.,* **22**:616–617.

8

BRAIN DEATH IN CHILDREN
The Philadelphia Experience

DEREK BRUCE

1. INTRODUCTION

Despite statements that the infant's or child's brain is more resistant to anoxia than is the adult brain, there is no evidence that this is a practical benefit to the child other than by extending the tolerance for a few minutes. Recent reports have suggested that the criteria for brain death in children should be different from those in adults (President's Commission for the Study of Ethical Problems in Medicine and Biomedical and Behavioral Research, 1982; Task Force for the Determination of Brain Death in Children, 1987). If the premature baby is excluded, there is no reason for the criteria to be different from those of the President's Commission. If the criteria are followed, the clinical diagnosis of brain death can be made safely in infants and children. Indeed, it is the author's experience that the clinical examination may define residual brain functions when, in fact, none exist, thereby erring on the side of suggesting that the possibility of survival may be present, when indeed it is not. It is not uncommon in children during their first year of life to find quite complex arm and leg movements, such as a bicycling type of activity, in the absence of intracranial blood flow.

2. DETERMINATION OF BRAIN DEATH

The primary step in the diagnosis of brain death is to determine that the patient does not have a reversible insult. For example, infants with bacterial meningitis may progress to the point of losing brainstem reflexes, yet have entirely normal cortical function and recover completely. These children are clearly not brain dead and can recover. But, there is no evidence that a history of prolonged hypoxia or ischemia, severe head trauma, or intracranial hemorrhage in association with a clinical examination compatible with brain death is any less reliable in infancy than it is

DEREK BRUCE • International Pediatric Neurosurgery Institute, Humana Advanced Surgical Institutes, Medical City Hospital, Dallas, Texas 75230.

in older children or adults. Thus, a good history identifying the causative proximal agent in the child's death is an essential first step in the diagnosis.

The next step is to be certain that the child has received no drugs that could influence the clinical examination. If there is any question, appropriate laboratory tests should be done to exclude drug effect.

Next, a complete neurological examination, including cold caloric responses, should be carried out and, if the examination is compatible with brain death, should be followed by an apnea test using standard methodology (Outwater and Rockoff, 1984; Rowland *et al.*, 1984). The Task Force for the Determination of Brain Death in Children (1987) suggests a period of 48 hr of observation in a child aged 7 days to 2 months, 24 hr for a child aged 2 months to 2 years, and 12 hr for a child over 2 years of age, with an electroencephalogram (EEG) at each end of the time frame. There is no reason for the prolonged observation in the younger child, if the conditions discussed above are satisfied. The clinical examination compatible with brain death, repeated 6 to 12 hr later, in the face of a known insult, is adequate proof of brain death.

In the absence of any clinical history, it may be impossible to establish brain death on purely clinical grounds. It is in such circumstances that ancillary tests for brain death are required. Ancillary tests of brain death are as applicable to children and infants as they are to the older patient. The EEG may be the least reliable in the premature or very young infant in whom EEG activity may be poorly developed and easily suppressed. Reliable studies show the presence of EEG activity in a situation of brain death and, on the other hand, a flat EEG with recovery. Thus, as commented on by Freeman and Ferry (1988), the use of the EEG is possibly the most questionable of the ancillary tests.

Measurement of intracranial pressure by any of several invasive techniques has been shown to be reliable and accurate. Thus, an intracranial pressure equal to systemic arterial pressure lasting longer than 1 hr should also be adequate proof of absent brain perfusion and death. When the systolic pressure of the arterial pulse wave is greater than that of the intracranial pressure pulse, cerebral blood flow (CBF) may occur in short bursts during systole. In this setting, the total absence of cerebral blood flow cannot be ensured. Thus, further observation for a longer period or the addition of some direct measurement of cerebral blood flow may be necessary before death is declared.

The techniques for measuring CBF, intracarotid xenon, intravenous xenon, or xenon inhalation, are not dependent on differences in anatomy or physiology between the adult and the infant, and there is no evidence that these techniques do not measure CBF in the child as reliably as in the adult. Thus, the finding of absent CBF in association with a clinical examination showing no cerebral or brainstem function constitutes adequate demonstration of death due to irreversible cerebral damage. Likewise, cerebral four-vessel angiography is an accurate indicator of absent CBF not modified by age. It is not infrequent, with this study, that no flow is seen through the carotids but rather a trickle of flow through the vertebral arteries. Finally, the use of cerebral radionuclide angiography has been shown to be applicable in children aged 2 months up; evidence given in this volume suggests that this is true, even, in the younger-aged child. Thus, there is no evidence that these ancillary tests do not adequately describe the status of CBF, and there is no evidence that an infant's or child's brain can tolerate 1 hr or more of total ischemia and recover any differently than can the adult brain.

To avoid precipitous declaration of brain death in early childhood, the criteria should be stringently applied. If there is any lingering doubt, all efforts to maintain the child should be continued and the studies repeated at some point in the future. The identification or certification of brain death in infancy and childhood should not present any major difficulties, but it should be done by physicians familiar with the neurological examination as well as with the diseases that occur in small infants.

3. ORGAN RETRIEVAL

Once death is declared, the child may then become a potential organ donor. How well the interface between life and death is handled by the medical professionals involved will often determine whether the parents agree to organ donation. What are the factors that will influence this period of time, hence the likelihood of agreement by the parents for their dead child to be an organ donor?

It is a worthwhile starting point to examine the frequency with which children's organs are harvested in the busy intensive care unit (ICU) setting. At the Children's Hospital of Philadelphia, the approximate number of ICU admissions is 1500 per year. There are some 50–70 deaths per year, yet the number of organ donors is very small, no more than 2–5 per year. While many of the children may not be satisfactory organ donors, it is certain that there are many more potential donors than the 4–10% obtained. In a similar but smaller pediatric ICU at St. Christopher's Hospital in Philadelphia, the number of organ retrievals is similar.

Table I shows the most frequent diagnoses of the children who become organ donors. The largest group are children who have suffered a hypoxic or ischemic brain injury. Most children in the group in whom cardiac arrest has developed have had the attack as a result of hypoxia secondary to primary respiratory problems rather than as the result of primary cardiac disease. Once sufficient hypoxemia or ischemia has occurred to produce cardiac dysfunction, cerebral damage is most likely to have already occurred. Thus, despite the potential ease of cardiac resuscitation, cerebral damage is likely to be present and irreversible. A few studies are available that review the outcome following pediatric arrest and resuscitation, but the available figures suggest that only 40% of emergency room or out-of-hospital arrests and 60% of hospital resuscitations result in the patient leaving the hospital alive. There is no information on the neurological condition of these surviving patients (Kettrick and Ludwig, 1983). Often the children that die are not considered organ donor candidates because of potential damage to the liver, kidneys, or heart as a result of the hypoxia or ischemia. This notion needs to be dispelled. The figures from other chapters in this volume also demonstrate that in children, hypoxic or ischemic insults are the most frequent cause of death in organ donors.

Why do so few pediatric patients become organ donors? In the author's experience, two

TABLE I.   Cause of Death in 23 Pediatric
Organ Donors

Cause of death	N
Head injury	
Motor vehicle	6
Fall	1
Cerebral hemorrhage	
Arteriovenous malformation	3
Subarachnoid	1
Anoxia	
Suffocation	4
Smoke inhalation	2
SIDS	2
Seizure	2
Drowning	1
Postcardiac surgery	1

major factors are involved: the medical personnel and the circumstances of death. Despite the President's Commission publishing its findings in 1981 and the passage of brain-death laws in many states, there are physicians and nurses who remain confused about brain death or who simply cannot accept that such an entity can be proved. These attitudes are in part related to the inability of physicians to accept that the patient has died. It is understandable but not realistic for the physician to feel that death constitutes a failure. There are disease states that we cannot correct. And it is appropriate to face the fact that the patient is dead and to refuse to stop cardio-pulmonary support, particularly because by the time cardiac death occurs, there is no possibility for organ donation. Thus, we have to alter the physician's attitude. If physicians have trouble accepting that there are two ways of being dead—cardiac death and brain death—the issue must be clarified. Otherwise, this dichotomous attitude will be passed on to the nursing staff and to the family. Such dichotomous feelings are frequently expressed by calling the patient dead but not "dead dead."

For the family, the differentiation between irreversible coma and death is a difficult one. The child looks no different on the day he or she is pronounced dead than on the day before, when the parents were led to believe there was still some possibility of recovery. There is no external evidence of a change from the state of coma to the state of death. If, in addition, the physicians and nurses have reservations about the definition of death, this will be passed on to the already confused parents, who are trying to cope with the initial grief of the predisposing event and are now having to face up to the realization that recovery is impossible and the life of their child over.

This less than certain feeling about brain death was a common concern among the parents of children who had died of brain death in the ICU at the Children's Hospital of Philadelphia. Many parents wanted to know whether they had done the right thing by accepting the decision to stop the respirator. It is not surprising that the uncertain attitude toward brain death found among the physicians and nurses was passed on to the parents. This is an area in which further education is vital to prevent feelings of guilt and questioning within the family and to permit the medical staff and attendants to pass on the certainty of their diagnosis to the family.

The combination of a dichotomous attitude to the acceptability of brain death and the feeling that death represents failure make this interface between life and death particularly traumatic for the medical personnel involved. Thus, once the physician considers the situation hopeless, there is a tendency for presence and support to be withdrawn. The nurses now are taking care of a patient they know to be dead, without the continued support of the physician. The parents may or may not have been told that the child is dead, but in either case will feel abandoned by the absence of their physician at a time when they most need to ask questions and require support.

If parents, in addition, are asked to make decisions about stopping the ventilator, they now feel an added burden. I believe it is quite inexcusable to ask the parents to make a decision about discontinuing the ventilator in a situation in which death has been declared. This approach makes no sense. Since the child is dead, there is no decision left for the parents to make other than whether they wish to consider their child as an organ donor. Discontinuing the ventilator is the physician's responsibility.

Another limiting factor to obtaining permission for organ donation is the rapidity of the events between the onset of the disease process and the declaration of death. If the parents have a chance to establish contact with the medical personnel over several days, a bond is formed that makes a discussion of organ donation more acceptable and easier. When the child is admitted and there is no evidence of cerebral function, it is extremely difficult to confront the family with the reality of the death of their child and at the same time discuss the question of organ donation. Yet if the request is not made, the family may be angry when they realize that organ donation would have been possible and they were not given the choice at the moment of stress. When the approach to this situation has been to admit the child to the ICU for aggressive therapy, no matter what the parents are told about the likelihood of nonrecovery, they cannot but believe that with all this effort is being expended, there is a chance of recovery. This must set up friction, since the nurses and doctors know the child is dead, yet the parents see a chance for recovery. The parents cannot begin to grieve until the doctor tells them in a most open fashion that the child is dead. The "correct" way to handle this problem should be based on the individual physician's own sense of what is moral and ethical rather than on the basis of how best to obtain permission for organ donation.

The final way in which the potential for obtaining permission for organ donation is lost results from the delay in obtaining any ancillary test for brain death that may be necessary and communicating these results to the parents as rapidly as possible. For example, if there is a question of brain death in a child in whom barbiturates are being employed, there is a need for a CBF study. This study should be obtained immediately and the results given as soon as the test is finished. There is no excuse for "waiting until Monday" or for obtaining an EEG Friday afternoon that will not be read until Monday. Once the medical personnel believe the child is dead, the parents must be included; otherwise, they will sense the withdrawal of concern by the physicians and nurses and be confused. They will feel abandoned and angry as they sense that some change has occurred of which they are not to be notified of until later. If the family feels abandoned for several days while the doctors are evasive, the former cannot be expected to have the faith required to accept that organ donations is being requested for altruistic and non-self-serving issues by the physicians. They are then likely to refuse organ donation.

Hippocrates said, "When there is a love of humanity, there will be a love of our profession." The parents must feel this love and concern before they can be expected to consider the benefits to others at a time of enormous personal loss. I would conclude by quoting from Freeman and Ferry (1988), "The diagnosis of pediatric brain death should remain a clinical one to be made at the bedside, by knowledgeable physicians who, in concert with grieving families, make the most agonizing of all life's events (the death of a child) as bearable as possible for all concerned." Only under these circumstances can we expect families to be receptive to the call that their dead child may be able to help someone else's child.

REFERENCES

Freeman, J. M., and Ferry, P. C., 1988, New brain death guidelines in children: Further confusion, *Pediatrics* **81**:301–303.

Kettrick, R. G., and Ludwig, S., 1983, *Resuscitation—Pediatric basic and advanced life support, in Pediatric Emergency Medicine* G. Fleisher and S. Ludwig, (eds.), pp. ????? Williams & Wilkins, Baltimore.

Outwater, K. M., and Rockoff, M. A., 1984, Apnea testing to confirm brain death in children, *Crit. Care Med.* **12**:357–358.

President's Commission for the Study of Ethical Problems in Medicine and Biomedical and Behavioral Research, 1982, Guidelines for the Determination of Death, *Neurology (NY)* **32**:395–399.

Rowland, T. W., Donnelly, J. H., and Jackson, A. H., 1984, documentation for determination of brain death in children, *Pediatrics* **74**:505–508.

Task Force for the Determination of Brain Death in Children, 1987, Guidelines for the Determination of Brain Death in Children, Am. *Neurol.* **21**:616–617.

9

Pediatric Brain Death and Organ Transplantation

John F. Edmonds and Sik-Nin Wong

1. INTRODUCTION

This chapter presents the criteria developed at a large Canadian pediatric hospital for the diagnosis of brain death, and our experience in reaching this diagnosis over a recent four year period. The historical development of Canadian guidelines is reviewed and future recommendations are presented.

2. DEVELOPMENT OF GUIDELINES

Following the publication of the Harvard criteria in 1968, the Canadian Medical Association in November 1968, published a series of criteria for the determination of death based on the findings of irreversible coma. These guidelines were revised in 1974 and 1975.

In 1976 the Law Reform Commission of Canada undertook an extensive research project on "The protection of human life", and in 1979 published its "Working Paper Number 23; The Criteria for the Determination of Death."

The Commission made the following recommendations:

1. That the Parliament of Canada adopt the following text:

A person is dead when an irreversible cessation of all that person's brain functions has occurred.

The cessation of brain functions can be determined by the prolonged absence of spontaneous cardiac and respiratory functions.

When the determination of the absence of cardiac and respiratory functions is made impossible by the use of artificial means of support, the cessation of the brain functions may be determined by any means recognized by the ordinary standards of current medical practice.

2. That the Government of Canada enter into agreements with the provincial Governments to

JOHN F. EDMONDS and SIK-NIN WONG · Intensive Care Unit, The Hospital for Sick Children, Toronto, Ontario M5G 1X8, Canada.

ensure the adoption of this text or a similar one throughout the country for all legal purposes in order to achieve suitable uniformity.

The recommendations presented in this Commission's working paper have as yet not been adopted by Canadian legislation.

In 1971, Dr. H. W. Bain, chairman of the Department of Paediatrics at the Hospital for Sick Children Toronto, appointed a committee "to make recommendations about the criteria necessary for the determination of death," and their recommendations were published in May 1971 and implemented by the Hospital. This committee was of the unanimous opinion that "death of the brain was synonymous with death of the person."

The following guidelines were suggested by that committee for the diagnosis of brain death:

(a) Unreceptivity and Unresponsivity of the Patient

There should be a total unawareness to externally applied stimuli and inner need and complete unresponsiveness. Even the most intensely painful stimuli should evoke no vocal or other response that can be attributed to cerebral function.

(b) No Movements or Breathing

Observation by physicians covering a period of at least one hour is adequate to satisfy the criteria of no spontaneous muscular movements or spontaneous respiration or response to stimuli such as pain, touch, sound or light.

When the patient is on a mechanical respirator, the total absence of spontaneous breathing may be established by turning off the respirator for three minutes and observing whether there is any effort on the part of the subject to breathe spontaneously.

However, the respirator may only be turned off for this time provided that at the start of the trial period the patient's carbon dioxide is within the normal range and provided also that the patient had been breathing not more than 40 percent oxygen for at least ten minutes prior to the trial.

(c) No Reflexes

Irreversible coma with abolition of central nervous system activity is evidenced in part by the absence of elicitable reflexes.

The pupils will be fixed and dilated and will not respond to a direct source of bright light. Since the establishment of a fixed, dilated pupil is clear-cut in clinical practice, there should be no uncertainty as to its presence. Ocular movement (to head turning and to irrigation of the ears with ice water) and blinking are absent. There is no evidence of postural activity. Swallowing, yawning, vocalization are absent. Corneal and pharyngeal reflexes are absent.

As a rule the stretch tendon reflexes cannot be elicited, i.e. tapping the tendons of the biceps, triceps, supinator pronator muscles, quadriceps and gastrocnemius muscles with the reflex hammer elicits no contraction of the respective muscles and plantar or noxious stimulation gives no response. However, in some instances the spinal cord may function even though the brain is dead. In these cases some reflex activity of the cord may be preserved.

(d) Electro-Cerebral Silence

Of great confirmatory value is the flat or isoelectric EEG. It is assumed that the electrodes have been properly applied, that the apparatus is functioning normally and that the person in charge is competent. It is prudent to have one channel of the apparatus used for an electrocardiogram. This channel will monitor the ECG so that if it appears in the electroencephalographic leads because of high resistance it can be readily identified. It also establishes the presence of the active heart in the absence of the EEG. It is recommended that another channel be used for a noncephalic lead. This will pick up space-borne or vibration-borne artefacts and identify them. The simplest forms of such a monitoring noncephalic electrode has two leads over the dorsum of the hand, preferably the right hand, so the ECG will be minimal or absent. Since one of the requirements of this state is that there is no muscle activity these two dorsal hand electrodes will not be bothered by muscle artefact. The apparatus should be run at the standard gain of 50 microvolts to 5 millimetres pen deflection. It should also be isoelectric at double the standard gain. At least ten full minutes of recording are desirable.

(e) Repeat Examination

  (i) All of the above tests should be repeated at least three hours later for cases in which there is obvious cause for the coma and where the patient is not hypothermic (temperature below 90°F (32.2°C)) and if there is no evidence of central nervous system depressants such as barbiturates.

 (ii) All of the above tests should be repeated at least 24 hours later for cases of coma of unknown origin.

(iii) The validity of such data as indications of irreversible cerebral damage depends on the exclusion of two conditions; hypothermia (temperature below 90°F(32.2°C)) and central nervous system depressants such as barbiturates.

   After brain death has been established, the death must be attested by three physicians before transplantation takes place and before any resuscitation apparatus is turned off. The attestation should be signed by the following people:

   a) The clinician in charge of the patient.
   b) A medical staff physician of the ICU.
   c) A clinician who is independent of both the patient and the doctors ordinarily in charge of the case. If possible this should be a member of the neurological staff.

These guidelines have remained unaltered since 1971. However, clinical practice has altered the implementation of some of the recommendations. A retrospective chart survey was therefore undertaken to establish our present practice in the area of brain death and organ transplantation.

3.   PRESENT PRACTICE

3.1.   Patients

The Hospital for Sick Children in Toronto is a tertiary care referral and teaching hospital with 580 pediatric beds. The hospital contains two major intensive care units (ICUs): the neonatal intensive care unit and the pediatric intensive care unit. The diagnosis of 'cerebral death' is rarely made in the neonatal ICU and the great majority of deaths occurring within that area are associated with irreversible multisystem failure due to hypoxia or congenital defects.

We conducted a retrospective survey of charts from patients admitted to the pediatric ICU over the period 1983–1986. The pediatric ICU has 18 beds and a full-time medical staff consisting of four critical care physicians. During these 4 years, from January 1, 1983, to December 31, 1986, the unit admitted 5136 patients, and a total of 562 deaths occurred.

The discharge reports were evaluated for children who sustained "a period of deep coma and absent brain stem reflexes before cardiac death." This screening definition produced 154 charts for further study. Two charts could not be traced, and 24 children were excluded from the survey as a more detailed chart review demonstrated that they were not considered "brain dead." Fifteen of these 24 cases were excluded because of spontaneous respiration, and the remaining 9 cases suffered cardiovascular death before the diagnosis of brain death was made. This analysis left 128 cases for whom a diagnosis of "brain death" was recorded on the chart.

3.2.   Staff Involved

The staff involved in making a diagnosis of brain death were full-time critical care physicians, neurologists, and neurosurgeons. In individual patients, the diagnosis of brain death was

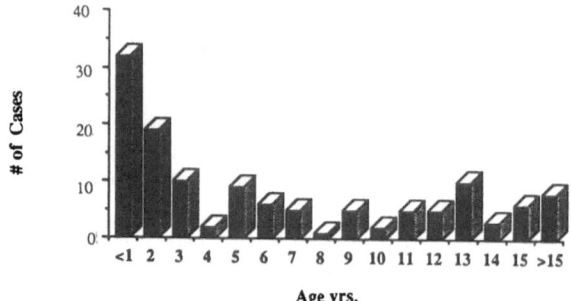

FIGURE 1. Age distribution in patients suffering brain death.

documented by four physicians in one case (1%), by three physicians in 23% of cases, by two physicians in 65% of cases, and by one physician in 11% of cases. In all cases, one of the physicians documenting the diagnosis of brain death was a critical care physician, a neurologist was involved in 66% of cases, and a neurosurgeon in 15%, and both neurology and neurosurgery were involved in 6% of cases.

3.3.   Age Distribution

The age distribution of the cases is presented in Fig. 1: 25% of the cases were under 1 year of age, 31% were between 1 and 5 years, 15% were between the ages of 6 and 10 years, and 29% were over 10 years of age.

3.4.   Etiology of Brain Death

The major cause of brain death in our group was a hypoxic insult to the brain. This insult was inflicted by the cessation of an oxygen supply to the brain either by asphyxiation, as in drowning or smoke inhalation, or by cerebral hypoxia from insufficient blood supply to the brain, as in cardiac arrest from aspiration. Other causes included head injury producing direct cerebral trauma, central nervous system (CNS) infections, intracranial vascular accidents, metabolic coma, such as Reye syndrome, and increased intracranial pressure from hydrocephalus (Fig. 2).

In children with a body weight of < 20 kg, hypoxia was the overwhelming etiological factor in the production of cerebral insults (Fig. 3).

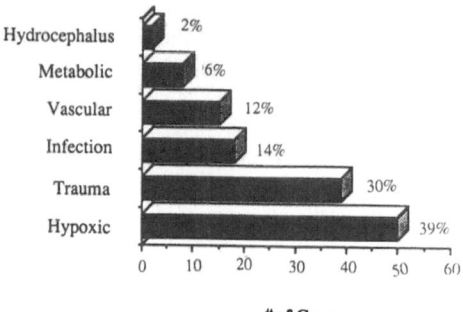

FIGURE 2. General etiology of the disease process causing brain death expressed as a percentage of all cases.

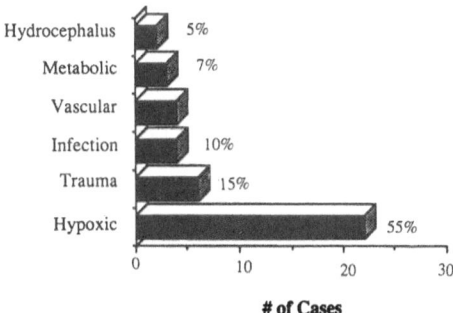

FIGURE 3. Etiology of the disease process causing brain death in children weighing less than 10 kg, expressed as a percentage.

3.5. Clinical Testing

The documentation of the clinical tests performed during the diagnosis of brain death is presented in Table I. The most consistent documentation consisted of the findings of apnea and of pupils fixed and dilated. Movements were documented in two patients during the diagnosis of "brain death." The presence of active spinal reflexes was documented in 50% of cases in which spinal reflexes were mentioned, and this occurred in 87% of cases. A conservative estimate is therefore of spinal reflexes present in 41% of cases of brain death in children.

3.6. Apnea Testing

The original criteria developed by our hospital in 1971 for apnea testing were designed to exclude the possibility of false-negative results by providing a stimulus to respiration from CO_2 retention and to exclude the possibility of respiratory depression from hyperoxia.

The guidelines stated: "However, the respirator may only be turned off for this time provided that at the start of the trial period the patient's carbon dioxide is within the normal range and provided also that the patient had been breathing not more than 40 percent oxygen for at least ten minutes prior to the trial."

Over the years, this test has been shown to produce hypoxia under some conditions; more

TABLE I.   Documentation of Clinical Testing: 128 Cases

Test/finding	No. recorded	Percentage	Atypical response
Spontaneous movement	106	83	2
Response to pain	102	80	0
Apnea	125	98	1
Muscle tone	75	59	1
Spinal reflexes	109	85	55 positive (50%)
Pupils	125	98	0
Corneal reflexes	120	94	0
Oculovestibular reflexes	78	61	0
Oculocephalic reflexes	104	81	0
Cough/gag	120	94	0

recent testing has maintained arterial oxygenation at a safe level with preoxygenation before the test and apneic oxygenation during the test. In the absence of this procedure, a significant percentage (36%) showed biochemical evidence of hypoxia during the test, with PaO_2 values of < 50 mm Hg. Apnea testing was documented with arterial blood gases (ABG) on 58 occasions; and 11 cases, the final $PaCO_2$ was < 50 mm Hg, and in most of these cases, the test was terminated at a time limit or at the clinical appearance of hypoxia.

3.7. Electroencephalograms

Our hospital criteria stated, ''Of great confirmatory value is the flat or isoelectric EEG.'' Our results show that electroencephalograms (EEGs) were performed in 122 cases (95%). The results (Table II) show that not all EEGs performed during the observation period were isoelectric. In two cases, the final EEG was not reported as isoelectric. One case was reported as containing ''occasionally low amplitude slow waves appeared with periodicity,'' and in the second case, the report documented ''A markedly abnormal record. There is burst suppression, with periods of electrocerebral silence lasting up to 20 seconds.'' Repeat EEGs were performed for a number of cases (Table II).

3.8. Exclusions

The validity of such data as indications of irreversible cerebral damage depends on the exclusion of two conditions: hypothermia [temperature below 90°F (32.2°C)] and CNS depressants such as barbiturates. The exclusion of hypothermia is a relatively simple matter; however, the exclusion of barbiturates is less simple.

Barbiturates are used in the management of seizures, and barbiturate coma has been advocated for the management of cerebral insults. Patients whose condition progressed to possible cerebral death may have received barbiturates for either of these indications. Our current practice is to accept a low to therapeutic phenobarbital level if the history and clinical findings are compatible with cerebral death or if the diagnosis can be confirmed by other means.

In 10 cases during this study period, the barbiturate levels were high; in 7 of these cases, the diagnosis of cerebral death was confirmed by the demonstration of absent cerebral perfusion using radionuclide angiography.

3.9. Radionuclide Angiography

Radionuclide angiography was used in a total of 24 cases during the study period. No flow was documented using this technique in 21 cases of 24 studied (88%). In those three cases with positive flow studies, the diagnosis of brain death was established by other criteria.

3.10. Outcome

In the 128 cases reviewed, the outcome depended on a number of factors. Spontaneous cardiovascular death occurred in 15%. In 11 patients, this was due to cardiovascular instability

TABLE II.   EEG Results

No. EEGs/patient	No. of cases	No. reported as isoelectric
1	38	36
2	68	66
3	16	16
	122	118

during the diagnosis of cerebral death and subsequent cardiovascular death. In 8 cases, ventilatory, as well as cardiovascular support, if necessary, was continued after the diagnosis of cerebral death was made, in accordance with parental wishes. The diagnosis of cerebral death is not necessarily easily accepted by some families; this may be on the basis of unfamiliarity with this entity, a denial of the facts, or in some cases religious or cultural beliefs.

Whatever the families' reasons, it has been our practice to observe their wishes when possible. The acceptance of this diagnosis may require considerable education of the family members and, not infrequently, a period of time to adjust to this reality. The diagnosis of cerebral death is a medical diagnosis made by a physician and does not rest with family members: however, the decision to terminate futile efforts to maintain the body after this diagnosis is made requires a degree of understanding and trust between physicians and family members. If the immediate family cannot accept this fact of death, we have continued support of the body either until the family is ready or until spontaneous cardiovascular death occurs. This practice may prolong support for a few days but, in our experience, is preferable to confrontation. Continued discussions with the family will usually resolve this conflict.

For most of our cases (56%), cardiorespiratory support was discontinued immediately after the diagnosis was made. The remaining 29% of cases were continued on support while arrangements were made for organ harvesting.

3.11. Organ Harvesting

Consent for organ donation was received in 44 cases (34%). In those potentially suitable cases in which no consent was received (65 cases), the reason for this lack of consent was not documented in 53 cases. Of these 53 cases, 24 were under 1 years of age and until recently would have been considered unsuitable for organ donation. In 10 cases, parents refused permission for organ donation, and in 2 cases the organs were unsuitable because of hypoxic or septic damage (Table III).

Of the 44 cases in which consent was obtained, 1 was lost due to "the absence of a suitable recipient." The organs actually harvested are shown in Table IV.

TABLE III. Outcome of Organ Retrieval in 128 Cases

Organ retrieval outcome	N	Percentage
Cardiovascular death		
Spontaneous	11	9
Prolonged support	8	6
	19	15
Consent for organ donation		
Organ donation	43	34
No recipient	1	1
	44	34
No consent for organ donation		
Refused	10	8
Unsuitable	2	2
	12	9
Undocumented		
<1-yr age	24	19
>1-yr age	29	23
	53	41

TABLE IV.   Organ Donation: 43 Cases

Organ	No. of organs harvested	
	On support	Postmortem
Kidneys	36	
Lungs	1	
Liver	11	
Heart	4	
Corneas	14	6
Heart valves	13	5

3.12.   Postmortem Examination

Postmortem examinations were performed on 82 cases (64%). The diagnosis of cerebral death is a clinical diagnosis, and the anatomical findings at postmortem examination do not reflect function. However, our cases demonstrated cerebral edema in 80% of cases examined, uncal and tonsillar herniation in 77%, neuronal eosinophilia in 51%, and necrosis of the tonsils in 18% of cases.

4.   THE FUTURE

4.1.   1987 Guidelines

The Canadian Medical Association issued a position paper in 1987 in which they "recognized the need for and the advisability of physicians' following recognized guidelines for the diagnosis of brain death," and they endorsed the guidelines of the Canadian Congress of Neurological Sciences.

The preamble to these guidelines stated that "brain death must be determined clinically by an experienced physician in accord with accepted medical standards. . . .   As knowledge advances it can be anticipated that further revisions will become necessary. Because of the major consequences of the diagnosis of brain death, consultation with other physicians experienced in 'he relevant clinical examinations and diagnostic procedures is usually advisable."

These published guidelines state:

The clinical diagnosis of brain death can be made when all the following criteria have been satisfied.

1 An aetiology has been established that is capable of causing brain death and potentially reversible conditions have been excluded.

2 The patient is in deep coma and shows no response within the cranial nerve distribution to stimulation of any part of the body. No movements such as cerebral seizures, dyskinetic movements, "decorticate" or decerebrate posturing arising from the brain are present (see 1a, below).

3 Brain-stem reflexes are absent (see 1b, below).

4 The patient is apneic when taken off the respirator for an appropriate time (see 1c, below).

5 The conditions listed above persist when the patient is reassessed after a suitable interval (see 2, below).

4.2.   Comments on These Guidelines

Although the purpose of this document is to state general principles and recommend guidelines rather than to outline a set of rules, certain features of the guidelines merit more detailed explanation:

1. Cessation of brain function. The clinical absence of brain function is defined as profound coma, apnea and the absence of brain-stem reflexes.

   (a) Coma. The patient should be observed for spontaneous behaviour and response to noxious stimuli. In particular, there should be no motor response within the cranial nerve distribution to stimuli applied to any body regions. There should be no spontaneous or elicited movements (dyskinesias, "decorticate" or decerebrate posturing, or epileptic seizures) arising from the brain. However, various spinal reflexes may persist in brain death.

   (b) Brain-stem reflexes. Pupillary light and corneal, vestibulo-ocular and pharyngeal reflexes must be absent. The pupils should be midsize or larger and must be unreactive to light. Care should be taken that atropine or related drugs that could block the pupillary response to light have not been given to the patient. The vestibulo-ocular reflexes should be tested with caloric stimulation while the head is 30° above the horizontal. In adults a minimum of 120 ml of ice water should be used. Grimacing or any other motor response to pharyngeal or tracheal suctioning is incompatible with brain death.

   (c) Apnea. Apnea was originally defined as lack of respiration when the patient was disconnected from the respirator for 3 minutes. This failed to consider whether an adequate $Paco_2$ level was present to trigger respiration. The $Paco_2$ threshold for respiratory stimulation in comatose patients may be elevated to as high as 50 to 55 mm Hg, and many patients on respirators have low $Paco_2$ levels that rise slowly (e.g., 2 to 3 mm Hg/min) when the respirator is stopped. In patients who fulfill the other clinical criteria of brain death, apneic oxygenation, described below, is a safe way of testing respiratory activity.

   If blood gas determinations are available, the $Paco_2$ should be 40 ± 5 mm Hg before testing for apnea begins. The patient should be preoxygenated (but not hyperventilated) with 100% oxygen for 10 minutes before testing. The respirator is then disconnected for 10 minutes while, to prevent hypoxemia, 100% oxygen is delivered at 6 L/min through an endotracheal cannula. This should produce a sufficient rise in $Paco_2$ to serve as a respiratory stimulant.

   If blood gas determinations are not available, an adequate test of brain-stem responsiveness to hypercarbia can be provided by ventilating the patient for 10 minutes with a 95% oxygen/5% carbon dioxide mixture before the 10-minute apneic oxygenation. In patients with severe respiratory disease, it is advisable to obtain the opinion of a respiratory physician to determine the safety and validity of this test for apnea.

   Testing for apnea without passive oxygenation is not recommended. In addition to its potential deleterious effects on the brain, the resultant hypoxemia can occasionally cause complex movements of the limbs and trunk, presumably owing to spinal cord ischemia, that could be confused with reflex movements of cerebral origin.

2. Irreversibility. Cessation of brain function is determined to be irreversible when potentially reversible causes have been excluded and the changes are judged to be permanent. Drug intoxication (particularly of barbiturates, sedatives and hypnotics), treatable metabolic disorders, hypothermia (core temperature less than 32.2°C), shock and peripheral nerve or muscle dysfunction due to disease or neuromuscular-blocking drugs must be excluded.

   Re-evaluation is essential to ensure that the nonfunctioning state of the brain is persistent and to reduce the possibility of observer error. Depending on the etiology, the interval between such examinations may be as short as 2 hours or as long as 24 hours; observation for at least 24 hours is usually recommended to confirm brain death due to anoxia/ischemia (e.g., postcardiac arrest). In situations where brain death is declared for purposes of organ transplantation, local regulations may stipulate specific intervals for reassessment.

Special circumstances

1. Infants and children. Brain death has not been sufficiently well studied in neonates, infants and young children to determine whether the clinical criteria listed above apply to these groups.
2. Inability to apply the clinical criteria. Some clinical situations such as uncertainty regarding etiology, inability to examine one or both eyes due to trauma, middle ear injuries, cranial neuropathies or severe pulmonary disease may preclude the valid application of the listed clinical criteria. In these circumstances, the only reliable means of confirming brain death is the absence of cerebral perfusion determined by cerebral angiography or radionuclide scintigraphy.

Laboratory tests

Although brain death can be established reliably by clinical criteria alone, special tests can be used to support and in some instances supplement the clinical diagnosis. The electroencephalogram assesses cerebral cortical function. Electrocerebral inactivity is confirmation of brain death only if all the clinical criteria apply and if established techniques are followed to ensure proper sampling of cortical activity. Visual, auditory and somatosensory evoked responses or other tests may eventually prove to be useful, but, at present, there are no standard guidelines for their use in assessing patients with suspected brain death.

The absence of intracranial perfusion, demonstrable by cerebral angiography or radionuclide scintigraphy, is reliable evidence of brain death. The mean arterial pressure should be greater than 80 mm Hg when cerebral perfusion is assessed. If cerebral angiography or radionuclide scintigraphy is used to determine the absence of cerebral perfusion, the procedure should be performed by an appropriately qualified specialist.

These guidelines were approved by the membership of the Canadian Neurological Society, the Canadian Neurosurgical Society, the Canadian Association for Child Neurology and the Canadian Society of Clinical Neurophysiologists, and are being studied by our Hospital.

5. DISCUSSION

As with all retrospective surveys, this presentation suffers from the deficiency of documentation. If a finding is not documented, this chapter assumes that the finding was not present— that assumption is not correct. Some findings will have been present, but will not have been documented.

The findings presented in this chapter are also subjected to the problems of definition; even though we are examining the topic of cerebral death, we are not only dealing with patients who have an unequivocal finding of total cerebral (including brainstem) death, but we are also dealing with patients in whom the cessation of life may be the criteria for discontinuation of treatment. The patient in whom there exists "small islands of electrical activity" (Fackler and Rogers, 1987), may fit the clinical criteria for a diagnosis of cerebral death and may be included in this discussion.

In spite of these deficiencies, we conclude that several important points can be made from this review.

1. Spinal reflexes are a common finding in children who are brain dead.
2. Although the demonstration of negative radionuclide angiographic cerebral flow studies is a reliable means of diagnosing brain death, the presence of a positive flow study does not exclude the diagnosis.
3. Well-conducted and well-documented testing of brainstem reflexes, including an apnea test, should be an important part of the diagnosis of brain death.

4. The entity of brain death does exist in infants and young children, and although we share the concern that this entity requires continued study and that the diagnosis needs to be made with caution in this group, we feel strongly that this caution should not override appropriate decision-making. To subject families to unwarranted periods of time after the death of a child, continuing to support the body without a decision being made, is not justified.

REFERENCES

Canadian Medical Association Statement on Death, 1968, *Can. Med. Assoc. J.* **99**:1266–1267.

A CMA Position., 1987, Guidelines for the diagnosis of brain death. *Can. Med. Assoc. J.* **136**:200A–200B.

Fackler, J. C., and Rogers, M. C., 1987, Is brain death really cessation of all intracranial function?, *J. Pediatr.* **110**:84–86.

10

PEDIATRIC BRAIN DEATH AND ORGAN TRANSPLANTATION

The Los Angeles Experience

J. GORDON MCCOMB

1. INTRODUCTION

An institutional approach to brain death was first undertaken at Childrens Hospital of Los Angeles (CHLA) by an Ad Hoc Committee during the 1970s. Subsequent modification of the initial guidelines has been an ongoing process by the Divisions of Neurosurgery and Neurology. CHLA does not now nor ever did have an official position on the criteria for brain death.

In California, the legal requirement for brain death is met if two licensed physicians are willing to attest to the fact. Initially, we limited the physicians participating in declaring brain death to those with clinical experience with the central nervous system (CNS), i.e., attending neurosurgeons and neurologists. Now, one of the two physicians is often an attending from the intensive care unit (ICU). Even though fully licensed in the State of California and by law, eligible residents and fellows do not participate in the official declaration of brain death.

2. CLINICAL CRITERIA

At CHLA written guidelines for establishing brain death have not been implemented, but the responsible clinicians use similar criteria of CNS unresponsivity that are widely accepted (Ad Hoc Committee on Brain Death, 1987; Ashwal and Schneider, 1987*a; b;* Black and Zervas, 1984; Kaufman and Lynn, 1986; Task Force for the Determination of Brain Death in Children, 1987). The more that is known about the patient, the clearer the etiology and the longer the period of observation, the better the certainty of the prognosis.

An initial good bedside test is to feel the temperature of the patient's head. If the head is cold and body is at normal temperature, rarely is there significant cerebral blood flow. Con-

J. GORDON MCCOMB • Division of Neurosurgery, Childrens Hospital of Los Angeles; Department of Neurosurgery, University of Southern California School of Medicine, Los Angeles, California 90027.

versely, a warm head does not guarantee adequate cerebral blood flow. If ventriculostomy is in place, the lack of cerebral profusion pressure (the mean arterial pressure minus the intracranial pressure) is indicative of brain death. If there is any uncertainty, or if the patient is a possible organ donor, a portable cerebral isotopic angiogram will be done to establish the lack of cerebral blood flow before the patient is declared brain dead.

3. CEREBRAL ISOTOPE ANGIOGRAPHY

In all cases in which organ transplantation is contemplated, the clinical examination is confirmed with a radiopharmaceutical cerebral blood flow study, using a portable gamma counter and computer system. The absence of cerebral blood flow establishes brain death regardless of the patient's age. However, we have rarely used isotopic angiography in the premature infant, as these patients as of yet have not been candidates for organ transplantation. We agree with Kaufman and Lynn (1986) that this test is easy for the family to understand and that it proves unequivocal brain death even in cases of altered metabolic states or hypothermia. The procedure we use is similar to that outlined by Goodman *et al.* (1985); it includes a single flow study that shows absence of flow above the intracranial portion of the internal carotid artery with no visualization of the arterial phase of the anterior and middle cerebral arteries, lack of arterial peak in the cerebral time–activity curves, and evidence of profusion of extracranial tissues only. We initially did not declare a patient brain dead if there was any visualization of the dural sinuses on the static scan. With the experience of more than 300 isotopic angiograms since 1980, there have been no survivors in this group of children, and we have subsequently discarded this requirement. Our findings are in agreement with those of Goodman *et al.* (1985), Ashwal and Schneider (1987), and Coker and Dillehay (1986).

4. ELECTROENCEPHALOGRAPHY

During the 1970s, we used the criteria of two isoelectric electroencephalograms (EEGS) 24 hr apart before declaring a patient brain dead. We found, as have many others (Fackler and Rogers, 1987), that it was often difficult to obtain two isoelectric EEGS because of artifacts even in the face of unequivocal clinical evidence of brain death. Improvements in EEG recording devices have significantly reduced the problem of artifact, making this problem less relevant.

In some cases, the patient would die before the 24 hr period had elapsed. Although the problem of getting EEGS at nights and weekends was once a problem, it no longer is. We largely abandoned the use of EEGs with the advent of portable cerebral isotopic angiography. If there is some minimal electrical activity on the EEG, but the isotopic cerebral angiography shows no evidence of cerebral blood flow, we still declare the patient brain dead.

5. NEONATAL BRAIN DEATH

We are in agreement with the statement by the Task Force for the Determination of Brain Death in Children (1987) that the usual criteria for brain death can be applied to the full-term infant (> 38 weeks) after the first week of life. Coulter (1987) as well as Ashwal and Schneider (1987a) pointed out that clinical evaluation and diagnostic studies may not be fully reliable in predicting brain death in the premature neonate. For example, the pupillary light reflex is reported to be absent before 29–30 weeks gestation, and the oculocephalic response is difficult to determine before 32 weeks (Ashwal and Schneider, 1987a). Coulter (1987) contends that the EEG and the evoked potentials are also unreliable in this patient population. Coulter (1987) has also presented several examples in which isotopic cerebral angiography indicated no cerebral blood flow, even though the patients survived with severe residual neurological deficit.

As, up to now, the premature neonate has not been a candidate for organ donation, the early establishment of brain death has not been a pressing problem. With the anticipated future use of neonatal organs, hence the growing need for organs to transplant as well as the great cost of supporting cardiorespiratory function after brain death, it is anticipated that more attempts will be made to establish unequivocal evidence of brain death when it is clinically suspected. With further technological refinements, better means of reliably detecting brain death in the premature neonate will be developed.

6. PERSISTENT VEGETATIVE STATE

As Kaufman and Lynn (1986) and Purvis (1987) noted, the need for organs far exceeds the present number of donors. Currently only those patients with total cessation of intracranial function can be declared brain dead, hence are suitable candidates for organ donation. Fackler and Rogers (1987) raise the question of whether it is necessary to have total cessation of brain function to declare brain death. Patients with such structural abnormalities as anencephaly, hydranencephaly, schizencephaly, and extensive multicystic encephalomalacia will never develop cognitive function and thus will remain in a persistent vegetative state, if they survive. Clinical diagnosis of anencephaly and appropriate imaging studies in the rest guarantee the neurological outcome of this group of patients. In one sense, they are brain dead, as they have no meaningful interaction with their environment; however, they do not fit the criteria for brain death, since brainstem function is still present. This group of patients is not currently considered for organ transplantation, and it would be necessary for society to widen the definition of brain death before this group of patients could be considered.

7. ORGAN TRANSPLANTATION

The Regional Organ Procurement Agency (ROPA) of Southern California is a transplant coordination team established by the Southern California Transplant Society to create a central network to educate, procure, preserve, distribute, and increase dramatically the availability of organs and tissues for transplantation (Procedural guidelines, Regional Organ Procurement Agency of Southern California, 1986).

ROPA receives referrals from more than 200 hospitals in the Southern California area. This referral system has been instituted for the following purposes:

1. To aid the hospital in protecting the rights of all parties—potential donor and family, hospital and staff, and potential recipients
2. To ensure that medico-legal criteria have been met
3. To ascertain that the patient is a suitable organ donor
4. To establish the necessary consents
5. To assist in donor maintenance
6. To ensure that the necessary tests (e.g., tissue typing, cross-matching) are performed
7. To ensure that the donor hospital will be reimbursed.

The determination of death must be made in accordance with accepted medical standards.

The physician certifying brain death must not have any affiliation with the transplant team.

This provision protects the rights of the potential donor by avoiding any conflict of interest by the physician involved.

Persons discussing donation with a family should be knowledgeable of the basic issues in organ donation:

TABLE I.   Cost of Organ Procurement

Organ	Cost	Comments
Kidneys	$8000	Total cost, of which 80% is paid by federal government
Liver[a]	$5000	Does not include surgical fee or transport costs
Heart	$5000	Does not include surgical fee or transport costs

[a]On a case-by-case basis, the governor of California can approve state funds for liver transplants in infants with biliary atresia.

TABLE II.
Childrens Hospital
of Los Angeles
Referrals to ROPA

Year	N
1983	4
1984	8
1985	16
1986	17
	45

TABLE III.   Organ Donations[a]

Age	Diagnosis	Organs
3 mo	Auto accident	Kidneys
11 yr	CNS hemorrhage (AVM)	Kidneys, pancreas
5 yr	Auto accident	Kidneys
9 yr	Auto accident	Kidneys
10 mo	Child abuse	Liver
10 yr	Drowning	Kidneys
2 yr	Primary brain tumor	Liver
14 yr	Auto accident	Kidneys, heart
3 yr	Auto accident	Kidneys
13 yr	Strangulation	Kidneys, liver
5 yr	Anoxia	Kidneys, liver
2 yr	Child abuse	Kidneys
8 yr	CNS hemorrhage (AVM)	Kidneys
2 yr	Child abuse	Kidneys, liver
16 yr	Brainstem infarct	Kidneys
10 yr	CNS hemorrhage (AVM)	Kidneys
3 yr	Drowning	Liver
15 yr	CNS hemorrhage (AVM)	Kidneys
2 yr	CNS hemorrhage (AVM)	Kidneys

[a]Total donations: 19.

TABLE IV. No Organ Donation

Age	Diagnosis	Reason
1 yr	Meningitis	Septicemia
4 mo	SIDS[a]	No waiting recipient
6 mo	Auto accident	No waiting recipient
5 mo	Child abuse	No waiting recipient
9 mo	Croup	No consent
1 yr	Asphyxiation	Donor arrested
2 yr	Accident	No coroner consent
1 yr	Child abuse	No coroner consent
2 yr	Child abuse	No waiting recipient
7 mo	SIDS	No waiting recipient
15 yr	Gunshot wound to head	Donor arrested
5 mo	Child abuse	No waiting recipient
17 yr	Encephalitis	? Infection
2 yr	Respiratory arrest	No consent
2 yr	Drowning	No coroner consent
2 yr	Child abuse	No coroner consent
1 yr	Child abuse	No coroner consent
2 yr	? Reye syndrome	No diagnosis
1 yr	Auto accident	Donor arrested
4 yr	Drowning	Donor arrested
2 yr	Meningitis	No consent
17 yr	Aspiration pneumonia	Donor arrested
5 wk	SIDS	Too young
3 yr	Seizure disorder	Donor arrested
5 yr	Reye syndrome	No consent
13 yr	Dysgerminoma	Malignancy

[a] SIDS, Sudden infant death syndrome.

1. Brain death
2. The critical need for organs
3. What is involved in accomplishing organ donation

Permission from the coroner should be obtained after declaration of death and family consent in the following situations:

1. Accidental causes
2. Homicide or suicide cases
3. Whenever there is any doubt about the cause of death

The family should be made aware that all costs incurred by the actual organ procurement will be paid for the ROPA. ROPA will reimburse the hospital for the following:

1. All costs incurred after declaration of death
2. All operating room costs
3. Any tests done to verify organ function

Table I lists the cost of organ procurement. Tables II–IV indicate the number of referrals by year and the outcome of such referral. There has been a steady increase in the number of referrals to ROPA from CHLA. Out of 45 referrals to ROPA, 19 (42%) resulted in organ donation.

REFERENCES

Ad Hoc Committee on Brain Death, The Children's Hospital, Boston, 1987, Determination of brain death, *J. Pediatr.* **110**:15–19.

Ashwal, S., and Schneider, S., 1987*a*, Brain death in children. I, *Pediatr. Neurol* **3**:5–11.

Ashwal, S., and Schneider, S., 1987*b*, Brain death in children. II, *Pediatr. Neurol* **3**:69–77.

Black, P. McL., and Zervas, N. T., 1984, Declaration of brain death in neurosurgical and neurological practice, *Neurosurgery* **15**:170–174.

Coker, S. B., and Dillehay, G. L., 1986, Radionuclide cerebral imaging for confirmation of brain death in children: The significance of dural sinus activity, *Pediatr. Neurol* **2**:43–46.

Coulter, D. L., 1987, Neurologic uncertainty in newborn intensive care, *N. Engl. J. Med.* **316**:840–844.

Fackler, J. C., and Rogers, M. C., 1987, Is brain death really cessation of all intracranial function?, *J. Pediatr.* **110**:84–86.

Goodman, J. M., Heck, L. L., and Moore, B. D., 1985, Confirmation of brain death with portable isotope angiography: A review of 204 consecutive cases, *Neurosurgery* **16**:492–497.

Kaufman, H. H., and Lynn, J., 1986, Brain death, *Neurosurgery* **19**:850–856.

Procedural Guidelines, Regional Organ Procurement Agency of Southern California, 1986.

Purvis, J. F., 1987, Organ transplantation and neurosurgeons, *Neurosurgery* **20**:650–651.

Task Force for the Determination of Brain Death in Children, 1987, Guidelines for the Determination of Brain Death in Children, *Arch. Neurol* **44**:587–588.

11

CLINICAL CRITERIA FOR PEDIATRIC BRAIN DEATH
The Washington Experience

DAVID C. MCCULLOUGH

1. INTRODUCTION

In this privileged nation, a death of a child is an exceptional event. It is a catastrophe that is unexpected, always tragic, and invariably appalling. The antecedent illness, shocking diagnosis, therapeutic failure, and terminal suffering of children with chronic disorders, such as cancer, developmental disabilities, and rare infectious conditions, are singularly morbid and disconcerting. But, in their own right, the swift and numbing experiences of accidental death represent a unique and contrasting experience. Accidents are the major contributor to pediatric mortality in the United States. Well-developed emergency care systems and life-support therapy often result in irreversible coma in juveniles with otherwise healthy bodies. Consequently, medical workers and parents may suddenly be confronted with revolting but inescapable decisions.

Physicians, nurses, and other health-care workers have a sacred responsibility to minister with skill and compassion, first to the dying child and next to the family. This is our duty and an obligation that must be accepted. It requires empathy and communication skills as well as maturity and discipline. Beyond the immediate concerns for patient and family, there is a social obligation with public health and economic implications. Partly due to concerns for the family, but also for social and economic reasons, there is obviously an impetus to define and institutionalize criteria for the definition of death.

In the contemporary multidisciplinary care setting treatment is often rendered by protocol and shared by specialty terms, which include numerous trainees. Subject to such systems, parents and family often suffer. Because the injured and dying child is most often the referral patient of high-technology tertiary care centers, it is imperative that workers in those facilities improve and

DAVID C. MCCULLOUGH • Department of Neurological Surgery and Child Health and Development, George Washington University School of Medicine, Washington, D.C. 20037; Department of Neurosurgery, Children's Hospital National Medical Center, Washington, D.C. 20010.

personalize services to families. As we do so we may also take a major step toward fulfilling important but less urgent societal obligations.

2. LEGAL REGULATIONS IN THE DISTRICT OF COLUMBIA

Before 1982, the definition of death in the District of Columbia simply required a physician's certification. That is, a person was deceased when a physician declared him so. There was no definition of death or a standard by which death could be determined in the D. C. code or in case law in this jurisdiction. The D. C. Anatomical Gift Act [D. C. Code, Section. 2-277 (B)] specified that the physician who determines that death has occurred "shall not participate in the procedure for removing or transplanting a part." The Uniform Determination of Death Act of 1982 (D. C. Law 4-68, Section 2, 28DCR 5045) (D. C. Code, 1984) was similar to definitions adopted by other states, deriving from the President's Commission of 1980. This law states "An individual who has sustained either (1) irreversible cessation of circulatory and respiratory functions; or (2) irreversible cessation of all functions of the entire brain including the brain stem; is dead. A determination of death must be made in accordance with the accepted medical standards." These represent the sum total of the regulations which have governed the author's practice over the last 18 years.

3. PERSONAL EXPERIENCE AND PROCEDURES

It is my belief that although the determination of death, communication, and counsel with the family may be shared with others in the medical profession, these duties are the basic personal responsibility of the attending physician. As a student, intern, and resident, I witnessed some very poor and some very good examples of the performance of this service. Learning from these, I have attempted to accept responsibility and to develop appropriate communication skills. With improved technology for life maintenance and the emergence of possibilities for organ transplantation, I have endeavored to retain this responsibility with an academic practice. Primarily for this reason, I cannot speak for any department or institution. Except for some recent statistical data obtained from the Children's Hospital National Medical Center, this communication is a personal account.

Initially in the course of my practice of pediatric neurosurgery, I was able to preside over all aspects of the situation of the dying child, including determination of brain death, family communication, removal of patients from life-support systems, and introduction of the transplant teams and coordinators. An early experience with brain death and transplantation guided by strict Harvard criteria (Beecher, 1968), resulted in an unpleasant encounter with the medical examiner's office. I had forgotten to inform that office prior to the organ recovery procedure and was soundly criticized by the coroner's representative. The case involved violent death due to gunshot wound through the brainstem.

It has not been my practice to remove patients from ventilator or other life-support measures without informed verbal permission of parents. I have not knowingly performed any procedures to hasten demise, even if suggested by colleagues or the patient's relatives. However, I have recommended and used strict criteria for brain death only in situations in which permission for organ donation was seriously considered or secured and in cases of violent death when prosecution was a consideration. In such situations, I have generally adhered to the Harvard criteria (Beecher, 1968).

When responsible family members (parents) have questioned the diagnosis of brain death or desired to persist with care indefinitely, I have performed procedures to evaluate for Harvard criteria with their permission. In most cases, the resolution of these conflicts occurs for reasons other than the explanations to parents. That is, the patient deteriorates further and cardiac arrest supervenes.

Thus far, I have not employed CO_2 measurements to define apnea (Kaufman and Lynn, 1986). After examining brain stem reflexes in a normothermic unintoxicated patient, I have resorted to one or two electroencephalograms, or alternatively, a single bedside radionuclide flow study (Goodman et al., 1968). If these tests supported the diagnosis of brain death, I have performed apnea testing in the process of removing the patient from the ventilator. I personally attend at the bedside, inviting the family to be present if they so desire. If a patient developed spontaneous breathing during this procedure, I would reinstitute respirator therapy, although I have never encountered this situation.

My procedure for requesting organ donation has been to suggest this possibility after describing the clinical situation. This applies only in cases in which I am the attending physician of record. If the response of parents is positive or at least exploratory, I invite the transplant coordinator or other team members to carry out further explanations. I do inform families that certain technical procedures will be required to confirm the diagnosis of brain death and that this will take at least several hours. During the recent era of high-dose barbiturate therapy for severe head injury, this was an agonizing process because of the time required to achieve acceptably low drug levels. Certainly organ donor candidates were lost because of the frustration or anger of parents.

Experience has demonstrated that veteran intensive care nurses have been most helpful in promoting organ donation through bedside family counseling. The dialogue that often develops through their intense involvement with patients not only comforts parents, but it also adds positive reinforcement for the concept of transplantation.

Recognizing that death presents more a spiritual than a psychological crisis, I have found that chaplains or pastoral care workers serve families more satisfactorily than psychologists and social workers. Moreover, there seems to be acceptance of pastoral counselors and frequent resentment of the involvement of psychological counselors. Often the clergy assists families in the resolution of conflicts relating to discontinuation of life-support systems and organ donation.

Except for cases of head injury, I have witnessed a decline in hospital deaths with the trend toward terminal home or hospice care since the middle 1970s. Most children with malignancy or severe birth defects are now taken home to die. Furthermore, with multidisciplinary and shared care, my direct involvement in patient and family therapy for the dying child has declined precipitously. On a 15-bed pediatric neurosurgical service with 450 admissions and more than 700 emergency room and inpatient consultations, an average of only seven patients expire each year.

4. STATISTICS AND PROCEDURES AT CHILDREN'S HOSPITAL

Institutional figures from Children's Hospital National Medical Center are fragmentary. This is a 240-bed acute tertiary care children's medical center with an extremely active trauma service. More than 400 children with head injuries are admitted each year. Most are assigned to a multidisciplinary trauma service. About 16% enter the intensive care unit (ICU). The mortality in head-injured children is approximately 3%. Among all diagnostic categories, determination of brain death is highest for head-injured patients at our hospital. Applying strict criteria, approximately 10 trauma patients suffer cerebral death annually and would be donor candidates for organ transplantation.

A survey of deaths and possible organ donor candidates among Children's Hospital patients was performed by the George Washington University Transplant Coordinator for the calendar year 1984, using Communicable Disease Center criteria for suitable donors. Among 156 deaths that year, 11 children were deemed to be "suitable" candidates. According to the record two families consented to organ donation and four refused. In five others, the prospect of organ donation was presumedly not presented or the suitability of the patient was not appreciated (Table I). A less detailed study for 1985 disclosed six donations of multiple organs from a similar population.

Conversely, in a study not completely compatible with the above survey, a recent review of electroencephalography (EEG) performed for determining brain death revealed 16 single procedures in 1985. Fifteen of those patients actually demonstrated isoelectric EEGs. During 1986, the experience was similar. Eighteen procedures were performed, and in 15 the tracings showed electrical silence.

Children's Hospital has no institutional policy for the determination and declaration of brain death. Perhaps because of competitive pressures within the community for the development of cardiac transplantation programs, a committee of the medical staff was appointed in 1986 to advise and draft institutional criteria for the declaration of brain death. Several senior physicians either participated in, or served as advisors to, the committee. The deliberations of that body were recently completed, but no officially sanctioned list of criteria has been adopted as hospital policy. The committee and its consultants were nearly unanimous in recommending ''suggested guidelines'' rather than rules or policy for determination and declaration of brain death. Central to the philosophy of these criteria (Table II) is the concept that the attending physician is responsible for the determination and declaration of brain death. Under the guidelines, the D. C. law is

TABLE I.   Survey of Potential Candidates for
Organ Donation: CHNMC, 1984

Potential candidates	N
Deaths	156
Organ donation candidates	11
Families solicited	6
Families consenting (donations)	2
Families refusing	4
Unsolicited	5

TABLE II.   Proposed Guidelines for Determination and Declaration of Brain Death:
CHNMC, 1987

Attending physician responsible
Standard for determining death in the District of Columbia outlined (D. C. Law 4-68, Section 2, 28 DCR
        5048)
Irreversible loss of all functions of brain and brainstem requires:
    Coma
        No spontaneous movements
        No spontaneous respirations
        No brainstem reflexes (pupillary, corneal, oculovestibular included)
        Absence of significant hypothermia or intoxication
Attending physician or immediate family may request any or all confirmatory tests:
    EEG
    Radionuclide flow study
    Brainstem evoked responses
    Cerebral arteriography
D.C. Medical Examiner's office should be informed when appropriate.
Formal medical consultation is encouraged.

reviewed. The criteria for irreversible loss of all function of brain and brainstem are defined, and appropriate confirmatory laboratory studies are listed. Formal medical consultation is suggested in cases in which there is uncertainty on the part of the attending physician. It is also stated that the attending physician should inform the medical examiner's office prior to the discontinuation of life support when appropriate or when questions of jurisdiction of that office arise. It is expected that these criteria will be approved and published as guidelines within the law, respecting the prerogatives and responsibilities of specific attending physicians.

5. OBLIGATIONS TO FAMILIES

With respect to my personal attitude on the subject of the dying child, brain death, and discontinuation of life support, the most serious conflict revolves around the family unit. Long periods of anguish and suffering occur while certain criteria are fulfilled and all the technical procedures are completed before discontinuation of life support. Although families often need a period of time to adjust to the reality and terror of their loss, few patients or parents are well served by a prolonged interval of technological maneuvers intended to fulfill protocol definitions or promote organ transplantation. Because these measures are at times necessary, the caring, communicating physician has serious professional obligations, which include the counsel and support of bereaved relatives.

6. CONCLUSION

The author's personal account of opinions and experience with respect to the dying child, determination of brain death, and solicitation of organ donation emphasizes the important therapeutic and communication responsibilities of the attending physician—first to the patient and then to the family. Acknowledged social obligations include consideration of organ donation and economic factors. Within the multidisciplinary care settings of high-technology tertiary referral institutions where care may be rendered under protocol by groups of physicians and numerous trainees, fundamental responsibilities to families may be neglected. Emphasis on the primary role of the attending physician is essential to the correction of this deficiency. Medical educators involved in patient care have the opportunity as well as the obligation to extend these family and public services by preceptorship.

REFERENCES

Beecher, H. K., 1968, A definition of irreversible coma: Report of the ad hoc Committee of the Harvard Medical School to examine the definition of brain death, *JAMA* **205**:337–340.
District of Columbia Code (annotated), 1981, 1984, Cummulative Supplement 6-2401.
Goodman, J. M., Heck, L. L., and Moore, B. D., 1985, Confirmation of brain death with portable radio-isotope angiography: A review of 204 consecutive cases, *Neurosurgery* **16**:492–497.
Kaufman, H. H., and Lynn, J., 1986, Brain death, *Neurosurgery* **19**:850–856.

12

Brain Death in Infants and Children
The Atlanta Experience

MARK O'BRIEN

1. INTRODUCTION

This chapter reports on the criteria for establishing brain death used at Henrietta Egleston Hospital for Children, Atlanta, Georgia. It also reviews the October 16, 1984, opinion of the Georgia Supreme Court in the case of *In Re: L.H.R.* addressing the issue of the circumstances under which life-support systems may be removed from an infant whose examination does not meet the criteria for establishing brain death.

2. BRAIN DEATH

2.1. Death and Brain Death

Traditionally, the cessation of heartbeat and respiration have been necessary conditions for the diagnosis of death, and it is recognized that these will remain the criteria for the diagnosis of death in most cases. However, modern life-support systems enable us to maintain both heartbeat and respiration by mechanical means. At times, it has become necessary to determine whether death has occurred in persons whose respiration and heartbeat are being mechanically sustained.

The term *brain death* means death diagnosed by neurological criteria. Once the criteria have been met, there have been no instances of prolonged survival despite the most vigorous resuscitative attempts. *Brain death* means the death of the patient.

2.2. The Georgia Law Regarding the Determination of Death

    (a) A person may be pronounced dead by a qualified physician if it is determined that the individual has sustained either (1) irreversible cessation of circulatory and respiratory func-

MARK O'BRIEN • Departments of Surgery and Pediatrics, Emory University School of Medicine; Neurosurgical Section, Henrietta Egleston Hospital for Children, Atlanta, Georgia 30322.

tion, or (2) irreversible cessation of all functions of the entire brain, including the brain
stem.

(b) A person who acts in good faith in accordance with the provisions of [the Georgia Law]
shall not be liable for damages in any civil action or subject to prosecution in any criminal
proceeding for such act.

(c) The criteria for determining death authorized in [the Georgia Law] shall be cumulative to
and shall not prohibit the use of other medically recognized criteria for determining death.

2.3. Criteria for Establishing Brain Death at Henrietta Egleston Hospital for Children

The guidelines for establishing brain death cited below are followed in all patients in whom
brain death is being considered. This would include potential organ donors. The criteria apply
only to the diagnosis of death. We are still unable to predict with certainty the outcome of
seriously brain damaged patients who do not meet these criteria, and it is not yet possible to
ascertain whether they will improve and to what extent they will improve. The decision as to
whether life-support systems should be maintained in such patients remains a matter of judgment
for the physician and family.

The criteria are as follows:

1. *Unresponsiveness:* There is total unresponsiveness to externally applied stimuli and inner
    need. Even the most intensely painful stimuli evoke no vocal or other purposeful re-
    sponses, not even a groan, cough, or gag.
2. *No movements or breathing:* Observations of the patient must establish that there are no
    spontaneous muscular movements or spontaneous respiration and none in response to
    stimuli, such as pain, touch, sound, or light other than on a spinal cord basis. After the
    patient is on a mechanical respirator, the total absence of spontaneous breathing may be
    established by turning off the respirator for 3 min and observing whether there is any
    effort on the part of the subject to breathe spontaneously. (The respirator may be turned
    off for this time provided that at the start of the trial period the patient's arterial P_{CO_2} is
    within the normal range, and provided also that the patient has been breathing room air
    for at least 10 min prior to the trial.)
3. *No cranial reflexes:* Irreversible coma with abolition of central nervous system (CNS)
    activity is evidenced in part by the absence of elicitable cranial reflexes. The pupils will
    be fixed and will not respond to a direct source of bright light. Ocular movements to head
    turning and to irrigation of the ears with ice water are absent. There is no evidence of
    postural activity (decerebrate, decorticate, or other). Swallowing, yawning, and vocali-
    zation are absent. Corneal, pharyngeal, and cough reflexes are absent. As a rule, deep
    tendon reflexes cannot be elicited, and plantar or noxious stimulation gives no response.
    Deep tendon reflexes occur at a segmental level, and their occasional preservation does
    not in itself negate the diagnosis of brain death.
4. *Electrocerebreal silence:* An electroencephalogram (EEG) recording demonstrating elec-
    trocerebral silence is of confirmatory value in the diagnosis of brain death, but the diag-
    nosis is a clinical one, and an EEG is not required for the diagnosis. However, if the
    patient is a potential organ donor, it is recommended that an EEG be obtained. If, for
    some reason, an EEG is not obtained in the case of a potential organ donor, one of the
    examining physicians must be either a neurologist or a neurosurgeon. An EEG should not
    be obtained to confirm brain death unless the clinical criteria for the diagnosis have al-
    ready been met. Only one EEG is sufficient unless there is some doubt as to whether or
    not electrocerebral silence truly exists with the initial recording. When an EEG is done,
    it must conform to the Minimal Technical Standards for Electroencephalogram in Sus-

pected Cerebral Death as proposed by the American Encephalographic Society *Guidelines in Electroencephalogram* 1980.

5. *No cerebral blood flow:* Optional tests demonstrating the absence of cerebral blood flow include cerebral arteriography and radioisotope flow studies.

6. *Timing and circumstances:* For the diagnosis of brain death to be established, the clinical assessment must be made by the attending physician, and he/she should have at least one consultation. Consultation should be freely sought with other attendings, i.e., neurologists or neurosurgeons. If the patient is a potential organ donor, no member of the organ transplantation team may participate in establishing the diagnosis.

The diagnosis of brain death depends on the exclusion of two conditions: hypothermia (temperature below 90° or 32.2°C) and CNS depressants such as barbiturates.

If the cause of the patient's adverse condition is not apparent, the responsible physician will obtain serum levels for intoxicants and administer an opiate antagonist such as naloxone prior to establishing the diagnosis of brain death.

3. THE CHRONIC VEGETATIVE STATE

3.1. The Problem

On occasion, a situation confronts the physician and the family in which a child is in a chronic vegetative state with no hope of cognitive function, but the examination does not meet the criteria for establishing brain death. The following case is an example. The history and the subsequent legal questions and their resolution are presented.

3.2. Case of LHR

A 4-month-old infant was admitted to Egleston Hospital for evaluation, having been transferred from a hospital in Savannah, Georgia. She was born at term and appeared to be perfectly normal. At 14 days of age, while being fed, she suddenly arched her back and became opisthotonic and comatose. She was admitted to a hospital in Savannah, at which time a computed tomography (CT) scan of her head showed cerebellar, intraventricular, and subarachnoid hemorrhage. An angiogram exhibited an arteriovenous malformation within her cerebellum. An emergency suboccipital craniectomy was performed. The brain was described as being under extreme pressure, and a large hematoma was removed from the left cerebellar hemisphere. Subsequently, the child never regained independent breathing and remained ventilator dependent. She then developed markedly increased intracranial pressure and required bilateral ventriculostomy for hydrocephalus. Following this, a *Pseudomonas* ventriculitis developed that was treated with antibiotics. Five weeks later, a ventriculoperitoneal shunt was placed. Ventriculomegaly persisted following the shunt despite adequate shunt function and no increase in intracranial pressure.

Examination on admission to Egleston Hospital indicated a comatose infant who was unable to breathe without continuous assistance from a respirator. She had no visual alerting. Her pupils were small and unresponsive to light. She never closed her eyes. Her fundi appeared unremarkable. There was adequate horizontal oculocephalic response but no vertical eye movements. She had bilateral facial paralysis. There was no gag reflex and no pharyngeal movement as well as pooling of secretions in the posterior pharynx. Her tongue did not move and did not respond to stimulation, and fasciculations were present. Head circumference was 40.5 cm, and the anterior fontanel was depressed. She showed intermittent random spontaneous movements of her arms and legs and withdrawal of the extremities to pain. Muscle tone was increased throughout with bilateral ankle clonus, knee clonus, and bilateral extensor plantar responses.

The outside CT head scan showed marked severe ventriculomegaly with surrounding cortical necrosis. Further information obtained was that the father, paternal grandfather, paternal grand uncle, and paternal great grandfather all had Osler–Weber–Rendue syndrome with small cutaneous angiomas, and the father and his two male children by a previous marriage had recurrent epistaxes. The paternal grandfather also had recurrent bleeding from the mouth.

Brainstem auditory evoked response was markedly abnormal. Wave 1 was obtained reproducibly from both sides at normal latencies, but waves 2–5 were absent bilaterally. This was strongly suggestive of structural disease of the brainstem bilaterally at the pontomedullary junction. The recording of wave 1 demonstrated an intact peripheral auditory function and excluded a technical error in recording the interpretation.

It was planned that the child would have a tracheostomy to facilitate care, but the parents at this point thought that further care would only result in prolongation of the life of a severely compromised infant who would never regain any function. The neurologist, the infant's parents, and the guardian *ad litem* appointed for the child all agreed that she should be removed from life-support systems. An ad hoc Infant Care Review Committee convened by the hospital to discuss the case concurred. (This committee consisted of two pediatricians, a registered nurse, a social worker, the hospital administrator, and the parent of a handicapped child.) Egleston Hospital filed a petition for declaratory relief on February 8, 1984. On February 9, after a hearing in DeKalb County Superior Court, the hospital and physicians were enjoined from interfering with the constitutional and common law rights of the child and from interfering with the wishes of L.H.R.'s parents and guardian to have life-support systems removed. After entry of this order, the life-support systems were removed, and the child died within 30 min.

The trial court *sua sponte* added the attorney general as a party to the suit and directed that he prosecute an appeal. The primary purpose for the appeal was to afford the Supreme Court an opportunity to set forth guidelines under what circumstances may life-support systems be removed from a terminally ill patient existing in a chronic vegetative state with no hope of development of cognitive function. The questions for decision were who may make treatment decisions and whether judicial intervention was required. On October 16, 1984, the Georgia Supreme Court affirmed the judgment, with all Justices concurring.

3.3. Summary of the Decision

On October 16, 1984 the Georgia Supreme Court published an opinion in the case of *In Re: L.H.R.*, in which a Georgia appellate court addressed for the first time the issue of the circumstances under which life-support systems may be removed. Although the patient involved in that case was an infant, the court's holding was not limited to infants. Set forth below is a summary of the main points of the decision, as well as some comments on the practical application of the decision.

3.3.1. What the Court Decided

L.H.R. was an infant female in a chronic vegetative state with a total absence of cognitive function. Her condition was described as "irreversible," with no hope of recovery. The infant's parents, her neurologist, and the guardian *ad litem* appointed for the child all agreed that she should be removed from life-support systems. The hospital convened an ad hoc committee to review the case, and this committee concurred in the decision. The hospital then filed a petition for declaratory relief, whereupon the trial court enjoined the hospital and physicians from interfering with the wishes of the child's parents to have life-support systems removed. Following the order, treatment was discontinued and the child died within 30 min.

On appeal, the Supreme Court did not spend much time discussing the threshold issue— whether an incompetent patient has the same constitutional right as a competent patient to refuse medical treatment. This question was quickly answered in the affirmative. Although the facts of this appeal only involved an incompetent infant, the court expanded its ruling to also cover incompetent adults who had not executed living wills. In the court's view, the critical questions remaining were (1) who may make these types of treatment decisions, and (2) whether judicial intervention is required prior to cessation of treatment. The court set forth the following guidelines for patients, families, hospitals, and physicians to observe prior to discontinuing life-saving treatment for incompetent patients:

1. The patient's attending physician must diagnose that the patient is terminally ill with no hope of recovery and that the patient exists in a chronic vegetative state with no reasonable possibility of attaining cognitive function.
2. Two physicians with no interest in the outcome of the case must concur in this diagnosis and prognosis.
3. Thereafter, a request to refuse or terminate treatment may be exercised by the "family" or legal guardian of an adult patient and by the "parents" or legal guardian of an infant.

Once these steps were completed, the court authorized the discontinuance of life-sustaining medical treatment. The court specifically rejected the necessity of prior judicial approval but noted that "courts remain available in the event of disagreement between the parties, any case of suspected abuse, or other appropriate instances." The opinion also concluded that no hospital ethics committee need be consulted, but the court did not wish to foreclose the use of such committees if desired by the hospital, physician or family. The opinion also declined to require the appointment of a legal guardian or guardian *ad litem* in situations in which family members are available.

Although requested to do so by the Georgia Hospital Association and others, the court declined to pronounce specifically that hospitals and physicians who discontinued or withheld medical treatment would be immune from civil or criminal liability. However, since this decision clearly authorized the cessation of treatment upon compliance with certain procedural guidelines, we would doubt any hospital or physician which complied with those guidelines in good faith would be found liable in any civil or criminal action. Nevertheless, hospitals may be prudent in obtaining a written release from liability and a written request for termination of treatment signed by the appropriate family members or the guardian.

3.3.2. What the Court Failed to Decide

The Supreme Court's opinion has several limitations, some of which are more subtle than others. For example, the opinion states: "We do not consider here the issue of *initiation* of treatment rather than its termination. . . ." This could mean that the court simply declined to rule whether the initiation of treatment on a terminally ill patient without proper consent would constitute a battery, as an Ohio court ruled earlier this year. On the other hand, some have expressed concern that the court's use of the term "initiation" could have symbolized its intent to exclude "do not resuscitate" orders from the scope of its decision since any decision whether or not to resuscitate involves a decision whether to "initiate" resuscitative treatment. It is hoped that the courts will not strain the interpretation of this term to include "do not resuscitate" orders.

The court also noted its opinion was not intended to address the "initiation or cessation of treatment for a terminally ill but *cognitive* child *or adult*. . . ." However, previous Georgia cases had already authorized the cessation of treatment for a terminally ill but competent adult (*Kirby v. Spivey,* 167 Ga. App. 751, 1983). Thus, we assume the court merely intended to exclude from the scope of its decision cognitive minors and those adults who are "cognitive" (aware) but not legally "competent" to make their own treatment decisions.

The court also declined to decide whether an ethics committee or prior judicial approval would be necessary "in cases in which the issue is *life*-prolonging rather than *death*-prolonging treatment for incompetent patients." Cautious hospitals might therefore be inclined to obtain court approval prior to discontinuing medical treatment in such situations.

The most troubling deficiency in the decision is found in the following disclaimer by the court: "We deal only with the termination of treatment of the terminally ill patient, adult or child, in a chronic vegetative state for whom there is no reasonable possibility of attaining [or regaining] cognitive function." Reading this sentence and other portions of the opinion literally, one concludes the court's holding is limited only to those patients who are both terminally ill and in an irreversible chronic vegetative state. However, many patients who are comatose and in an irreversible vegetative state might not be considered terminally ill by some standards. Indeed, there is no evidence in the record to conclude that L.H.R. herself was "terminally ill" other than the fact that she died soon after life-support systems were removed. Presumably, patients in a condition similar to L.H.R.'s would meet the standard for being considered "terminally ill," but the court's failure to define this term could cause legal difficulties in the future for patients in dissimilar conditions.

Additional complications arise when this decision is viewed in conjunction with the living will statute. The court's opinion appears only to address the withdrawal of treatment from "the incompetent adult who has made no living will. Thus, if the adult had executed a valid living will before becoming incompetent, the hospital should consider the guidelines of the living will statute. O.C.G.A. SS31-32-1, *et seq.* Under the statute's restrictive definition of "terminal condition," a living will can only be effectuated if (1) death is "imminent," and (2) the patient suffers from a condition "which, regardless of the application of life-sustaining procedures, would produce death" [O.C.G.A. S31-32-2(10)]. In other words, an incompetent adult in L.H.R.'s condition would not meet the definition of "terminal condition," since application of a respirator might prevent death indefinitely. The court's decision, therefore, does not provide the same protection for adults who have executed living wills and those who have not. It is hoped that subsequent court decisions will address this unfortunate inconsistency.

3.3.3. Some General and Practical Observations

In summary, while prior legal authority existed in Georgia to discontinue care for competent adults and those incompetent adults who had signed living wills, the *L.H.R.* case addresses the previously uncharted area of noncognitive minors and those incompetent adults who had not executed living wills.

As a result of this and other cases, Georgia has now established a legal precedent to authorize the discontinuance of life-sustaining treatment upon a competent adult's request as to his own person and upon an incompetent adult when requested by a family member or guardian. While a competent adult's request to discontinue treatment may be implemented without any prior procedural steps, the court in *L.H.R.* has required certain procedural safeguards prior to withholding medical treatment from an incompetent adult or noncognitive minor. If an adult patient has executed a living will and is in a "terminal condition" as defined in the living will statute, separate procedural safeguards need to be followed as outlined in the statute (see O.C.G.A. SS31-32-1, *et seq.*).

We also have some practical observations in light of this decision. First, since the court did not choose to define or limit the term *family,* this provides hospitals with some flexibility in dealing with this difficult issue. However, we would advise that if a disagreement arises between family members, judicial intervention should be sought as a protective measure.

Second, we would not interpret this decision to authorize the withholding of appropriate nutrition, hydration, and medication from an incompetent patient, since a court might conclude that such measures are life-prolonging rather than death-prolonging. Furthermore, in light of the court's dichotomy between treatment that prolongs death rather than life, we would suggest that the hospital's medical record contain a physician's recitation that continued maintenance of routine life-support treatment would prolong the patient's death rather than his or her life. Finally, since the court requires the concurrence of two physicians with no interest in the outcome, we would advise those hospitals with few physicians on their staff to make preliminary arrangements now with physicians in neighboring communities for emergency consultations when necessary.

In summary, we believe that the Supreme Court has taken a great step forward in protecting the rights of patients, their families, hospitals, and physicians in these sensitive and difficult situations. Although further litigation may be necessary to address other issues involved in this area, we are generally pleased with the progress represented by this latest decision.

REFERENCES

Ashwal, S., and Schneider, S., 1987, Brain death in children. I, *Pediatr. Neurol.* 3:5–11.

Ashwal, S., Smith, A. J. K., Torres, F., Loken, M., and Chou, S. N., 1977, Radionuclide bolus angiography: A technique for verification of brain death in infants and children, *J. Pediatr.* 91:722–728.

Coker, S. B., and Dillehay, G. L., 1986, Radionuclide cerebral imaging for confirmation of brain death in children: The significance of dural sinus activity, *Pediatr. Neurol.* 2:43–6.

Dear, P. R. F., and Godfrey, D. N., 1985, Neonatal auditory brainstem response cannot reliably diagnose brainstem death, *Arch. Dis. Child.* 60:17–19.

Drake, B., Ashwal, S., and Schneider, S., 1986, Determination of cerebral death in the pediatric intensive care unit, *Pediatrics* 78:107–112.

Green, J. R., and Lauber, A., 1972, Recovery of activity in young children after ECS, *J. Neurol Neurosurg. Psychiatry* 35:103–107.

Holzman, B. H., Curless, R. G., Sfakianakis, G. N., Ajomone-Marsan, C., and Montes, J. E., 1983, Radionuclide cerebral perfusion scintigraphy in determination of brain death in children, *Neurology (NY)* 33:1027–1031.

In re L.H.R., 253 GA 439, 321 SE2d 716 (1984).

McMenamin, J. B., and Volpe, J. J., 1983, Doppler ultrasonography in the determination of neonatal brain death, *Ann. Neurol.* 14:302–307.

Mizrahi, E. M., Pollock, M., and Kellaway, P., 1985, Neocortical death in infants: Behavioral neurologic and electroencephalographic characteristics, *Pediatr. Neurol.* 1:302–305.

Moshe, S. L., and Alvarez, L. A., 1986, Diagnosis of brain death in children, *J. Clin. Neurophysiol.* 3:239–249.

Outwater, K. M., and Rockoff, M. A., 1984, Apnea testing to confirm brain death in children, *Crit. Care Med.* 12:357–358.

Parvey, L. S., and Gerald B., 1976, Arteriographic diagnosis of brain death in children, *Pediatr. Radiol.* 4:78–82.

Rowland, T. W., Donnelly, J. H., and Jackson, A. H., 1984, Apnea documentation for determination of brain death in children, *Pediatrics* 74:505–508.

Rowland, T. W., Donnelly, J. H., Jackson, A. H., and Jamroz, S. B., 1983, Brain death in the pediatric intensive care unit, *Am. J. Dis. Child.* 137:547–550.

Schwartz, J. A., Baxter, J., and Brill, D. R., 1984, Diagnosis of brain death in children by radionuclide cerebral imaging, *Pediatrics* 73:14–18.

Steinhart, C. M., and Weiss, I. P., 1985, Use of brainstem auditory evoked potentials in pediatric death, *Crit. Care Med.* 13:560–562.

13

Brain Death in Children
The Loma Linda Experience

SANFORD SCHNEIDER

> *O' shut the door! And when*
> *Thou hast done so,*
> *Come weep with me past hope,*
> *Past cure, past help!*
> Juliet
> *Romeo and Juliet*
> William Shakespeare

1. INTRODUCTION

The brain-dead child is past cure, hope, and help. Discontinuing respiratory support for this child is simply an affirmation that death has already occurred. Maintenance of life-support systems after unequivocal documentation of brain death is futile and inhuman. Life-support systems cease to be life sustaining after brain death. After documenting brain death, the extraordinary action is not terminating, but continuing, life-support systems. Obviously, an error in this decision-making process is fatal and intolerable. The diagnosis of brain death in children has evolved independently in many centers without universal agreement as to criteria. Discussion is limited to our present-day neurologic management of suspected brain death in children at Loma Linda University School of Medicine.

2. PEDIATRIC POPULATION AT RISK

Before focusing on the criteria currently used to determine brain death in children, it is necessary to review the critically ill pediatric patient population that is being assessed for brain death. Between 1980 and 1985, 61 patients were admitted to the pediatric intensive care unit (ICU) at Loma Linda University Medical Center with an initial diagnosis of brain death (Drake

---

SANFORD SCHNEIDER • Department of Pediatrics and Neurology, Division of Child Neurology, Loma Linda University School of Medicine, Loma Linda, California 92350.

et al., 1986). All patients required assisted respiration, and 41% required vasopressors to stabilize blood pressure. Newborns were not included in this study, as they are maintained in a separate neonatal ICU. The mean age of our patients was 34 months with the ranges shown in Table I; 54% of these patients were admitted with a diagnosis of near-drowning, child abuse, or closed-head trauma (Table II).

A literature compilation of an additional 195 children cited in 17 references is quite similar and noted in Table III (Ashwal and Schneider, 1987). Closed-head trauma (25%), near-drowning (12%), asphyxia (9%), and nonaccidental trauma (6%) constitute 52% of the total 195 children reviewed. Thus, accidental and nonaccidental trauma constitute the largest population of brain-dead children maintained on life-support systems. The acuteness of the initial diagnosis indicates that families of most of our ICU patients will have had no expectation or emotional preparation to deal with the catastrophic knowledge that their child is brain dead and will not survive.

TABLE I. Age at
Diagnosis of Brain
Death[a]

Age	N
<2 mo	7
2–12 mo	16
1–5 yr	28
6–10 yr	4
10–18 yr	6
	61

[a]From Drake *et al.* (1986).

TABLE II. Primary Hospital Admission Diagnosis of 61
Children with Suspected Brain Death[a]

	Children	
Diagnosis	N	%
Drowning	13	21.3
Nonaccidental trauma	10	16.4
Closed-head trauma	10	16.4
Aspiration/asphyxia	5	8.2
Septic shock	4	6.6
Meningitis/encephalitis	3	4.9
CNS hemorrhage	3	4.9
Hemorrhagic disease of the newborn	1	
Arteriovenous malformation	1	
Acute lymphocytic leukemia	1	
Sudden infant death syndrome (SIDS)	3	4.9
Prematurity	2	3.3
Postsurgery	2	3.3
Strangulation	2	3.3
Neuroblastoma	1	1.6
Severe dehydration	1	1.6
Asthma	1	1.6
Fulminant hydrocephalus	1	1.6

[a]From Drake *et al.* (1986).

TABLE III.   Primary Admission Diagnosis in Children with
Suspected Brain Death[a,b]

Diagnosis	N	%
Closed-head trauma	45	23
Near-drowning	24	12
Asphyxia	18	9
Nonaccidental trauma	12	6
Infection–meningitis (9), encephalitis (5), abscess (2)	16	8
Metabolic disease: Reye syndrome (8), acute encephalopathy (2), hepatic failure (2), adrenogenital syndrome	13	7
Near-miss SIDS	10	5
CNS hemorrhage	7	4
Aspiration	5	2
Strangulation/suffocation	5	2
Hydrocephalus	4	2
Cardiac arrest: epiglotitis, status epilepticus cardiac disease, unknown	4	2
Smoke inhalation	3	2
Intra-/postoperative	2	1
Miscellaneous: asthma, dehydration, malignant (1 each); hyperthermia, neuroblastoma, myelodysplasia, hemolytic uremic syndrome, prosthetic valve emboli, air embolus, exsanguination	9	5
Newborn: asphyxia (9), meningitis (1), aspiration (1)	11	6
Premature—intraventricular hemorrhage (3), asphyxia (2), meningitis (2)	7	4
Total number of patients	195	100

[a] From Ashwal and Schneider (1987).
[b] Data extracted from 16 sources.

3.   DETERMINATION OF BRAIN DEATH

What criteria are valid for the determination of brain death? As with any critically ill child, historical information, neurological examination, and appropriate laboratory tests will determine the potential for survival.

3.1.   Patient History

Understanding the pathophysiology that results in a comatose respirator-dependent child is the most important contribution of the attending physician. The historical and clinical events will usually establish a diagnosis. For a variety of disorders, death in childhood is a natural progression for which there is no effective therapy. For these patients, initiation or continuation of ventilator support is inappropriate. Therefore, the first and most important step in deciding whether brain death has occurred is to determine the events that resulted in respirator intervention.

3.2. Clinical Examination

Evaluation of the child is similar to that of the adult with some limitations, particularly in the preterm infant. Brainstem function, including lack of spontaneous respiration, pupillary activity, corneal response, oculocephalic (doll's eyes), and if necessary vestibulo-ocular (caloric) responses, needs to be assessed. Total cessation of brainstem function as an irreversible indicator of brain death in children has not been extensively studied, and it may be different from that in adults, particularly in immature infants. (McMenamin and Volpe, 1983). Therefore, we commonly expand the clinical evaluation with an apnea challenge and then carry out laboratory testing, usually including electroencephalography (EEG) and one study to assess cerebral blood flow, to fully document neocortical brain death.

3.3. Determination of Apnea

Lack of spontaneous respiration is one of the most important criteria in assessing brain dysfunction and ultimately brain death. This is usually evaluated by discontinuing respirator support and allowing a measured rise in Pa_{CO_2}. Studies in childhood are relatively limited (Outwater and Rockoff, 1984, Rowland et al., 1984). High oxygen tension is maintained by supplying 100% tracheal oxygen during the apnea challenge. CO_2 tension is allowed to rise 60 mm Hg before terminating the test if patient does not initiate respiration spontaneously.

3.4. Electroencephalography

Most patients suspected of brain death will have at least one EEG, using the guidelines for electrocerebral silence (ECS) formulated by the American EEG Society (1986). Return of cortical activity from ECS is an exceptional occurrence, but it has been reported (Green and Lauber, 1972). Persistence of low-voltage EEG activity does not preclude a diagnosis of brain death, and rarely such activity may not correlate with absent cerebral blood flow studies (Ashwal and Schneider, 1979).

3.5. Cerebral Blood Flow Studies

This volume contains many chapters that describe the rationale and application of a number of techniques for determining the adequacy of cerebral blood flow. One or more of these techniques should be used by a physician who has assimilated the patient's history and, who has thoroughly examined the patient's brainstem function. At Loma Linda University School of Medicine, we now rely on two methods of estimating cerebral blood flow: radionucleotide isotope angiogram scanning and, more recently, xenon-computed tomography (XeCTCBF).

Radionucleotide angiography has proved a sensitive index of the adequacy of cerebral blood flow (Korein et al., 1977; Holzman et al., 1983; Schwartz et al., 1984). XeCTCBF permits the measurement of regional blood flow (ml/min/100 g) by contrasting the density of a routine CT scan with a second CT scan while the patient is being ventilated on a mixture of oxygen and xenon rather than oxygen and air. Computer analysis of density changes permits instant determination of regional cortical blood flow. Normal gray matter cerebral blood flow in children is 60–80 ml/min/100 gs. In our studies of brain-dead children with electrocerebral silence (ECS) by EEG, XeCTCBF showed flow values of less than 50 ml/min/100g centrally and virtually no flow at the cortex (Thompson et al., 1986). In comatose children with partial brainstem dysfunction, minimum EEG cortical activity, and positive cerebral blood flow by radionucleotide isotope scanning, we have demonstrated values of 20–80 ml/min/100 g by XeCTCBF. Values below 15 ml/min/100 g imply irreversible cortical injury. We are now completing XeCTCBF studies that may be predictive in determining the potential for recovery and the minimal neocortical perfusion necessary to prevent a persistent vegetative state in children.

3.6. Specific Recommendations

Every institution dealing with the complex care of comatose children needs to determine its own specific medical and ethical guidelines for evaluating suspected brain death death until universally accepted standards are available. Table IV summarizes our current protocol for determining brain death in children. Our management includes the stabilization of patient and environment, evaluation of the depth of coma, and tests of brainstem integrity by pupillary light reflex, corneal response, oculocephalic response, and oculovestibular responses (caloric). Neurological examination is followed by an apnea challenge raising the $Paco_2$ level to > 60 mm Hg. If the patient meets the above clinical criteria for brain death, we simultaneously exclude sedating drugs and metabolic dysfunction by appropriate blood and urine studies.

If these metabolic and drug tests are acceptable and clinical evaluation persistently demonstrates absent brainstem function, the diagnosis of brain death is substantiated in one of the following ways:

1. A 24-hr period of absent brainstem function
2. One cerebral blood flow study, usually radionucleotide isotope scanning, although Xe-CTCBF may clinically be more informative
3. Two ECS EEG at least 12 hr apart.

TABLE IV.   Decision-Making in Suspected Brain Death: Comatose Child

Evaluation

No purposeful responses to external environment, excluding spinal reflexes

Apnea—no spontaneous respiration to Pco_2 60 mm Hg

Normothermic: normotensive without volume depletion

Absent brainstem reflexes: pupillary, oculocephalic, corneal auriculo-ocular, vestibulo-ocular (caloric), gag (exclude if intubated)

Brain death status

Negative	Positive
Continue observation; monitor and support vital functions.	Toxins, drugs, or metabolic disorders are excluded.
Await drug and metabolic screens; then reassess.	If A, B, or C, patient can be declared brain dead.
	A. Clinical re-examination remains unchanged over 24 hr with continued coma, absent brainstem reflexes, and apneic despite Pco_2 challenge to 60 mm Hg.
	B. One cerebral perfusion study (isotope, cerebral angiography, or xenon CT) shows no significant flow.
	C. Two EEGs, 12–24 hr apart, demonstrate electrocerebral silence.

This protocol is applicable to the 7-day-old term infant or older child but does not have a significantly enlarged data base to apply to the newly born or premature infant. The use of cerebral blood flow studies permits a rapid and probably infallible diagnosis, although single isolated clinical oddities of return of EEG function (Green and Lauber, 1972) and restoration of absent radionucleotide flow (Hartshorne *et al.*, 1984) have been reported. Cerebral blood flow studies by radionucleotide scanning or XeCTCBF will accelerate the ability to formulate decisions and potentially speed recovery of donor organs before ischemic damage.

4. PARENTAL CONFLICTS, CONCERNS, AND INTERACTIONS

Obviously, parents do not readily accept the possibility that their child is near death. The vast majority of clinical situations are acute: trauma, near drowning, and asphyxia. Parents are not prepared to deal with the concept of discontinuing respirator support in these painful situations, much less discuss organ donation. This emotional devastation must be recognized by the treating physician. If the initial prognosis is grim, this should be realistically discussed without undue delay. It is crucial that the physician use knowledge and experience in helping the parents understand the clinical diagnosis, the dilemmas of treatment, and the anticipated outcome. The diagnosis should be established quickly, and it should be realized that knowledge of etiology and pathophysiology of the child's coma is far more useful than any specific laboratory test in discussing prognosis with parents. The physician must be willing to address every question raised by parents, relatives, and friends that seemingly conflicts with these discussions. It is important to explain that return of deep tendon reflexes and withdrawal in the brain dead patient is mediated at the spinal cord level and is not due to improvement of cortical function. Families must always be part of the decision-making process but should not be made to feel responsible for the ultimate decision to discontinue respiratory support. Most parents do not want their child to exist as a profoundly brain-damaged, comatose, respirator-dependent child who will ultimately succumb to infection or cardiac arrest. Parents will depend on physician guidance in this decision-making process. The physician must not coerce or be indecisive toward these grieving families but should remain both sympathetic and supportive. The physician's personal feelings, ethics, and religious beliefs should not be used in discussions with parents grieving over the impending death of their recently well child. Since the finality of discontinuing respirator support is so emotionally traumatic, the responsible physician must be available and responsive to the needs and inevitable feelings of guilt experienced by the parents. During these discussions regarding the futility of continued support, the possibility of potential donation may be raised. If the child is not a potential donor (infection, prolonged ischemia), the reason that donation is not possible should be discussed, so the parents do not feel later that organ donation was overlooked.

5. TRANSPLANTATION CONCERNS

Transplantation of organs is not new, as renal transplantation has been in existence for more than 30 years. However, transplantation of heart, lung, and liver, particularly in infants, is recent, and experience in donor collection is only now beginning to accumulate. New situations arise for which there are no present solutions. Anencephalics, theoretically ideal donors, are not used due to the difficulty in declaring the brainstem dead before irreversible hypoxia has occurred in other body organs. Similarly, infants with spinomuscular atrophy (Werdnig–Hoffman syndrome) cannot be declared brain dead while maintained on respirators despite their inevitable death. Thus, donor organs will continue to be largely supplied by acute trauma victims under the circumstances previously described.

A recently completed study at Loma Linda University School of Medicine reviewed 50 brain-dead children for suitability as cardiac donors (Doroshow *et al.*, 1986). Prior to death, these patients were screened by echocardiograms (ECGs) and fractionated creatinine kinase determinations. Thirty-three hearts were carefully examined postmortem, 19 of which would have been suitable for transplantation. Prolonged cardiac arrest did not generally preclude selection as a donor. Near-drowning patients tended to be poor cardiac donors, while child-abuse victims were excellent potential donors.

Brain death from child abuse is a relatively unique circumstance, due in part to the fact that consent for organ donation will probably come from the abuser(s). In addition, the consent of the local coroner or medical examiner (and possibly their presence at donor surgery) must be obtained after declaring the child brain dead, while continuing to maintain cardiac function by mechanical ventilation. Transplant surgeons, child neurologists, and pediatricians need to establish an advanced working relationship with their respective coroners to ensure that this type of donation may occur. This is particularly important, since child abuse unfortunately remains as one of the common causes of brain death in young children.

It is our experience that parents are more willing to permit donation if discussion is initiated early in the process of declaring a child brain dead. The dialogue should be initiated and continued by the responsible physician. An extremely zealous approach should be avoided, as this may solidify parental guilt, and a belief that their child's suffering will continue if organs are removed after death. The National Organ Transplant Act of 1987 requires hospitals in the United States to have a mechanism in place for requesting donation of organs.

After a child considered suitable for organ donation is declared brain dead, the parents, previously briefed on the value of organ donation, should be requested to allow donation. An adamant refusal should be accepted without further cajoling parents who have been adequately informed and educated in the need for pediatric donor organs. If the parents concur, as many will, arrangements should be made with a transplant team to remove the organ(s) or transfer the respirator dependent body to a transplant center. Donor parents should never bear any of the expense of organ removal or transportation or increased funeral costs.

Public education needs to replace isolated individual media pleas for organs. All parents need to understand that their children may possibly need to be an organ donor, as well as a recipient.

> Give me my Romeo, and when he shall die,
> Take him and cut him but in little stars,
> And he will make the face of heaven so fine,
> That all the world will be in love with night.
>   Juliet
>   *Romeo and Juliet*
>   William Shakespeare

ACKNOWLEDGMENTS. Studies and protocols mentioned within this chapter have been developed in association with my colleagues Dr. Stephen Ashwal, from the Division of Child Neurology, Dr. Joseph Thompson, from the Division of Neuroradiology, and Dr. Leonard Bailey, from the Division of Cardiothoracic Surgery at Loma Linda University School of Medicine.

REFERENCES

American Electroencephalographic Society, 1986, *Guidelines in EEG 1-7 (Revised 1985)*, J. Clin. Neurophysiol. **3**:131–168.

Ashwal, S., and Schneider, S., Failure of electroencephalography to diagnose brain death in comatose patients, *Ann Neurol.* **6**:512–517.

Ashwal, S., and Schneider, S., 1987, Brain death in children. I, *Pediatr. Neurol.* **3:**5–11.

Doroshow, R. W., Saurel, G. W., and Ashwal, S., 1986, Availability and selection of pediatric cardiac donors, presented at the *Fifty-ninth American Heart Association, Dallas, Nov. 1986.*

Drake, B., Ashwal, S., and Schneider, S., 1986, Determination of cerebral death in the pediatric intensive care unit, *Pediatrics,* **78:**107–112.

Green, J. R., and Lauber, A., 1972, Recovery of activity in young children after ECS, *J. Neurol. Neurosurg. Psychiatry* **35:**103–107.

Hartshorne, M. S., Ramirez, R., and Cawthon, M. A., 1984, Multiple imaging techniques. CSF shunted Arnold Chiari malformation with false negative brain death radionucleotide angiograms, *Clin. Nucl. Med.* **9:**650–653.

Holzman, B. H., Curless, R. G., and Sfakianakis, G. N., 1983, Radionucleotide cerebral perfusion scintigraphy by determining brain death in children. *Neurology (NY)* **33:**1027–1031.

Korein, S., Braunstein, P., and George P., 1977, Brain Death. I. Angiographic correlation with a radioisotope bolus technique for evaluation of cerebral blood flow, *Ann. Neurol.* **2:**195–205.

McMenamin, J. B., and Volpe, J. J., 1983, Doppler ultrasonography in the determination of neonatal brain death, *Ann. Neurol.* **14:**302–307.

Outwater, K. M., and Rockoff, W. A., 1984, Apnea testing to confirm brain death in children, *Crit. Care Med.* **12:**357–358.

Rowland, T. W., Donnelly, J. H., and Jackson, A. H., 1984, Apnea documentation for determination of brain death in children, *Pediatrics* **74:**505–508.

Schwartz, J. A., Baxter, J., and Brill, D. R., 1984. Diagnosis for Brain Death in Children by Radionucleotide Imaging. *Pediatrics,* Vol. 73:14–18, 1984.

Thompson, J. R., Schneider, S., and Ashwal, S., 1986, Comparison of cerebral blood flow measurements by xenon computed tomography and dynamic brain scintigraphy in clinically brain dead children, presented at the *Thirteenth Symposium Neuroradiogicum, Stockholm, June 24, 1986,* abst. 179.

14

BRAIN DEATH IN CHILDREN
Task Force Guidelines

DAVID A. STUMPF

1. INTRODUCTION

Several organizations simultaneously began to address the issue of brain death guidelines in children. A Task Force was thus formed, with representatives from various societies and organizations (Table I). The Task Force met in Chicago (November 1985), New Orleans (April 1986), and Boston (October 1986), and was called Task Force on Brain Death in Childhood. A conference call in November 1986 finalized the document. Between these discussions, feedback was requested by the parent organizations and other interested parties. Thus, a consensus was sought.

The Task Force was not interested in pontification; it based the statement on published clinical data. The Task Force strove to be succinct in an effort to encourage the statement's use. We stuck to the issue, brain death, and avoided tangents into other areas, such as the persistent vegetative state and transplantation issues.

The Task Force sought to prepare a flexible document that would allow for variations in hospital resources and clinical situations, as well as accommodate changes inherent in technological advancements. The Task Force was careful not to impair physicians ability to discontinue supportive care in other situations. It is appropriate to terminate supportive measures in many hopeless situations in which the patient is not brain dead. The Task Force subsequently sent the document back to the parent organizations, where it was formally reviewed and endorsed as indicated. The organizations have published the document in their respective journals.

2. TASK FORCE DOCUMENT

2.1. Guidelines for the Determination of Brain Death in Children

Most states now have laws on brain death, and the American Medical Association, the American Bar Association, the National Conference of Commissioners on Uniform State Laws, the

DAVID A. STUMPF • Department of Pediatrics and Neurology, Northwestern University Medical School, The Children's Memorial Hospital, Chicago, Illinois 60614.

TABLE I.   Task Force Committee Membership

George J. Annas, J.D.
Boston University School of Medicine
American Bar Association

Patrick F. Bray, M.D.
University of Utah School of Medicine
American Academy of Neurology

Donald R. Bennett, M.D.
College of Medicine, University of Nebraska
American Neurological Association

Lester L. Lansky, M.D.
University of Illinois School of Medicine, Chicago
American Academy of Pediatrics

Edwin C. Myer, M.D.
Medical College of Virginia
Richmond, Virginia
Child Neurology Society

Russell C. Raphaely, M.D.
Children's Hospital of Philadelphia
American Academy of Pediatrics

Sanford Schneider, M.D.
Loma Linda Medical School
American Academy of Neurology

David A. Stumpf, M.D., Ph.D.
Northwestern University School of Medicine
Child Neurology Society

Joseph J. Volpe, M.D.
Washington University School of Medicine
American Neurological Association

Karin Nelson, M.D.
National Institute of Neurological, Communicative Diseases and Stroke

Endorsed by the following organizations (listed alphabetically):
   American Academy of Neurology
   American Academy of Pediatrics, Section on Neurology
   American Neurological Association
   Child Neurology Society

President's Commission for the Study of Ethical Problems in Medicine and Biomedical and Behavioral Research, and our task force have all endorsed the following language regarding the determination of death:

> An individual who has sustained either (1) irreversible cessation of circulatory and respiratory functions, or (2) irreversible cessation of all functions of the entire brain, including the brainstem, is dead. A determination of death must be made in accordance with accepted medical standards.

There are no unique legal issues in determining brain death in children as compared to adults. The unique issues are all medical ones, and relate directly to the more difficult task of confirming brain death in young children.

Current criteria of brain death avoid application of these standards to "young children." The report of the Presidential Commission outlines criteria valid in children over 5 years of age. It is generally assumed that the child's brain is more resistant to insults leading to death, although this issue is controversial and lacks convincing clinical documentation (Schwartz *et al.*, 1984; Moshe and Alvarez, 1986).

The criteria outlined are useful in determining brain death in infants and children. In term newborns (> 38 weeks gestation), the criteria are useful 7 days after the neurologic insult. The newborn is clinically difficult to evaluate after perinatal insults. This relates to many factors including the difficulties of clinical assessment, the determination of the proximate cause of coma, and the certainty of the validity of laboratory tests. These problems are accentuated in a premature infant. However, after an interval, currently suggested as the first 7 days after the insult in a term newborn, the extent and reversibility of neurological injury can be determined by the physical examination and laboratory studies.

2.2. Clinical History

The critical initial assessment is the clinical history and examination. The most important factor is determination of the proximate cause of coma to insure absence of remediable or reversible conditions. Most difficulties with the determination of death on the basis of neurological criteria have resulted from overlooking this basic fact. Especially important are detection of toxic and metabolic disorders, sedative–hypnotic drugs (Powner, 1976), paralytic agents, hypothermia, hypotension, and surgically remediable conditions. The physical examination is necessary to determine the failure of brain function.

2.3. Physical Examination Criteria

1. Coma and apnea must coexist. The patient must exhibit complete loss of consciousness, vocalization, and volitional activity.
2. Absence of brainstem function as defined by:
   a. Midposition or fully dilated pupils which do not respond to light. Drugs may influence and invalidate pupillary assessment.
   b. Absence of spontaneous eye movements, those induced by oculocephalic and caloric (oculovestibular) testing.
   c. Absence of movement of bulbar musculature including facial and oropharyngeal muscles. The corneal, gag, cough, sucking, and rooting reflexes are absent.
   d. Respiratory movements are absent with the patient off the respirator. Apnea testing using standardized methods can be performed (Rowland *et al.*, 1984; Outwater and Rockoff, 1984) but is done after other criteria are met.
3. The patient must not be significantly hypothermic or hypotensive for age.
4. Flaccid tone and absence of spontaneous or induced movements, excluding spinal cord events such as reflex withdrawal or spinal myoclonus should exist.
5. The examination should remain consistent with brain death throughout the observation and testing period.

2.4. Observation Periods According to Age

The recommended observation period depends on the age of the patient and the laboratory tests utilized.

   7 days to 2 months: The Task Force recommends two examinations and electroencephalograms (EEGs) separated by at least 48 hr.

2 months to 1 year: The Task Force recommends two examinations and EEGs separated by at least 24 hr. A repeat examination and EEG are not necessary if a concomitant radionuclide angiographic (CRAG) study demonstrates no visualization of cerebral arteries.

Over 1 year: When an irreversible cause exists, laboratory testing is not required and the Task Force recommends an observation period of at least 12 hr. There are conditions, particularly hypoxic–ischemic encephalopathy, in which it is difficult to assess the extent and reversibility of brain damage. This is particularly true if the first examination is performed soon after the acute event. Therefore, in this situation, the Task Force recommends a more prolonged period of at least 24 hr of observation. The observation period may be reduced if the EEG demonstrates electrocerebral silence or the CRAG does not visualize cerebral arteries.

2.5. Laboratory Testing

2.5.1. Electroencephalography

Electroencephalography (EEG) to document electrocerebral silence should, if performed, be done over a 30-min period, using standardized techniques for brain death determinations (American Encephalographic Society, 1986). In small children, it may not be possible to meet the standard requirement for a 10-cm electrode separation. The interelectrode distance should be decreased proportional to the patient's head size. Drug concentrations should be insufficient to suppress EEG activity.

2.5.2. Angiography

A cerebral radionuclide angiogram (CRAG) confirms cerebral death by demonstrating the lack of visualization of the cerebral circulation. A technically satisfactory CRAG that demonstrates arrest of carotid circulation at the base of the skull and absence of intracranial arterial circulation can be considered confirmatory of brain death, even though there may be some visualization of the intracranial venous sinuses (Goodman *et al.*, 1985; Drake *et al.*, 1986; Holzman *et al.*, 1983). The value of this study in infants under 2 months is under investigation. Contrast angiography can document lack of effective blood flow to the brain.

2.5.3. Techniques under Investigation

The Task Force recognizes that other tests, including xenon computed tomography (CT) (Thompson *et al.*, 1986), digital subtraction angiography (Vatne *et al.*, 1985; Lee *et al.*, 1984), visualization of cerebral arterial pulsations by real-time cranial ultrasound, Doppler determination of cerebral blood flow velocity (McMenamin and Volpe, 1983), and evoked potentials, are under investigation.

REFERENCES

American Electroencephalographic Society, 1986, Guidelines in EEG 1–7. (revised 1985), *J. Clin. Neurophysiol.* **3**:131–168.

Drake, B., Ashwal, S., and Schneider, S., 1986, Determination of cerebral death in the pediatric intensive care unit, *Pediatrics* **78**:107–112.

Goodman, J. M., Heck, L. L., and Moore, B. D., 1985, Confirmation of brain death with portable isotope angiography: A review of 204 consecutive cases. *Neurosurgery* **16**:492–497.

Holzman, B. H., Curless, R. G., Sfakianakis, G. N., Ajmone-Marsan, C., and Montes, J. E., 1983, Radionuclide cerebral perfusion scintigraphy in determination of brain death in children, *Neurology (NY)* **33**:1027–1031.

Lee, B. C., Voorhies, T. M., Ehrlich, M. E., Lipper, E., Auld, P. A., and Vannucci, R. C., 1984, Digital intravenous cerebral angiography in neonates, *Am. J. Neuroradiol.* **5**:281–286.

McMenamin, J. B., and Volpe, J. J., 1983, Doppler ultrasonography in the determination of neonatal brain death, *Ann. Neurol.* **14**:302–307.

Moshe, S. L., and Alvarez, L. A., 1986, Diagnosis of brain death in children, *Clin. Neurophysiol.* **3**:239–249.

Outwater, K. M., and Rockoff, M. A., 1984, Apnea testing to confirm brain death in children, *Crit. Care Med.* **12**:357–358.

Powner, D. J., 1976, Drug-associated isoelectric EEGs. A hazard in brain-death certification, *JAMA* **236**:1123.

President's Commission for the Study of Ethical Problems in Medicine and Biomedical and Behavioral Research, 1981, Guidelines for the Determination of Death, *JAMA* **246**:2184–2186.

Rowland, T. W., Donnelly, J. H., and Jackson, A. H., 1984, Apnea documentation for determination of brain death in children, *Pediatrics* **74**:505–508.

Schwartz, J. A., Baxter, J., and Brill, D. R., 1984, Diagnosis of brain death in children by radionuclide cerebral imaging, *Pediatrics* **73**:14–18.

Thompson, J. R., Ashwal, S., Schneider, S., Hasso, A. N., Hinshaw, D. B., Jr., and Kirk, G., 1986, Comparison of cerebral blood flow measurements by xenon computed tomography and dynamic brain scintigraphy in clinically brain dead children, presented at the *Thirteenth Symposium of Neuroradiologicum, Stockholm, Sweden, June 24, 1986*, p. 179 (abst.).

Vatne, K., Nakstad, P., and Lundar, T., 1985, Digital subtraction angiography (DSA) in the evaluation of brain death. A comparison of conventional cerebral angiography with intravenous and intraarterial DSA, *Neuroradiology* **27**:155–157.

15

Validity of Radionuclide Cerebral Angiography for Diagnosing Brain Death in Infants

Julius M. Goodman, Larry L. Heck,
Stephen K. Nugent, and Michael S. Turner

1. INTRODUCTION

Since 1969, we have been using intravenous (IV) radionuclide cerebral angiography (RCA) as a confirmatory test for brain death in both children and adults (Goodman and Heck, 1977; Goodman et al., 1969, 1985). However, a recent highly respected consensus report (Report of the Medical Consultants on the Diagnosis of Death, 1981) has advised caution in using adult-based criteria for determining brain death in children, implying that a young child with a severe neurological insult may have greater recovery potential than an adult in a similar situation. In order to respond to concerns raised about the validity of RCA in diagnosing brain death in very young patients, we have reviewed our recent results with this technique in infants under 2 years with suspected brain death.

Our data indicate that a portable radionuclide flow study that shows unequivocal arrest of the carotid circulation at the base of the skull and absence of intracranial arterial circulation is a valid diagnostic test for brain death in infants, including neonates. When the nuclear imaging criteria of brain death are present in a patient of any age, we contend that arbitrary waiting periods for repeat neurological examinations, routine drug screening, mandatory consultations, and electrophysiological studies are unnecessary for further substantiation of irreversibility.

Julius M. Goodman • Indianapolis Neurosurgical Group, Neuroscience Section, Methodist Hospital of Indiana; Division of Neurosurgery, Indiana University Medical Center, Indianapolis, Indiana 46202-1206. Larry L. Heck • Section of Nuclear Radiology, Methodist Hospital of Indiana, Indianapolis, Indiana 46202-1206. Stephen K. Nugent • Pediatric Intensive Care Unit, Methodist Hospital of Indiana, Indianapolis, Indiana 46202-1206. Michael S. Turner • Indianapolis Neurosurgical Group, Neuroscience Section, Methodist Hospital of Indiana, and Division of Neurosurgery, Indiana University Medical Center, Indianapolis, Indiana 46202-1206.

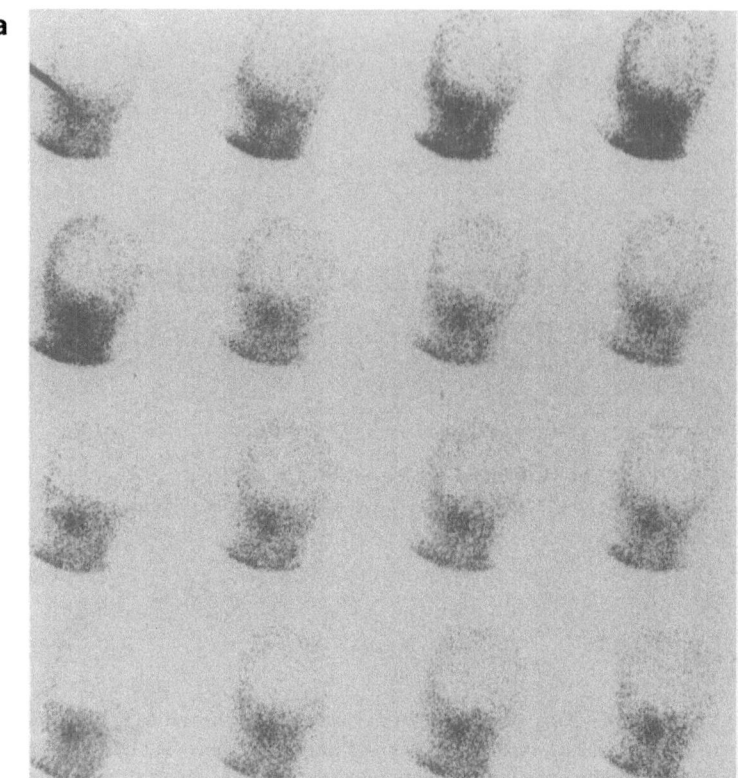

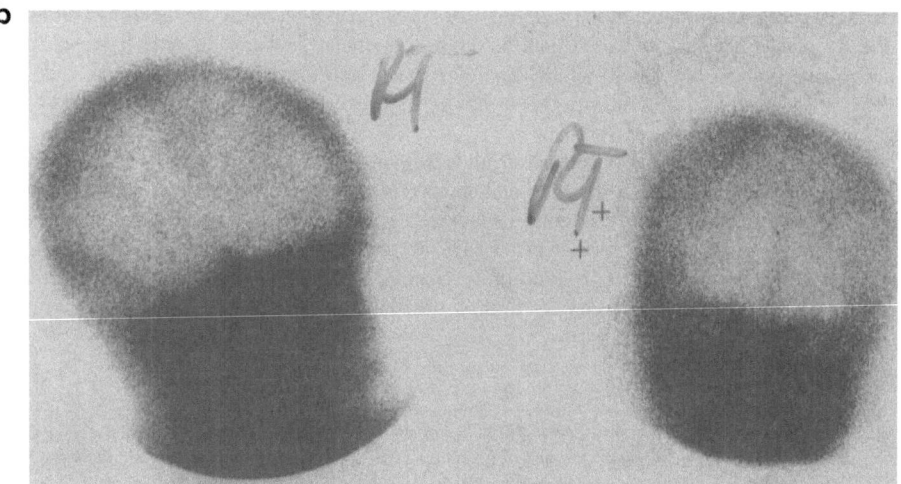

FIGURE 1. A 7-month-old with head injury. (a) Flow study showing arrest of carotid circulation at base of skull with no intracranial arterial circulation. (b) On static scan, there is slight filling of sagittal and lateral sinuses.

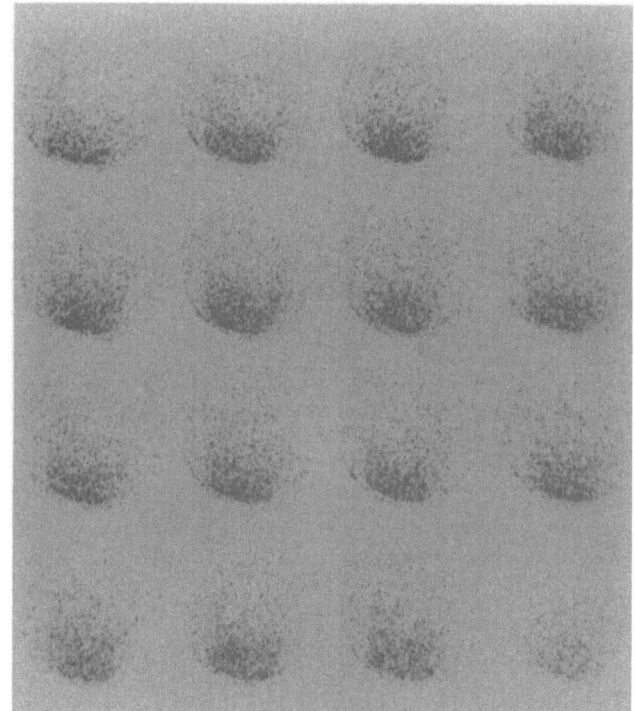

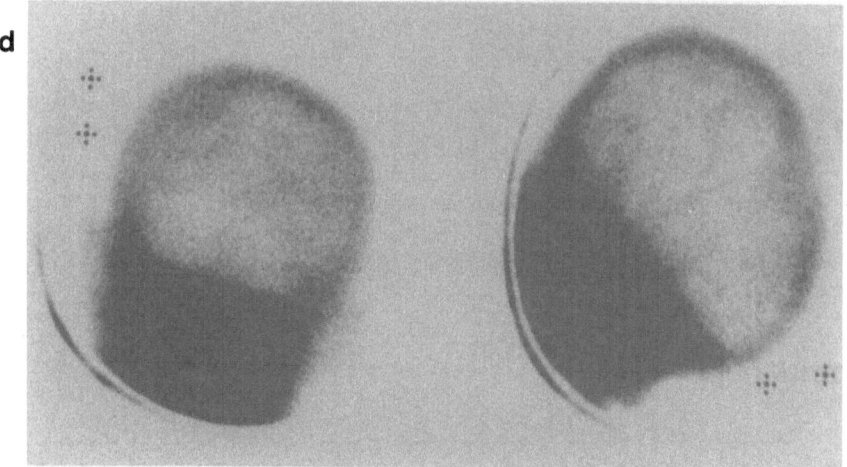

(c) On repeat scan, 24 hr later, there is still no arterial circulation. (d) Venous structures no longer seen.

2. MATERIAL

The medical records, computed tomography (CT) scans, nuclear scans, and autopsy reports of 30 consecutive infants below age 2 years, who had radionuclide flow studies compatible with brain death, were reviewed. The nuclear images had been performed at the bedside in the pediatric

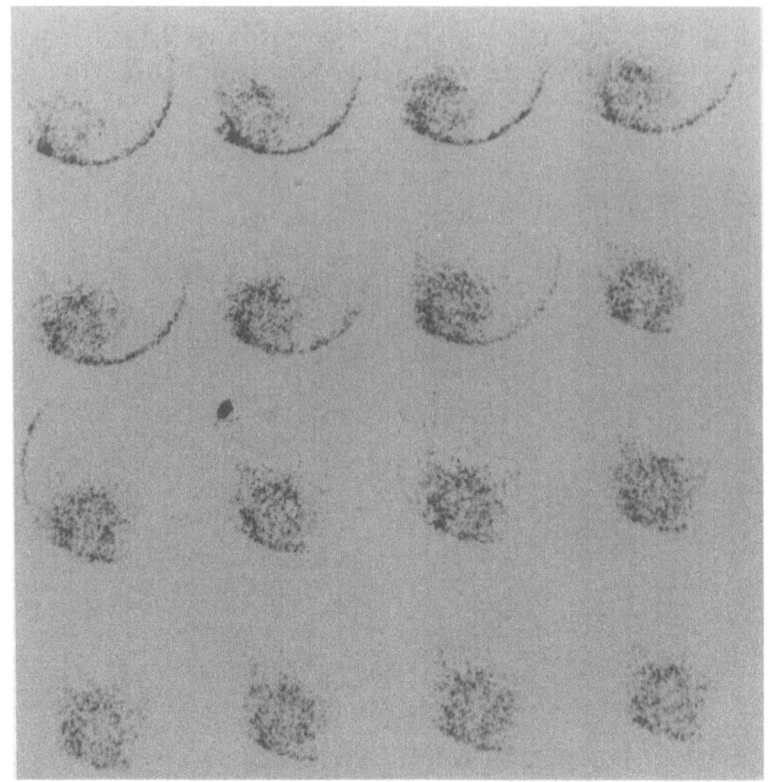

FIGURE 2. Radionuclide cerebral angiograms in a 2-month-old with head injury. (a) No arterial flow on dynamic image.

intensive care unit (ICU) at the Methodist Hospital of Indiana, Indianapolis, between 1979 and 1987. The patients' ages, which ranged from newborn to 23 months, are shown in Table I. The etiologies of brain death are listed in Table II. During the same period, we encountered five other infants with suspected brain death who had normal isotope angiograms. These cases were also reviewed.

3. TECHNIQUE

After the diagnosis of brain death was suspected by clinical assessment, a radionuclide brain scan was performed as soon as was practical and convenient. The time from clinical recognition of brain death to imaging ranged from 30 min to 12 hr. A portable gamma camera was used following the technique of Goodman and Heck (Goodman and Heck, 1977; Goodman *et al.*, 1985). Pictures were taken every 2–3 sec after rapid injection of ^{99m}Tc-labeled human serum albumin containing 10 μCi of activity (flushed with 20 ml of saline through a three-way stopcock). Upon completion of this dynamic study, lateral and anterior 400,000-count static images were obtained to assess activity in the sagittal and transverse sinuses. If the ^{99m}Tc was not injected as a good IV bolus or if other technical factors interfered with the quality of the images, the RCA was read as nondiagnostic and the procedure was rescheduled. The scans were interpreted by a nuclear radiologist who was not involved in the management of the patient. If the imaging criteria

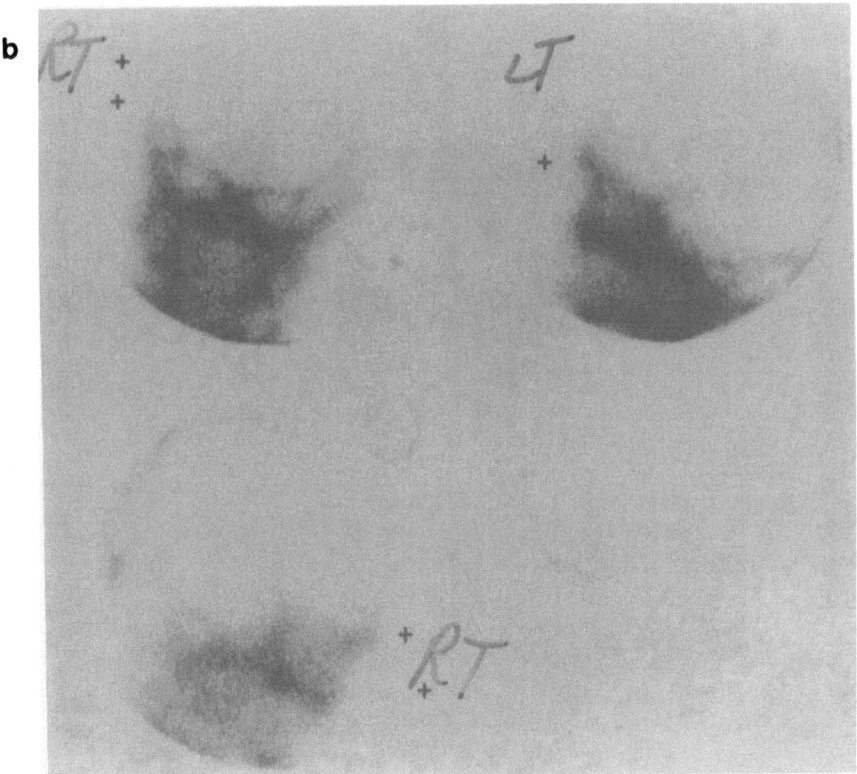

(b) Faint visualization of lateral sinus on static image. Ventilator stopped. Respirator brain noted at postmortem examination.

TABLE I. Age of Infants with Brain Death

Age (months)	N
1	3
2	3
3	2
4	2
5	1
7	2
8	2
9	2
10	1
11	1
13	1
15	1
16	3
17	2
19	2
21	1
23	1
	30

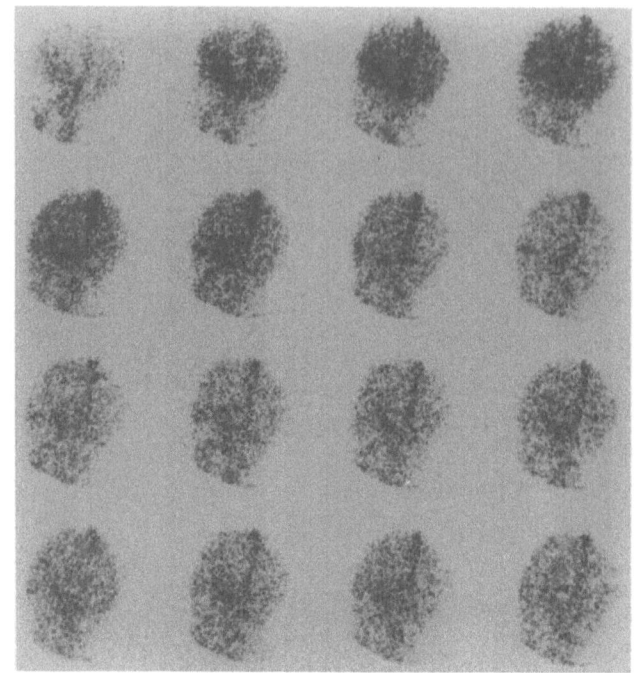

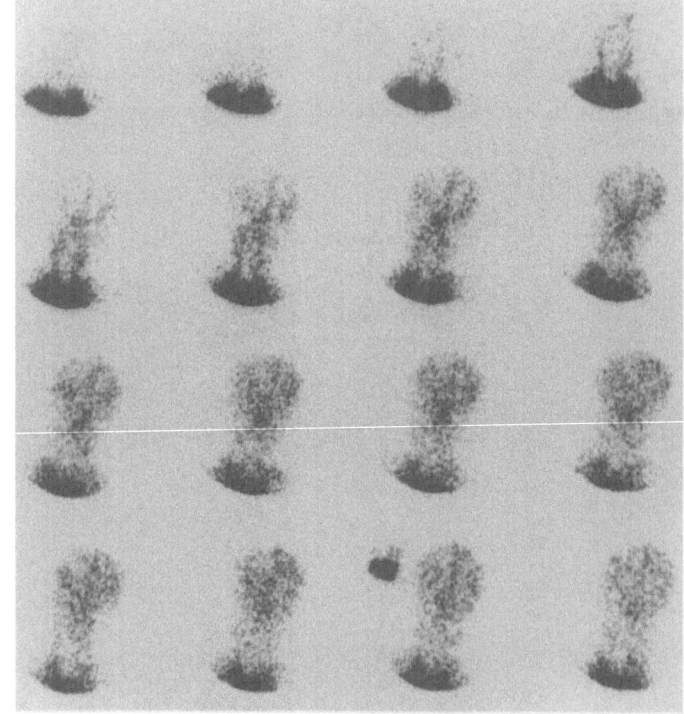

FIGURE 3. A 2-month-old with diffuse head injury and split sutures. Intracranial pressure (ICP) monitored. (a, b) Dynamic scans 1 day apart showing normal arterial circulation.

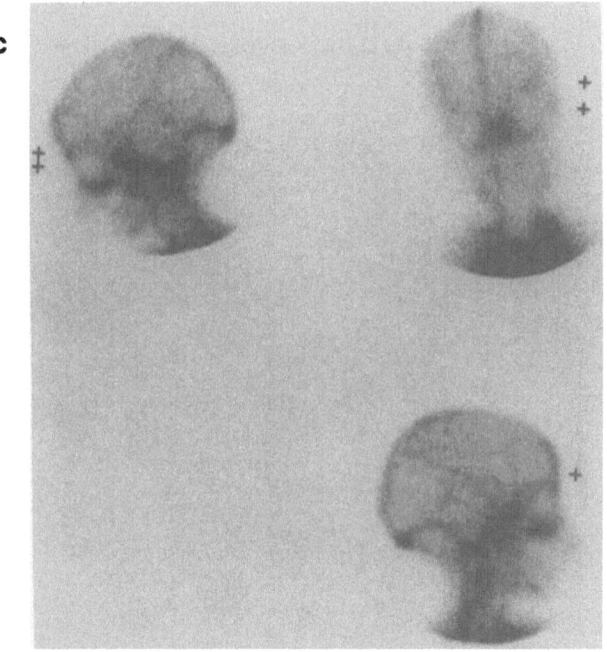

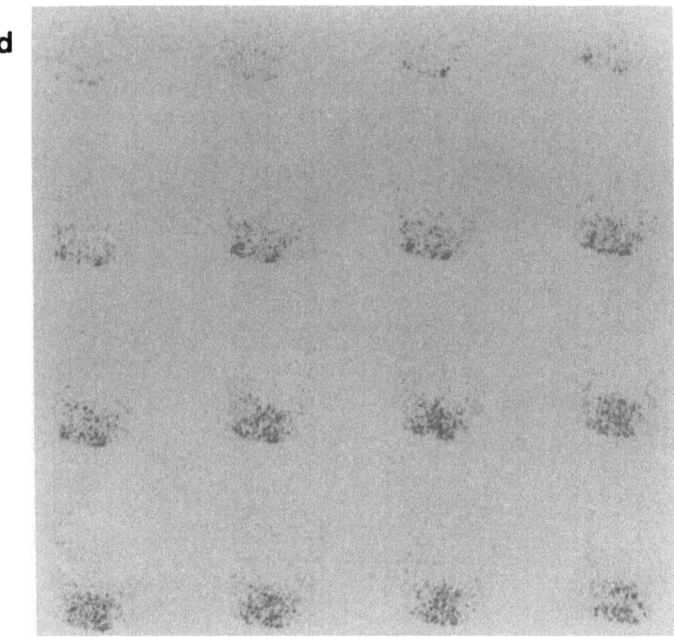

(c) Second static scan showing sinuses. (d, e) Dynamic and static scans 1 day later, when ICP became greater than mean arterial pressure.

e

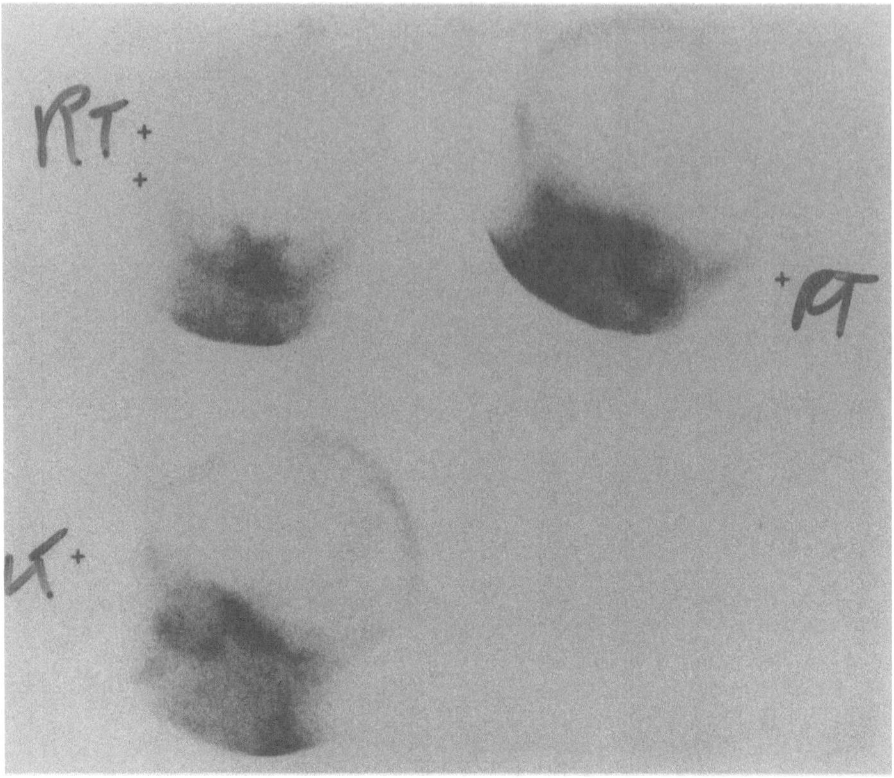

FIGURE 3. (*Continued*)

TABLE II.   Etiology of
Brain Death

Cause	N
Birth trauma	2
Trauma	13
SIDS	2
Anoxia	6
Meningitis	6
Sepsis	1
Total:	30

of brain death was not present on the nuclear scan and the attending physician, after reassessing the patient, still believed the clinical diagnosis of brain death was correct, scans were performed again at intervals of about 12–24 hr, until a diagnostic study was obtained. A wait of at least 12 hr is necessary before a flow study can be repeated to allow adequate disappearance of the last dose of ^{99m}Tc from the circulation, particularly if human serum albumin is used.

4. RESULTS

Scans were confirmatory of brain death in 30 patients. According to a strict protocol adhered to before 1984 (Goodman and Heck, 1977; Goodman *et al.*, 1969), the diagnosis of brain death by isotope aniography required the complete absence of all intracranial arterial, as well as venous, flow. An initial scan in seven infants met the criteria, and death was confirmed, but five infants had some venous sinus filling, and treatment was continued. Two of the five infants died before the scans could be repeated, but the other three had subsequent scans that showed no arterial flow and also absence of the previously visualized venous structures (Fig. 1).

Our radiographic criteria for diagnosing brain death were revised in 1984 (Goodman *et al.*, 1985). Brain death was diagnosed when there was unequivocal arrest of the carotid circulation at the base of the skull, as well as absence of intracranial arterial circulation, even though some of the venous structures could still be visualized (Fig. 2). Since modifying the criteria, brain death has been declared in 18 infants who had no arterial flow on the RCA. Images in seven of these patients did show some visualization of venous sinuses.

Autopsies were obtained in 14 of 30 (47%) of patients with scans confirmatory for brain death. Features characteristic of brain death were present in 12 patients. Two infants showed no gross or microscopic changes of postmortem autolysis on retrospective review of the autopsy material. One patient was a 2-month-old abused child who had a closed head injury. While receiving high doses of barbiturates in an effort to lower intracranial pressure (ICP), RCAs on two successive days showed normal flow (Fig. 3). On the third day, the patient's ICP exceeded mean arterial pressure. No arterial or venous flow was seen on the third flow study, and the ventilator was stopped shortly thereafter (Fig. 3). On sectioning of the brain, there was severe edema of the white matter as well as frontal and temporal cortical contusions but no herniation. The other patient without autolysis was a 19-month-old who sustained a severe head injury in a motor vehicle accident. Although he had no mass lesions, the ICP exceeded mean arterial pressure. The child was pronounced brain dead on the basis of an RCA less than 24 hr after injury, and mechanical ventilation was discontinued. The consistency of the brain at autopsy was normal, but there was marked swelling with transtentorial and tonsillar herniation.

Brain death was confirmed by RCA in five infants while there was still visualization of venous sinuses. The respirator was discontinued, and postmortem changes of brain death were present in each case. Lack of cerebral perfusion by RCA was noted in two newborn infants with brain trauma (Figs. 4 and 5). One underwent autopsy and respirator brain was found.

Between 1979 and 1987, we encountered five other infants suspected of being brain dead who had normal flow studies. In two, the clinical diagnosis of brain death was erroneous. A 23-month-old head-injured child with superimposed hypoxic encephalopathy appeared clinically brain dead but had a normal flow study. A subsequent repeat neurological examination showed a flicker of pupillary response. Treatment was continued, but the infant died shortly thereafter of sepsis. A 15-month-old was thought to be brain dead while under treatment with coma-producing levels of barbiturates for intractably high ICP. A nuclear flow study was normal, and this child survived.

Three infants with successful cardiopulmonary resuscitation following prolonged apnea met all the clinical criteria of brain death, but had normal RCAs. A 5-five-week-old girl with sudden infant death syndrome (SIDS) had five normal flow studies and was subsequently declared brain dead on clinical grounds with confirmation by two flat electroencephalograms (EEGs). A 6-week-old with SIDS had a normal RCA but died of an arrhythmia before the flow study could be repeated. A 2-month-old had two normal flow studies. The ventilator was finally stopped after repeated neurological examinations and two flat EEGs convinced the clinicians that brain death had occurred. Autopsies were not done in these SIDS cases. However, two infants with SIDS in the series of 30 patients did have confirmatory flow studies showing lack of cerebral perfusion.

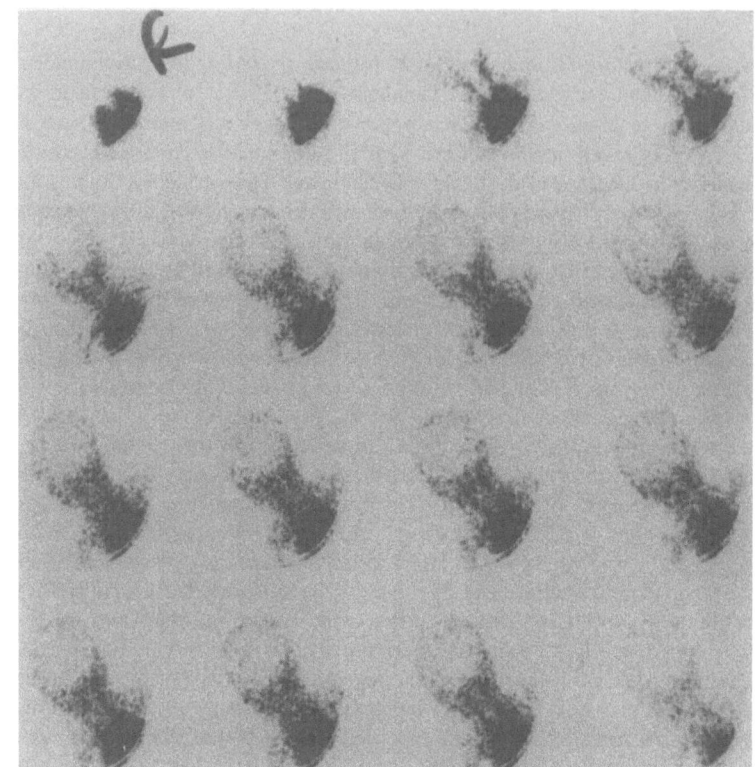

FIGURE 4. Scans consistent with brain death in a newborn. (a) Dynamic. (b) Static.

5. DISCUSSION

When a single RCA shows arrest of the carotid circulation at the base of the skull and unequivocal absence of intracranial arterial circulation, we as well as others are convinced that death has occurred regardless of the age of the patient and irrespective of metabolic abnormalities or drug intoxications (Drake *et al.*, 1986; Goodman *et al.*, 1985; Schwartz *et al.*, 1983, 1984; Tsai *et al.*, 1982). Some clinicians (Ad Hoc Committee on Brain Death, 1987; Drake *et al.*, 1986; Holzman *et al.*, 1983) who also appreciate the value of RCA in brain death still recommend EEGs and other confirmatory tests even when the RCA shows no flow. In our experience, further testing is unnecessary. We have not seen, nor are we aware of any patient of any age who has had no flow on an RCA who has subsequently had return of flow or who has survived.

The present study included 30 consecutive cases of brain death from a variety of causes in infants under age 2 that showed no flow on RCA. There were no mitigating circumstances to persuade us that these young patients should have been handled differently from adults. The brains of 14 of these patients were examined at autopsy. All but two infants with severe head trauma showed the characteristic softening and necrosis of brain death. One infant with elevated ICP had two normal RCAs. No flow was seen on the third RCA performed shortly after the ICP exceeded mean arterial pressure. Ventilation was then discontinued. At autopsy there was diffuse swelling of the white matter but no autolysis. The second infant also had ICP above mean arterial pressure when the RCA showed no flow. He was pronounced dead less than 24 hr after injury. There was

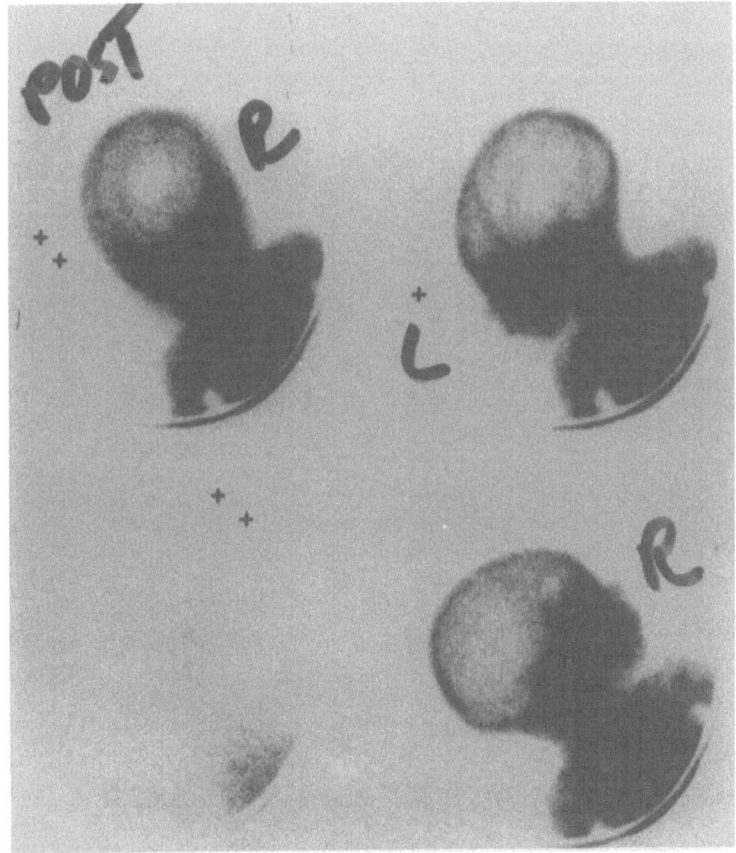

FIGURE 4. (*Continued*)

diffuse swelling and transtentorial and tonsillar herniation, but the typical changes of brain death were not seen. The lack of autopsy confirmation of brain death in these two infants does not detract from the validity of the RCA in confirming brain death. Both patients had ICP sustained above mean arterial pressure, which in itself may be considered a confirmatory sign of brain death (Holzman *et al.*, 1983; Korein, 1986). Also, time must elapse before the postmortem changes of brain death take place (Korein, 1986). It is estimated that approximately 12 hr without cerebral perfusion is required before the autolytic process becomes apparent (Leestma *et al.*, 1984). The ventilators for both infants described above were discontinued shortly after confirmation of brain death by RCA. If ventilation had been supported longer, it is reasonable to assume that autolysis would have occurred.

Practically every published protocol for brain death emphasizes the neurological examination, but we believe, in certain circumstances, confirmation by portable RCA should be undertaken before the conventional clinical tests are performed. For example, a patient in this series was thought to be brain dead while under treatment for very high ICP. Had barbiturates and mechanical ventilation been discontinued in order to test for apnea and other brainstem reflexes, the infant would probably have succumbed to raised ICP. Treatment was continued because of the normal scan, and the infant survived. Holzman and co-workers (1983) describe a similar case. Because

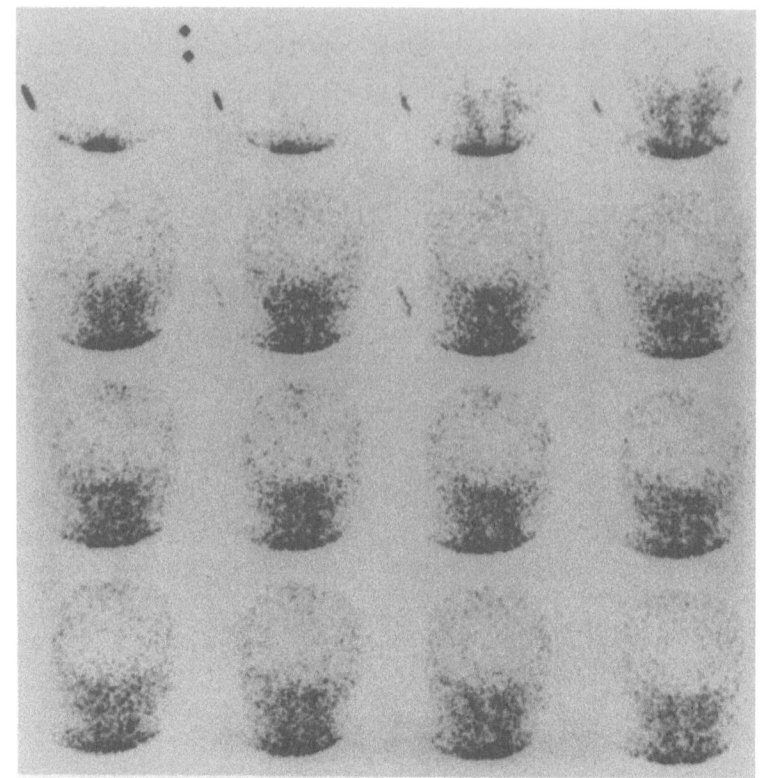

FIGURE 5. Scans consistent with brain death in another newborn. (a) Dynamic. (b) Static.

sedative drugs and metabolic abnormalities may cause reversible electrocerebral silence but do not influence the RCA (Goodman *et al.*, 1985; Holzman *et al.*, 1983; Nordlander *et al.*, 1973), we were comfortable in diagnosing brain death in nine infants in this series while they were receiving large doses of barbiturates.

Although our recent experience in newborns is limited, we would not hesitate to accept an RCA showing no arterial flow as confirmatory of brain death, as occurred in two patients in this series. In our earlier experience, we had encountered several premature infants with classic findings of brain death who had persistently normal flow studies. We attributed this phenomenon to the easily expandable premature skull. The EEG may also be misleading in such cases (Ashwal and Schneider, 1979), and the determination of brain death may have to be made on clinical grounds.

Unfortunately, autopsies were not performed in the three infants with SIDS who were resuscitated. All three had normal flow studies but met the generally accepted clinical and EEG criteria of brain death. These cases do not detract from the value of RCA in the determination of brain death because the error is on the side of continuing life support. However, these three cases were a surprise to us, because in our large 16 years of experience with older children and adults, we have never encountered a patient with clinical brain death who did not ultimately develop the characteristic lack of cerebral perfusion on sequential radionuclide scans.

Although a proponent of bolus radionuclide flow studies for the determination of brain death, Korein (1986) recently criticized radionuclide angiography with gamma camera imaging because

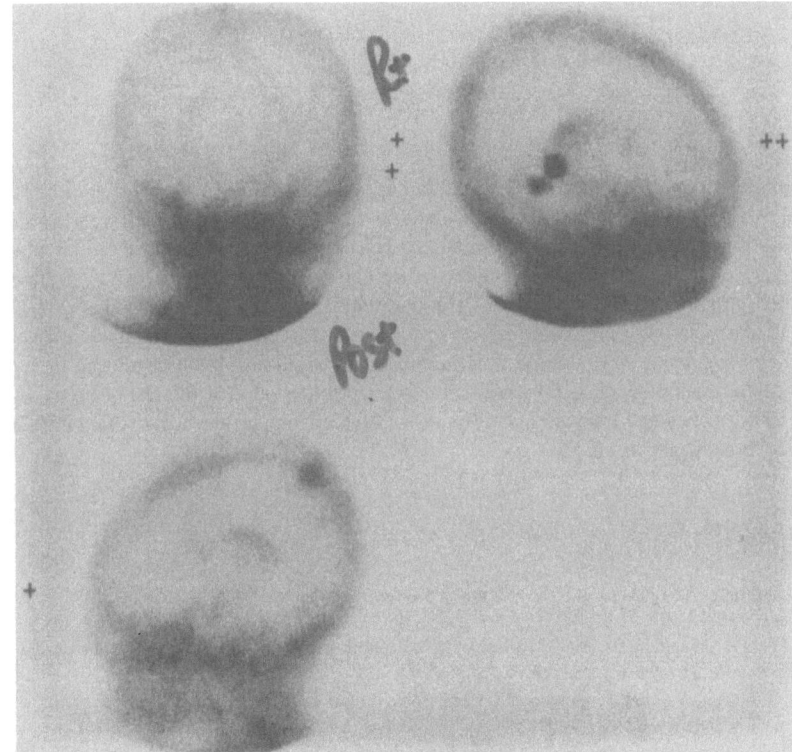

FIGURE 5. (*Continued*)

of the high radiation dose and the difficulty in interpreting the studies sometimes experienced by nuclear radiologists. In reality, the isotope dosage is the same as that used in an ordinary nuclear brain scan and is harmless. It is true that the significance of persistent venous sinus visualization in the absence of arterial circulation created confusion among some radiologists and frustration among clinicians. However, since the radiographic criteria for interpreting the scans have been more clearly defined (Goodman *et al.*, 1985; Schwartz *et al.*, 1984), the radionuclide image characteristic of brain death is quite simple to interpret and is rarely equivocal. We know of no other condition that has been reported to have a similar scan appearance (Mishkin, 1975).

While four-vessel cerebral angiography has been held as the standard against which other tests of blood flow in brain death should be judged (Lynn, 1983), we consider RCA a better test. Not only is it portable, safer in a potentially salvageable patient, less expensive, and well correlated with no flow on conventional angiography (Goodman *et al.*, 1985; Korein, 1986; Schwartz *et al.*, 1984), but the test uses the IV route for injection of radionuclide. In a recent pediatric case report (Fackler and Rogers, 1987), cerebral angiography showed extremely slow filling of the vessels near the base of the brain, while other tests, including bolus radionuclide angiography, were confirmatory of brain death. We speculate that the intracranial vessels filled as a result of the pressure head in the carotid arteries as the contrast was being injected. Much to the consternation of the attending physicians, that child was maintained on a ventilator for an unreasonable period of time. It is unlikely that such a dilemma would have occurred had RCA been used instead of conventional angiography.

6. SUMMARY

A single portable radionuclide cerebral angiogram in an infant suspected on clinical grounds of having brain death is diagnostic of that condition when there is unequivocal arrest of the carotid circulation at the base of the skull and failure to visualize the intracranial arterial circulation. We believe that further tests to confirm irreversibility and arbitrary waiting periods are unnecessary before life support can be discontinued. It is not necessary for levels of sedative drugs to return to normal. An occasional premature infant with brain death and young infants who have suffered anoxia may have persistently normal flow in the setting of clinical brain death, but the error is on the side of continuing support, thus not detracting from the value of the test. Almost one half of patients in this series had autopsies, the findings of which support the validity of the technique in diagnosing brain death in infants.

REFERENCES

Ad Hoc Committee on Brain Death, The Children's Hospital, Boston, 1987, Determination of brain death, *J. Pediatr.* **110**:15–19.

Ashwal, S., and Schneider, S., 1979, Failure of electroencephalography to diagnose brain death in comatose children, *Ann. Neurol.* **6**:512–517.

Drake, B., Ashwal, S., and Schneider, S., 1986, Determination of cerebral death in the pediatric intensive care unit, *Pediatrics* **78**:107–112.

Fackler, J. C., and Rogers, M. C., 1987, Is brain death really cessation of all intracranial function?, *J. Pediatr.* **110**:84–86.

Goodman, J. M., and Heck, L. L., 1977, Confirmation of brain death at bedside by isotope angiography, *JAMA* **238**:966–968.

Goodman, J. M., Mishkin, F. S., and Dyken, M., 1969, Determination of brain death by isotope angiography, *JAMA* **209**:1869–1897.

Goodman, J. M., and Heck, L. L., and Moore, B. D., 1985, Confirmation of brain death with portable isotope angiography: A review of 204 consecutive cases, *Neurosurgery* **16**:492–497.

Holzman, B. H., Curless, R. G., Sfakianakis, G. N., Ajmone-Marsan, C., and Montes, J. E., 1983, Radionuclide cerebral perfusion scintigraphy in determination of brain death in children, *Neurology (NY)* **33**:1027–1031.

Korein, J., 1986, Brain states: Death, vegetation, and life, in: *Anesthesia and Neurosurgery* (J. E. Cottrell and H. Turndorf, eds), pp. 293–351, CV Mosby, St. Louis.

Leestma, J. E., Hughes, J. R., and Diamond, E. R., 1984, Temporal correlates in brain death. EEG and clinical relationships to the respirator brain, *Arch. Neurol.* **41**:147–152.

Lynn, J., 1983, Diagnosis of brain death. (Letter.) *JAMA* **250**:612.

Mishkin, F., 1975, Determination of cerebral death by radionuclide angiography, *Radiology* **115**:135–137.

Nordlander, S., Wiklund, P. E., and Asard, P. E., 1973, Cerebral angioscintigraphy in brain death and in coma due to drug intoxication, *J. Nucl. Med.* **14**:856–857.

Report of the Medical consultants on the Diagnosis of Death to the President's Commission for the Study of Ethical Problems in Medicine and Behavioral Research, 1981, Guidelines for the determination of death, *JAMA* **246**:2184–2186.

Schwartz, J. A., Baxter, J., Brill, D. and Burns, J. R., 1983, Radionuclide cerebral imaging confirming brain death, *JAMA* **249**:246–247.

Schwartz, J. A., Baxter, J., and Brill, D. R., 1984, Diagnosis of brain death in children by radionuclide cerebral imaging, *Pediatrics* **73**:14–18.

Tsai, S. H., Cranford, R. E., Rockswold, G. L., and Koehler, S., 1982, Cerebral radionuclide angiography. Its application in the diagnosis of brain death, *JAMA* **248**:591–592.

16

Detection of Blood Flow to the Brain by Radionuclide Cerebral Imaging

Jan Arthur Schwartz, David Brill, and John Baxter

1. INTRODUCTION

The Guidelines for the Determination of Death provide two separate diagnostic pathways, the clinical pathway and the irreversible ischemic pathway, by which diagnosis of clinically suspected brain death may be confirmed (President's Commission for the Study of Ethical Problems in Medicine and Biomedical and Behavioral Research, 1981).

2. THE CLINICAL PATHWAY

The clinical pathway is the diagnostic tract by which a stabilized patient (normothermic, normotensive, and nonintoxicated) with suspected brain death is evaluated by serial neurological examination over a period of time. A subsequent laboratory study, usually electroencephalogram (EEG) or radionuclide cerebral imaging (RCI) scan, is generally used to confirm the clinical findings.

The primarily clinical pathway is the most commonly utilized sequence of testing for brain death diagnosis in children. A recent statement by the American Neurological Society and the American Academy of Pediatrics supports practice wherein the diagnosis of brain death is adequately secured primarily by clinical examination (Report of the Special Task Force, 1987.)

In our experience, the strictly or primarily clinical diagnosis of brain death in the pediatric intensive care unit (PICU) is frequently fraught with confounding factors *(vide infra)* and may be unduly prolonged. The difficulty in brain death determination by strictly clinical diagnosis is best illustrated by the case of trauma victims. For these patients, proper clinical examination requires the withdrawal of life-sustaining therapies specific to brain support. Apnea testing, for example,

JAN ARTHUR SCHWARTZ • Departments of Anesthesiology and Pediatrics, Geisinger Clinic, Geisinger Medical Center, Danville, Pennsylvania 17822. DAVID BRILL • Department of Nuclear Imaging, Division of Radiology, Geisinger Clinic, Geisinger Medical Center, Danville, Pennsylvania 17822. JOHN BAXTER • Department of Special Procedures, Division of Radiology, Geisinger Clinic, Geisinger Medical Center, Danville, Pennsylvania 17822.

is begun by the acute elevation of $Paco_2$ to levels that are known to increase cerebral blood flow (CBF) and intracranial hypertension and thereby adversely affect the cerebral perfusion, and outcome of a brain-injured patient (Jastremski et al., 1978). Discontinuing critical support, including pharmacological therapies that ablate neurological responses (i.e., barbiturates and neuromuscular relaxants) before any objective assessment of their effectiveness seems to be unnecessarily hazardous if alternative diagnostic techniques are available. If the therapies are life-sustaining, why discontinue them at a time when the potential of a hoped-for survival is most uncertain?

From a practical standpoint, the neurological assessment of young children, particularly newborns, for determination of irreversible cessation of brain function can be unreliable (Volpe, 1987). Survival of children has been reported after demonstration of clinical brain stem failure or with isoelectric EEGs (Monte and Conn, 1980; Pasternak and Volpe, 1979). Similarly, EEG artifact may obscure the diagnosis of brain death in children who by all other neurological criteria, including subsequent postmortem examination, have died (Ashwal and Schneider 1979). While these were children under 2–6 months of age, the reports illustrate the desirability of a more generally accurate prediction of patient outcome before any therapeutic withdrawal is considered.

3.   THE IRREVERSIBLE ISCHEMIC PATHWAY

The irreversible ischemic pathway of brain death diagnosis involves the radiological determination of cessation of blood flow to the brain of a patient whose body temperature exceeds 32.2°C (President's Commission, 1981).

3.1.   Cerebral Arteriography

Irreversible brain ischemia classically has been demonstrated by four-vessel carotid and vertebral arteriography. In this situation, the laboratory study is diagnostic rather than confirmatory; i.e., the test result is by itself sufficient to render a diagnosis. Blood-flow studies indicating no blood flow to the brain provide the clinician with specific and irrefutable information about the prognosis for patient survival. Distinguished from the clinical examination and EEG, whose results are affected by a variety of drugs and peculiar clinical circumstances (Power, 1976), the evaluation of CBF by arteriogram is not obscured by other clinical therapies or medical conditions.

Dye-contrast arteriography is the radiologic test classically accepted as sufficient for brain-death diagnosis. The test itself, i.e., vessel cannulation and dye injection, appears to be safe vis-à-vis the injured brain (Mani, 1977). Circumstances surrounding the performance of the test, however, are frequently undesirable for the critically injured patient. Performance of the study requires that the patient be transported from an intensive care area to the radiology laboratory. Indeck et al. (1987) recently reported a 63% incidence of morbidity during intrahospital transport of patients from critical care areas for laboratory studies and clinical therapies.

Arterial desaturation and hypotension occurred commonly during transport. It is not possible to study a patient maintaining the head in an elevated mid-position. Insofar as management of position, ventilation, and blood pressure represents the mainstay of brain-oriented intensive-care therapy, the use of an alternative radiological diagnostic test to detect CBF, that can be used at the bedside, is particularly desirable.

3.2.   Radionuclide Cerebral Imaging

Radionuclide cerebral imaging (RCI) has been employed in the confirmation of brain death diagnosis for nearly twenty years (Goodman et al., 1969; Goodman and Heck, 1977, 1985). The study is portable and can be perfomred in the ICU. Radionuclide is injected intravenously. A gamma scanner at the bedside provides images (Fig. 1) as the material passes through the common

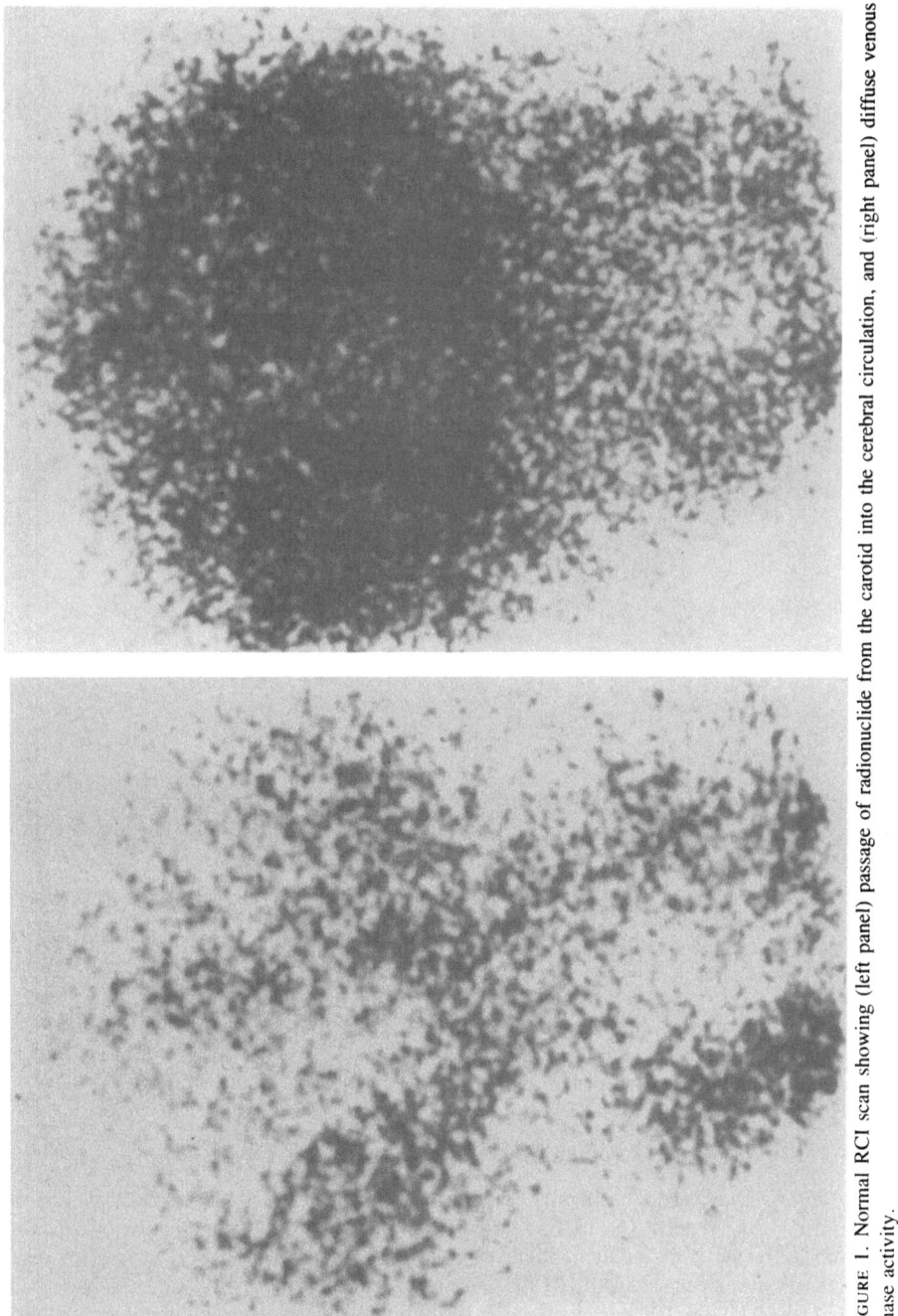

FIGURE 1. Normal RCI scan showing (left panel) passage of radionuclide from the carotid into the cerebral circulation, and (right panel) diffuse venous phase activity.

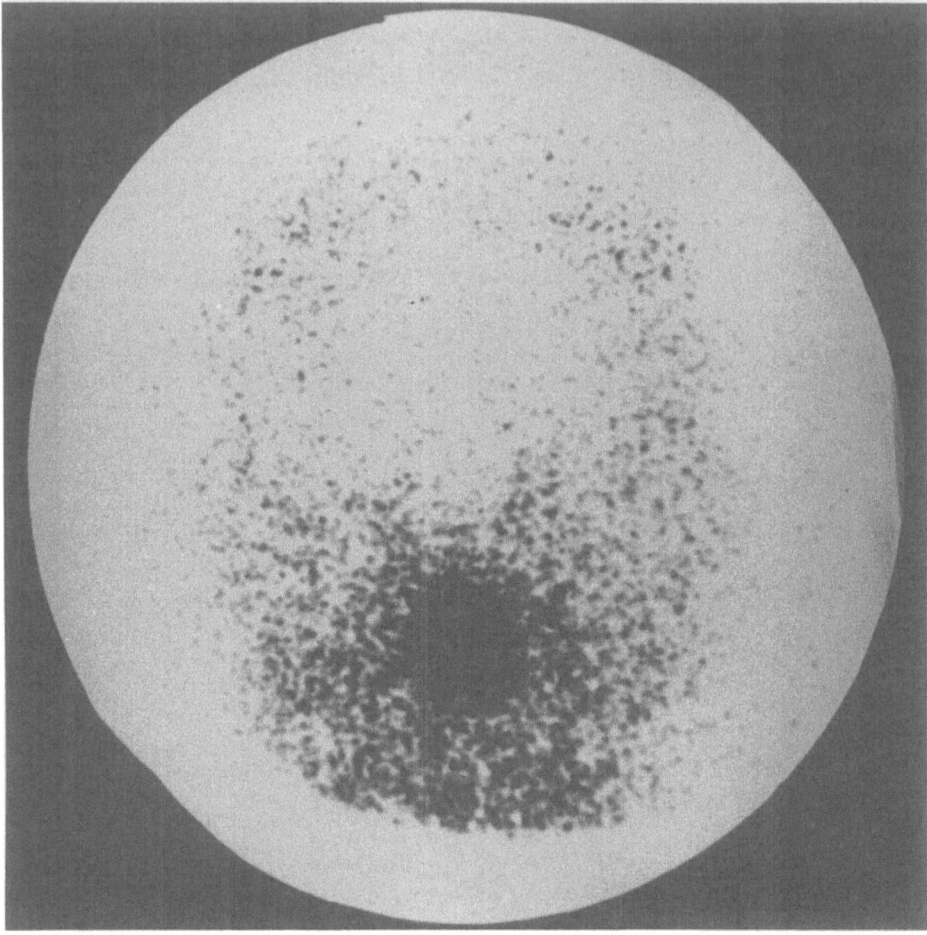

FIGURE 2. Abnormal static phase RCI scan. No radionuclide material is detected within the intracranial vault. The central "hot point" reflects circulation to the patient's nose, which serves to confirm the entrance of radionuclide up the level of the common carotid artery.

carotid arteries and into the central cerebral circulation; and within 10–20 min after the injection, diffuse activity is seen throughout a perfused brain. Failure to detect activity within the arterial system of the brain (Fig. 2) is consistent with a clinical examination demonstrating brain death.

3.2.1. RCI in the General Patient Population

The RCI scan has been a commonly used diagnostic tool for a variety of neurological problems. A false-negative result (no CBF detected in a patient with clear alternative evidence of blood flow) has never been reported. More than 40,000 patients with clinical syndromes other than brain death have been studied by RCI at Geisinger Medical Center in Danville, Pennsylvania, and Methodist Hospital in Indianapolis since 1970. In this very large population of neurologically impaired but functioning patients, the pattern of no CBF seen in brain death has never been identified.

3.2.2. RCI in Patients with Clinically Suspected Brain Death

We have reported 100% correlation between the demonstration of no CBF by RCI and by four-vessel contrast arteriography in both adults and children (Schwartz *et al.*, 1983, 1984). In our population, all patients with no CBF demonstrated by arteriography demonstrated no cerebral arterial filling by RCI. The RCI scans of nearly 25% of these patients, however, demonstrated some persistent nuclear uptake into the sagittal or other venous sinus (Fig. 3) after 20 min. Goodman *et al.*, (1985) confirmed these findings. They have further observed that the isolated identification of static venous activity on RCI scan in the absence of demonstrable arterial structures is inevitably followed by failure to identify any intracranial vascular structures (arterial or venous) during subsequent RCI.

The source of the venous sinus activity appears to be through the normal route of blood flow into the head. In severely limited CBF states, the radionuclide passes without detection through the arterial system; over 15–30 min, it collects to detectable levels as it pools in a relatively static

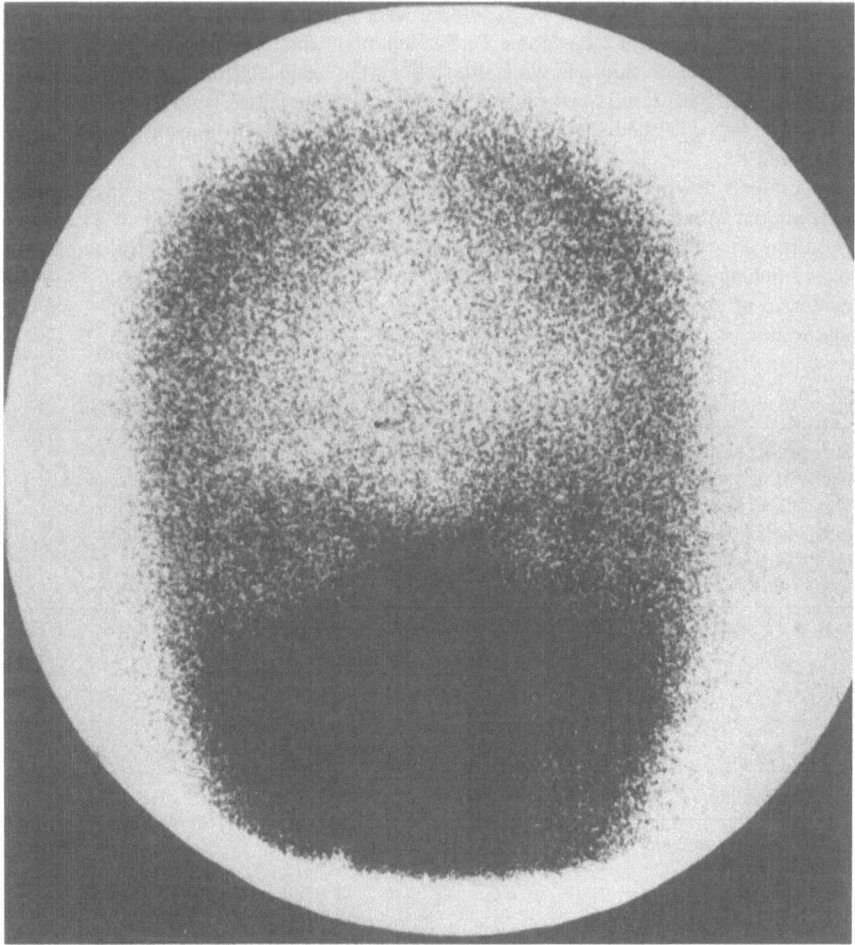

FIGURE 3. Abnormal static phase RCI scan. Radionuclide material is not diffusely distributed but detected only within venous sinuses.

venous system. Undetected arterial flow with venous pooling by RCI is entirely consistent with what we know about CBF in brain-dead patients. Xenon cerebral blood flow (XcCBF) measurement, a highly sensitive reearch method, has demonstrated severely diminished (11–16% of normal) but persistent CBF in brain-dead patients (Muizelaar and Obrist, 1985).

The observations of our groups would therefore support the view that the RCI scan is more sensitive than is arteriography for detection of CBF. Within the context of clinical brain-death diagnosis and demonstration of irreversible ischemia, the tests appear to be of equal specificity and sensitivity.

3.2.3. A National Collaborative Study

In 1982, the Departments of Anesthesiology, Nuclear Imaging and Special Procedures at the Geisinger Clinic initiated a study through the membership of the American College of Nuclear Physicians (ACNP) to review the national experience with RCI evaluation of patients with clinically suspected brain death. Individual contributors from the ACNP and the authors of publications that have previously evaluated RCI scanning were asked to review and verify RCI reports and specific aspects of patient data (Table I). Patients or institutions that were unable to obtain specifically retrieved scan results and clinical histories were excluded from our review. A total of 1172 complete RCI scan results and clinical histories were submitted from 34 institutions. We present here the first published summary of this collaborative effort. The results are summarized in Tables II and III.

Arterial blood flow to the head was undetectable in 856 scans. Venous filling, despite no detectable arterial flow, was noted in 117 of scans. Arteriography, obtained in 112 patients, always confirmed the RCI. No patient in whom arterial blood flow could not be detected survived. The isolated finding of static phase venous activity in 14% of patients did not affect the outcome when evaluated by subsequent RCI, four-vessel arteriography, or cardiovascular collapse prior to additional testing.

TABLE I.   RCI Scanning Confirming Clinically Suspected Brain Death[a]

1. Number of RCI scans performed for brain-death diagnosis
2. Number of RCI scans indicating conventional brain-death confirmation (no arterial or venous activity)
3. Number of RCI scans indicating no arterial flow but some residual venous activity
4. Number of RCI scans showing no-flow and/or venous phase activity only that were confirmed by four-vessel arteriography
5. Clinical history of any patients with no flow or venous activity only on RCI scan who survived

[a] A summary of the questionnaire distributed through the American College of Nuclear Physicians.

TABLE II.   Tabulated Review of RCI Undertaken in Patients with Clinically Suspected Brain Death[a]

Patient group	No flow	Ven act only	Artiograms
42 Newborns–2 mo	30	2	6
88 2 mo–19 yr	63	15	17
1042 Adults	646	101	99
1172 Scans	739	118	112

[a] No flow, no visualized cerebral arterial or venous sinus activity detected; Ven act only, venous phase activity seen after failure to detect any cerebral arterial filling.

TABLE III. Forty-two Neonates with Clinical
Brain Death: Tabulated Review of Pediatric RCI
Scan Results and Patient Survival Statistics

RCI scan result	Patients	Survivors
No flow	30	None
Ven act only	2	None
Normal	10	5

Pediatric Experience. A total of 130 children under 19 years of age, including 42 newborn infants under 2 months of age were reviewed. Most children (83/130) studied with RCI were additionally evaluated by either four-vessel arteriography (23/130) and/or by EEG (60/130). In nearly all cases, children diagnosed with brain death underwent postmortem examination. The diagnosis was confirmed pathologically in all instances.

The experiences with CBF studies in the neonatal group were particularly interesting (Table III). As in the adult group, all patients with no detected (arterial) CBF died. However, normal CBF by RCI was detected in five neonatal patients with clinical brain death confirmed by EEG, clinical examination, and postmortem examination. The unusual finding of normal CBF was confirmed by arteriography in two patients.

4. SUMMARY

The use of portable RCI studies for brain-death diagnosis provides the practitioner with a safe and accurate prediction of outcome. Therapy critical to brain support need not be discontinued during the diagnostic evaluation, and the patient need not be transported away from the controlled ICU environment. By comparison with conventional arteriography, RCI appears to be a more sensitive detector of CBF. Incorrect identification of brain death by RCI is unknown.

Brain death diagnosed by a no-flow RCI is very clear, but CBF appears to be better maintained in some brain-dead newborn infants than in older patients. The clinically brain-dead neonate may have detectable CBF. In this group, comprehensive clinical examination and occasionally multiple diagnostic laboratory studies may be necessary to confirm the clinical impression.

REFERENCES

Ashwal, S., and Schneider, S, 1979, Failure of electroencephalography to diagnose brain death in comatose children, *Ann. Neurol.* **6:**512–517.

Goodman, J. M., and Heck, L. L., 1977, Confirmation of brain death at the bedside by isotope angiography, *JAMA* **238:**966–968.

Goodman, J. M., Mishkin, F., and Dyken, M., 1969, Determination of brain death by isotope angiography, *JAMA* **209:**1869–1872.

Goodman, J. M., Heck, L. L., and Moore, B. D., 1985, Confirmation of brain death with portable isotope angiography: A review of 204 consecutive cases, *Neurosurgery* **16:**492–497.

Indeck, M., Peterson, S., and Brotman, S., 1987, Risk, cost, and benefit of transporting patients from the ICU for special studies, *Crit. Care Med.* **15:**350.

Jastremski, M., Powner, D., Snyder, J., Smith, J., and Grevnik, A., 1978, Problems in brain death determination. *Forensic Sci.* **11:**201–212.

Mani, R. L., 1977, Angiography of cerebrovascular occlusive disease: Current concepts, in: *Diagnostic Ra-diology 1977* (A. R. Margulis and C. A. Gooding, eds.), pp. 741–760, CV Mosby, St. Louis.

Montes, J. E., and Conn, A. W., 1980, Near-drowning: An unusual case, *Can. Anaesth. Soc. J.* **27:**172–174.

Muizelaar, J. P., and Obrist, W. D., 1985, Cerebral blood flow and brain metabolism with brain injury, in: *Central Nervous System Trauma Status Report* (D. P. Becker and J. T. Povlishock, eds.), pp. 123–137, William Byrd Press, Richmond, Virginia.

Pasternak, J. F., and Volpe, J. J., 1979, Full recovery from prolonged brainstem failure following intraventricular hemorrhage. *J. Pediatr.* **95:**1046–1049.

Powner, D. J., 1976, Drug-associated isoelectric EEGs, a hazard in brain-death certification, *JAMA* **236:**1123.

Report of the Medical Consultants on the Diagnosis of Death for the President's Commission for the Study of Ethical Problems in Medicine and Biomedical and Behavioral Research: Guidelines for the Determination of Death, 1981, *JAMA* **246:**2184–2186.

Report of the Special Task Force, 1987, Guidelines for the Determination of Brain Death in Children, *Pediatrics* **80:**298–299.

Schwartz, J. A., Baxter, J., and Brill, D. R., 1984, Diagnosis of brain death in children by radionuclide cerebral imaging, *Pediatrics* **73:**14–18.

Schwartz, J. A., Baxter, J., Brill, D. R. and Burns, J. R., 1983, Radionuclide cerebral imaging confirming brain death, *JAMA* **249:**246–247.

Volpe, J. J., 1987, Brain death determination in newborn, *Pediatrics* **80:**293–297.

17

THE EEG IN THE DETERMINATION OF BRAIN DEATH IN PEDIATRIC PATIENTS
The NIH Study

DONALD R. BENNETT

1. INTRODUCTION

The National Institute of Health Collaborative Study of Cerebral Survival (CS) remains the largest prospective study on the outcome of patients with cerebral unresponsivity and apnea. One purpose of this investigation was to formulate a set of criteria that would identify a dead brain in an otherwise living body. Although patients under 1 year of age were excluded and only 43 of the 503 patients enrolled were between the ages of 1 and 9 years, the electroencephalographic (EEG) results of this study are relevant to the pediatric brain-death issue. Therefore, the EEG experiences and findings are reviewed and correlated with clinical data as well as with other investigations. Where potential problems or differences in the pediatric age group are seen, they are so commented on. Since the CS report was published, it has been criticized, and some of the criticisms are justified, particularly the working definition of apnea. However, the CS study serves as a prototype for future investigations.

Since Fishgold and Mathis (1959) reported that scalp recordings in patients in "coma dé-passé" (Mollaret and Goulon, 1959) showed absence of demonstrable EEG potentials, the role of EEG in confirming the brain-dead state has been the subject of heated debates, oral as well as written (Mollaret and Goulon, 1959). In the United States, many still favor its use; however, in the United Kingdom, it is considered nonessential.

The key issues in the controversy are the sensitivity and specificity of the EEG diagnosis of electrocerebral inactivity (ECI), previously called electrocerebral silence (ECS), in the determination of brain death (entire brain, including brainstem). These terms have been defined, and the technical guidelines for recording this abnormality have been published by the American EEG

DONALD R. BENNETT • Department of Neurology, University of Nebraska College of Medicine, Omaha, Nebraska 68105; Department of Neurology, Creighton University School of Medicine, Omaha, Nebraska 68105-1065.

Society (Minimal Technical Standards, 1986) and the International Federation of Societies for Electroencephalography and Clinical Neurophysiology (1977).

Electrocerebral inactivity indicates a marked disturbance of cortical and subcortical neuronal electrical generators. It does not indicate that all cells in the cortex and subcortical structures are nonfunctioning, nor does it imply irreversibility. It is not disease specific. Although measuring primarily the cerebral hemisphere and some subcortical electrical activity, it has a high degree of correlation with the severity of total brain dysfunction. However, the EEG, considered in isolation, can not diagnose brain death. It is only one part of the diagnostic criteria, the most important being the determination of the cause of coma to ensure the absence of remedial or reversible conditions. The guidelines for the Determination of Brain Death in Children (1987) emphasize that "most difficulties with the determination of death on the basis of neurological criteria have resulted from overlooking this basic fact" and also that the physical examination is necessary to determine the failure of brain function.

2. LIMITATIONS OF THE EEG

2.1. Technical

There are no published technical guidelines for the recording of ECI in the pediatric age group, particularly the very young. In the 1980 American EEG guidelines for the EEG recording and Suspected Cerebral Death, mention is made that since the National Institutes of Health (NIH) study did not include children, "comparable data on which to base recommendations for this young age group do not exist."   To date, this society has not recommended guidelines for the pediatric patient. I would suspect that a lack of uniformity exists between EEG laboratories in selecting the montages for determining ECI in children. There are several potential EEG problems, particularly in the young infant (prematures are excluded in this discussion).

The first is ensuring that the interelectrode distance is ≥ 10 cm. Because of the infant's head size, this may not always be possible to achieve in all derivations. If not, does an interelectrode distance, for example, of 8 cm versus 10 cm make that much difference? Additional potential problems with interelectrode distances and symmetry of the derivations, particularly in the newborn, are skull molding, cephalohematomas, various bony defects, other craniospinal anomalies, as well as congenital malformations of the brain such as hydranencephaly and microcephaly. However, the presence of these conditions should be known by the electroencephalographer before he or she interprets the tracing. The duration of recording needs to be determined. The American EEG guidelines for suspected cerebral death require at least 30 min duration of ECI. Whether this period should apply to children, particularly young infants, has not been established; however, the author believes that a period of 30 min is sufficient, although others recommend 1 hr (Moshe and Alvarez, 1986). It is crucial that the American EEG Society as well as the Internal Federation develop guidelines for the technical standards in recording ECI in children, particularly young infants.

The second difficulty has to do with artifacts. In the CS study, 5.2% of the 2256 EEGs were classified as unsatisfactory, although in some cases, the electroencephalographer could definitely state that brain waves were present (Bennett et al., 1976). The major technical problems were artifacts. In 23% of the recordings, special efforts were required to correct them. The major sources of artifact were muscle, electrocardiogram (ECG), and movement, particularly respirator artifact. As both the technicians and electroencephalographers gained experience, particularly with the use of Pancumonium bromide in abolishing scalp muscle activity, the incidence of unsatisfactory records decreased toward the end of the study. The author would suspect that EEG artifacts will also be troublesome in the pediatric age group, particularly in the newborn as well as young infants. Additional channels will be required other than the two recommended by the American EEG Society to monitor extracerebral potentials such as those from eye movements, submental muscle activity, respirator artifacts, and body movements.

The third difficulty is that pediatric electroencephalography perhaps requires more technical and interpretive expertise than does the adult EEG. Chatrian (1986) estimated that of the 5500 employed EEG technicians, only about 26% were certified by the American Board of Registration for Electroencephalographic Technicians in 1984. Even for those certified, sufficient contact with pediatric patients, particularly in busy newborn or pediatric intensive care units (ICUs), may be limited. Thus, the test should only be used in those hospitals in which expertise is available. No one would take issue with the statement by Pampiglione et al. (1978) that "no EEG investigation at all is better than unreliable and misleading services."

2.2. Reader Concordance

In the CS study, 303 of the 2250 EEGs were selected by the project coordinator for review by a panel of expert electroencephalographers (Bennett, 1978). These records were selected at random because the project coordinator disagreed with the interpretation, or because he found the records to be interesting. The overall agreement rate was only 78%. For records interpreted as ECS by the center electroencephalographer, the concurrence was 86%; for those called equivocal, 67%; and for those showing brain activity, 82%. However, the project coordinator estimated that if all the records had been reviewed, the percentage concurrence would be approximately 98%. This concordance rate should also be the same in pediatric brain death suspects, provided proper expertise is available. In this regard, Chatrian (1986) also noted that the number of physicians certified by the American Board of Qualification for Electroencephalography, mostly neurologists, was only 533 in 1984.

3. ECI–CLINICAL CORRELATIONS

3.1. Etiology

In the CS study, approximately 55% of the primary causes for the unresponsive and apneic state were intracranial insults secondary to cerebrovascular disease, particularly hemorrhage and brain trauma. Of the systemic causes, cardio and/or respiratory arrest was by far the leading cause. Primary intracranial insults accounted for approximately 75% of the initial EEGs diagnosed as showing ECS (Bennett, 1978). From a review of selected papers on pediatric brain death in children (i.e., Furgivele et al., 1984; Holzman et al., 1983; Schwartz et al., 1983; Rowland et al., 1983; Drake et al., 1986), particularly in newborns and young infants, it appears that systemic causes, such as neonatal asphyxia, near sudden infant death syndrome (SIDS), septicemia, metabolic derangements, and Reye syndrome, are the major causes for the suspected brain-death state. It was the patients with systemic causes for unresponsivity and apnea who were the most troublesome, both clinically and electroencephalographically, in the CS study. It was because of this uncertainty that the Presidential Commission recommended that with anoxic injury, an observation period of 24 hr is generally desirable (Presidential Commission Guidelines for the Determination of Death, 1981). In the Guidelines for the Determination of Brain Death in Children (1981), observation periods were extended in the young age group.

3.2. Vital Signs

In the Presidential Commission Guidelines for the Determination of Brain Death (1981), hypothermia and shock were two of the complicating conditions requiring correction before a diagnosis of brain death could be made. For hypothermia, a core temperature below 32.2°C was used. This figure is purely arbitrary. The core temperature that will result in an ECS record is not known. Prior (1973) mentioned that ECI will probably not occur until the core temperature is below 20°C. Knowing the temperature that will cause ECS is important, particularly in infants whose thermal systems are not well regulated and in patients unresponsive secondary to cold water drownings. The same applies to blood pressure values for hypotension and ECI.

3.3. Apnea

The criteria for determining apnea in the CS study has been replaced by more objective tests. Therefore, it is not scientifically correct to compare the data from the CS study with those for the pediatric age group. However, I would suspect that with the tests used today, there would be a high degree of correlation with ECI.

3.4. Unresponsivity

All patients in the CS study with ECS were unresponsive. There are rare case reports of patients who awaken from coma, although they are apparently unaware of their surroundings and do not behave in a purposeful manner (neocortical death or apallic syndrome). In this state, the EEG may show ECI. This results from the cerebral insult producing primary and subcortical damage with relative preservation of brainstem function. This syndrome has been reported in infants. Of interest is the report of Pollack and Kelleway (1978). In three infants, two of whom had unremitting ECI and the third only a late return of equivocal electrocerebral activity, they noted that all three infants cried and grimaced. They invariably became quiet when held and comforted, although their cries showed a relative lack of modulation and variability. These infants were generally loud and vigorous. Pollack and Kelleway (1978) "believe that their apparent interaction with their environment was also subcortical in origin."

In the Guidelines for the Determination of Death (1981), it was written but not referenced, that "the brains of infants and young children have increased resistance to damage and may recover substantial functions even after exhibiting unresponsiveness on neurological examination for longer periods compared with adults." That this is so has not been confirmed by clinical or basic research investigations. If this assumed plasticity is correct, it is possible that the apallic syndrome may be more common in infants and young children than in adults. This is perhaps suggested by the recent report by Coulter (1987).

3.5. Brainstem Reflexes

In the CS study, 187 patients showed ECI in their initial EEG. In 144 of these patients, 10 cephalic reflexes were tested and were found to be absent (Bennett, 1978). A pupillary reflex was present in three patients, a corneal in one, and an oculocephalic and oculovestibular in one each. In the remaining patients, all 10 reflexes were not tested for various reasons, some of these legitimate, such as traumatic injuries about the head and face; 7% of the 5030 reflexes (503 patients × 10 reflexes) were not tested. Either the pupillary, corneal, oculocephalic, vestibular, and pharyngeal reflexes, which physicians would ordinarily test, were not examined in 56 patients. Interobserver agreement on the neurological examination was not evaluated in the CS study. To have all neurologists and neurosurgeons agree on the presence or absence of a neurological sign would be a happening. In investigating interobserver assessment and agreement of ocular signs of coma, Van Den Berge et al. (1979) found the assessment of the pupil reaction to light as well as the quality of pupils "to be satisfactory" but more disagreement on assessing spontaneous eye movements and oculocephalic reflexes. The author would suspect that the agreement on signs in infants would be even more difficult. Certainly, the examination has to be performed by a physician qualified in this field. As Fletcher (1982) stated, "most of us assume, that, except in occasional borderline cases, the signs we observe are present and those we do not observe are absent." Thus, if one accepts the concept of brain death as cessation of all functions of the brain including the brainstem, the EEG serves as a useful safeguard, since ECI shows a high degree of correlation with the absence of brainstem reflexes. Also noteworthy in the CS study is that in the 303 cases whose initial EEGs showed definite brain waves, 137 patients had all 10 cephalic absent. Thus, the absence of brainstem reflexes has little correlation with ECI, whereas the reverse is true.

3.6. Morbidity and Mortality

In the CS study, only two patients with ECI survived both drug intoxications. That sedatives and hypnotics can cause reversible ECS has been known for some time. Since barbiturates are used perhaps more in pediatrics than in adult patients in the management of increased intracranial pressure as well as in the treatment of status epilepticus, the question is: What should the blood level be before an ECI recording can be considered totally related to the primary neurological insult and not secondary to a medication? Stated another way: Can hypnotic or sedative drugs in therapeutic or subtherapeutic blood concentrations produce ECI in a patient with an already damaged brain? There are no answers. Because of this uncertainty, a declaration of brain death cannot be made until the drugs are undetectable in the blood or until blood flow studies are performed.

3.7. Imminent Death

Of the 187 patients whose initial EEG showed ECS, 75 were declared brain dead, and resuscitation was discontinued. With the exception of the two survivors, 79% of the other patients suffered cardiac standstill within 24 hr of the first ECS record. One patient survived 144 hr before somatic death. Of the 241 patients with definitive brain waves on the initial EEG, 48 recovered sufficiently to be discharged from the study. The remaining patients died, although the duration of life was more prolonged, in some cases up to 4 weeks. In a study of 94 consecutive patients at the University of Utah Medical Center (D. R. Bennett, unpublished data) (67 entered in the CS study) 36 patients showed ECI on their initial EEG examination. The mean time from entry until death of these patients, was 22 hours, with a range of 1 hr to 5 days. By contrast, 52 patients, 25 of whom survived, showed definite brain activity in all their EEGs. The mean time from entry for the 27 who died was 9 days, with a range of 1 hr to 39 days. Of 6 patients who showed initial activity in their EEGs and then subsequent ECI, all died. The mean time of entry until death was 58 hr, with a range of 27–96 hr. In the patients with definite ECI, 28% were declared brain dead, and resuscitative efforts were discontinued. In the remaining patients, somatic death occurred. Thus, in patients with nonremediable conditions, an ECI record has a high degree of prediction of imminent death. It has been suggested that infants and young children who satisfy the clinical and the EEG criteria for brain death survive longer before cardiac standstill. There is no definitive evidence to support this.

4. ECI–NEUROPATHOLOGICAL CORRELATIONS

The neuropathology concordance rate in the CS study was only 66% (Walker et al., 1975). In 48% of patients with records showing ECI showed the morphological changes of a respirator brain. In 9% of cases with respirator brain, biological activity was present in the last EEG, usually obtained within 6 hr of death. Approximately 12 to 36 hr is necessary for the development of the neuropathological findings of a respirator brain in the adult. Neuropathological studies correlating ECI in the pediatric age group, particularly the young infant, have not been performed.

5. ECI–CEREBRAL BLOOD FLOW STUDIES

This subject is addressed in Chapter 13, this volume. It would appear that although there is a very good correlation with the various techniques used to evaluate blood flow and ECS, occasional cases will show ECS with positive studies, although these are far from normal. The reasons for this are unclear at this time.

6. CONCLUSION

The EEG results of the CS study have been reviewed. Questions concerning the use of this data, both technical as well as clinical, in the diagnosis of brain death in children were raised. The answers await further investigation.

REFERENCES

An Appraisal of the Criteria of Cerebral Death, 1977, A Summary Statement. *JAMA,* **237:**982–986.
Bennett, D. R., 1978, The EEG in the determination of brain death, *Ann. NY Acad. Sci.* **315:**110–120.
Bennett, D. R., 1981, Brain death. (Letter.) *Lancet.* **1:**106.
Bennett, D. R., Hughes, J. R., Korein, J., Merlis, J. K., Suter, C., 1976, *Atlas of Electroencephalography in Coma and Cerebral Death,* Raven, New York.
Chatrian, G. E., 1986, Electrophysiologic evaluation of brain death: A critical appraisal, in: *Electrodiagnosis in Clinical Neurology,* M. J. Aminoff, (ed.), Underhill, Livingston, New York.
Coulter, D. L., 1987, Neurologic uncertainty in newborn intensive care, *N. Engl. J. Med.* **316:**840–844.
Drake, B., Ashwal, S., and Schneider, S., 1986, Determination of cerebral death in the pediatric intensive care unit, *Pediatrics* **78:**107–112.
Fishgold, H., and Mathis, P., 1959, Obnubilations, Comas et stupeurs. *Electroencephalogr. Clin. Neurophysiol. Suppl.* **11:**1–124.
Fletcher, C. M., 1982, The clinical diagnosis of pulmonary emphysema—An experimental study, *Proc. R. Soc. Med.* **45:**577–584.
Furgivele, T. L., Frank, M., Riegle, C., Wirth, F., and Earley, L. C., 1984, Prediction of cerebral death by cranial sector scan, *Crit. Care Med.* **12:**1–3.
Guidelines for the Determination of Brain Death in Children, 1987, *Neurology (NY)* **37:**1077–1078.
Guidelines for the Determination of Death, 1981, *JAMA* **246:**2184–2186.
Holzman, B. H., Curless, R. G., Sfakianakio, G. N., Ajmone-Marsan, C., and Montes, J. E., 1983, Radionuclide cerebral perfusion scintigraphy in determination of brain death in children, *Neurology (NY)* **33:**1027–1031.
The International Federation of Societies for Electroencephaloghraphy and Clinical Neurophysiology, 1983, EEG Instrumentation Standards, (rev. 1977). Report of the Committee on EEG Instrumentation Standards of the International Federation Societies for Electroencephalography and Clinical Neurophysiology, Elsevier, Amsterdam.
Minimum Technical Standards for EEG Recordings in Suspected Cerebral Death, 1986, *J. Clin. Neurophysiol.* **3:**144–149.
Mollaret, P., and Goulon, M., 1959, Le coma dépassé (mémoire préliminaire), *Rev. Neurol.* **101:**3–15.
Moshe, S. L., and Alvarez, L. A., 1986, Diagnosis of brain death in children, *Jo. Clin. Neurophysiol.* **3:**239–249.
Pallis, C., and MacGillivray, B., 1980, Brain death in the EEG. (Letter.) *Lancet* **2:**1085.

Pampiglione, G., Chaloner, J., Harden, A., and O'Brien, J., 1978, Transitory ischemia/anoxia in young children and the prediction of quality of survival, *Ann. NY Acad. Sci.* **315**:281–292.

Pollack, M. A., and Kelleway, P., 1978, Cortical death with preservation of brainstem function. Correlation of clinical, electrophysiologic and CT scan findings in 3 infants and 2 adults with prolonged survival, *Trans. Am. Neurol. Assoc.* **103**:36–38.

Prior, P. F., 1973, *The EEG in Acute Cerebral Anoxia,* Excerpta Medica. Amsterdam.

Rowland, T. W., Donnelly, J. H., Jackson, A. H., and Jamroz, S. B., 1983, Brain death in the pediatric intensive care unit, *Am. J. Dis. Child.* **137**:547–550.

Schwartz, J. A., Baxter, J., Brill, D., and Burns, J. R., 1983, Radionuclide cerebral imaging confirming brain death, *JAMA* **249**:246–247.

Television verdict on brain death. (Editorial.), 1980, *Lancet* **2**:841.

Van Den Berge, J. H., Schouten, H. J. A., Boomstra, S., Van Drunnen Little, S., and Braakman, R., 1979, Interobserver agreement in assessment of ocular signs in coma, *J. Neurol. Neurosurg. Psychiatry* **42**:1163–1168.

Walker, A. E., Diamond, E. L., and Moseley, J. I., 1975, The neuropathological findings in irreversible coma. A critique of the "respirator brain," *J. Neuropathol. Exp. Neurol.* **34**:296–323.

18

ROLE OF EEG IN BRAIN DEATH DETERMINATION IN CHILDREN
The Bronx Experience

SOLOMON L. MOSHÉ, LUIS A. ALVAREZ,
and BEVERLY A. DAVIDOFF

1. INTRODUCTION

The cessation of heartbeat and respiration has traditionally been considered the standard by which a person can be declared legally dead. The rapid expansion of medical technology has enhanced our ability to save life and at times to maintain cardiac and respiratory functions in patients that in the past would have failed. The technological progress led to the development of a new standard for the determination of death, namely the cessation of all brain functions (Harvard Medical School, 1968).

The concept of brain death as an indicator of the end of life arose from the notion that when the brain stops functioning irreversibly, somatic death, including cardiac death, will inevitably follow. This conclusion is supported by the findings of the National Collaborative Study (1977); 99% of patients who exhibited three basic factors denoting evidence of profound and total brain failure, i.e., (1) cerebral unresponsiveness, (2) apnea, and (3) electrocerebral silence (ECS) on the electroencephalogram (EEG), died. Over the years, the brain death standard has been accepted among medical and legal circles, as well as by laypersons, as a basis for establishing death (Beresford, 1984; Black, 1978a; Chatrian, 1980; Margolick, 1984; Setzer, 1985; Ventura and Mason, 1985; Vernon and Holtzman, 1986).

In 1980, the National Conference of Commissioners on Uniform State Laws adopted the Uniform Determination of Death Act (UDDA) adding the brain-death standard to the cardiac and respiratory standards (President's Commission, 1981). To date, 39 states and the District of Columbia have laws adopting the cessation of brain function as compatible with the end of life as

SOLOMON L. MOSHÉ • Departments of Neurology and Pediatrics, Albert Einstein College of Medicine and Montefiore Medical Center, Bronx, New York 10467.   LUIS A. ALVAREZ • Department of Neurology, Albert Einstein College of Medicine and Montefiore Medical Center, Bronx, New York 10467.   BEVERLY A. DAVIDOFF • Administration, Bronx Municipal Hospital, Bronx, New York 10461.

we currently know it. In six other states, the brain-death standard has been established by judicial decision (cited from the report of the New York State Task Force, 1986).

The acceptance of the UDDA is of great importance both medically and legally. It recognizes common standards that can be applied to every individual of either sex, irrespective of religious beliefs and age.

2. CRITERIA FOR THE DETERMINATION OF BRAIN DEATH IN CHILDREN

The guidelines proposed by the medical consultants on the diagnosis of death to the President's Commission (1981) included the recommendation that "physicians should be particularly cautious in applying neurological criteria to determine death in children younger than 5 years." This recommendation has been widely adopted by many institutions and is frequently included in hospital brain-death protocols. On certain occasions, very strict guidelines are added, such as those included in the brain-death protocol of one of the largest municipal hospital systems in the country, the Health and Hospital Corporation in New York City. These guidelines were prepared by Corporation staff in conjunction with an ad hoc committee of experts assembled for this purpose. The protocol reads as follows:

> For children under 3 years of age, it is strongly recommended that a time period of at least 72 hours elapse from the onset of the prerequisite condition to pronouncement of brain death. Three different brain function examinations should be performed. Confirmatory test of lack of cerebral circulation should be performed in all cases. Caution should be exercised in interpreting clinical condition of children and interpreting ancillary confirmatory tests, including EEGs.

It should be noted that in this protocol the cutoff age is 3 years.

We argued previously (Moshé and Alvarez, 1986) that it is unclear whether there exists a physiological basis to the argument that "the brains of infants and young children have increased resistance to damage and may recover substantial functions even after exhibiting unresponsiveness on neurological examination for longer periods compared with adults" proposed by the medical consultants to the President's Commission (1981) (see also Schwartz *et al.*, 1984). To date, there is no evidence that a child who has met the brain death criteria designated for adults (Table I) has survived (Moshé and Alvarez, 1986). The accuracy of the clinical examination can be enhanced by the use of appropriate confirmatory tests such as the EEG or cerebral blood flow (CBF) studies.

3. THE ROLE OF ELECTROENCEPHALOGRAPHY

The EEG is a portable test that does not require any invasive procedures and is readily available in most centers. Fischgold and Mathis (1959) first demonstrated that ECS in the EEG

TABLE I.   Clinical Criteria of Brain Death
for Adults

No spontaneous activity
No response to loud noise
No pupillary light reflexes
Absent oculocephalics and oculovestibular reflexes
Absent corneal and oropharyngeal reflexes
No cardiac response to eyeball compression
No decorticate or decerebrate posturing
No spontaneous respirations
Observation >6 hr

indicates absence of cerebral function. In this respect, the EEG contributes significantly to the clinical examination, which can correctly assess brainstem function but not necessarily cerebral function. Since an intact brainstem is necessary for the expression of cortical responses (Allen *et al.*, 1980), accurate evaluation of cortical function may not be accomplished solely by clinical examination in patients with significant brainstem dysfunction. This phenomenon was demonstrated in recent reports of patients with severe Guillain-Barré syndrome who appeared to be clinically brain dead but had EEGs showing electrocerebral activity (Drury *et al.*, 1985; Langedorf *et al.*, 1986). This is the reason why in addition to clinical demonstration of brain death, confirmation of absence of cerebral function by ancillary tests, principally by EEG and CBF studies, is required in most brain-death protocols worldwide (for review, see Walker, 1985).

3.1. EEG Recording

Electrocerebral silence, electrocerebral inactivity, flat EEG, isoelectric EEG, and equipotential EEG are synonymous terms (Bennett *et al.*, 1976; Chatrian, 1980; Walker, 1985) used to define the absolute absence of electrocerebral activity, which is the electrographic manifestation of cerebral death (Fig. 1). Because the technical aspects of the EEG recording are extremely important, the American EEG Society (AEEGS, 1979) has offered Minimal Technical Standards for EEG Recording in Suspected Cerebral Death, as did the International Federation of Societies for Electroencephalography and Clinical Neurophysiology (Chatrian, 1980; Walker, 1985). These recommendations, summarized in Table II, have been well accepted and are now used as standard in determination of ECS.

A typical montage used for the determination of ECS that satisfies the recommendations of AEEGS is depicted in Fig. 1. The application of the AEEGS guidelines to young infants raises an apparent contradiction. The significantly smaller head size in this age group makes it practically impossible to use the International 10–20 system and still apply the recommended interelectrode distances of 10 cm. However, in infants and children, the diminished thickness of the skull results in a much better conduction of EEG activity to surface electrodes, so that the wider interelectrode distances required in adults may not be necessary. It was recently proposed (Chapter 14, this volume) that in small infants the interelectrode distance should be decreased proportionally to the patient's head size.

The AEEGS has also recommended that the duration of the EEG recording should be at least 30 min. The consensus document evolved by pediatric neurologists (Chapter 14, this volume) espouses this recommendation for young infants, including premature and newborn babies. Since there are no data for this age group, we have advocated longer EEG recordings (1 hr) in the

TABLE II. EEG Guidelines for the Determination of Electrocerebral Silence[a]

A minimum of eight scalp disc electrodes
Interelectrode distances of 10 cm
Interelectrode impedances of 100–10,000 Ω
Sensitivity increased from 7.5 to 2 μV/mm
Time constant of 0.3–0.4 sec during part of the recording
Duration of recording at least 30 min
EMG monitor
ECG monitor
Each electrode touched separately to create an artifact potential and to confirm the integrity of the system
EEG tested for reactivity during the recording with auditory, visual, and painful stimuli
Recording made only by a qualified technologist

[a]Modified from the guidelines proposed by the AEEGS (1979).

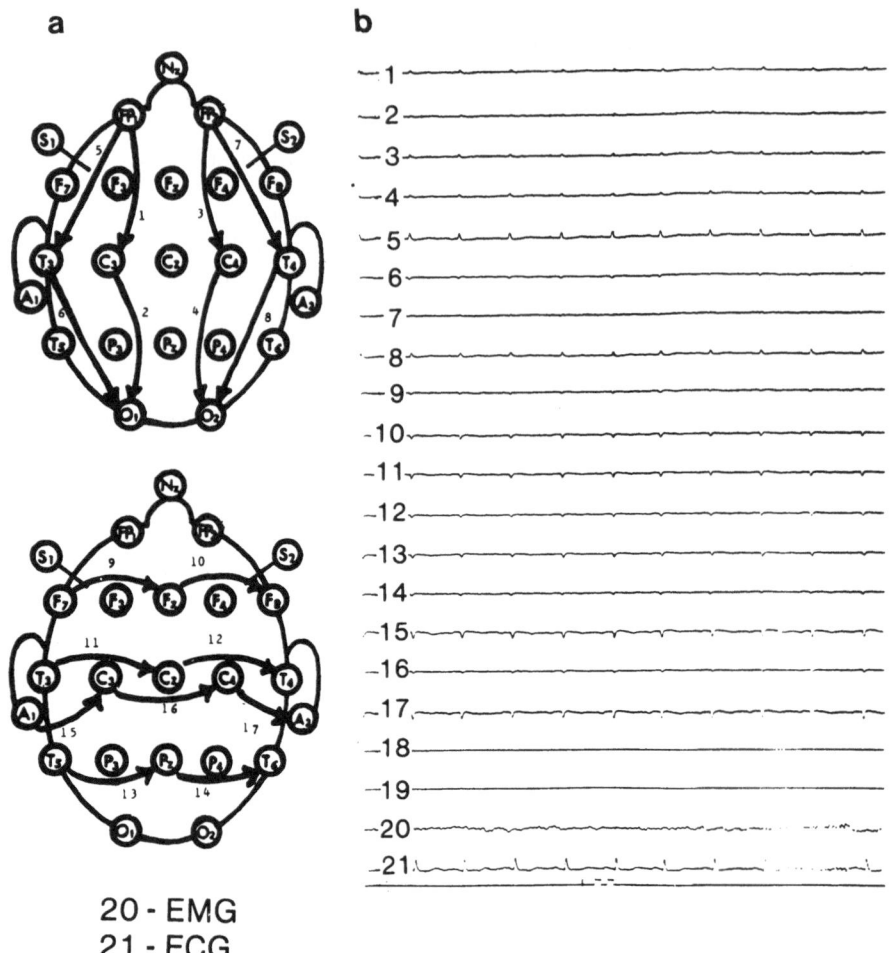

20 - EMG
21 - ECG

FIGURE 1. (a) Representative EEG montage that can be used for the recording of ECS. This montage was designed according to the guidelines suggested by the AEEGS. (b) EEG recording exhibiting ECS. Sensitivity 2μV/mm except for ECG, 75 μV/mm; low linear frequency filter 0.3 Hz.

newborn period (Moshé and Alvarez, 1986; Alvarez *et al.*, 1988); 1-hr recordings are routinely obtained in babies in order to establish the lack of EEG cycling (Tharp, 1980).

3.2. Causes of Electrocerebral Silence

The guidelines for determination of brain death require the exclusion of conditions that may mimic brain death. A similar statement is applicable to the interpretation of ECS. Several conditions can produce reversible ECS (Table III) and, in fact, these constitute the major and probably only limitations of the EEG as an ancillary test in the determination of cerebral death.

The most frequent cause of reversible ECS is overdose with a central nervous system (CNS) depressant, whether accidental or iatrogenic (Bennett, 1980; Powner, 1976; Walker, 1985). Other causes include hypothermia (Arfel and Weiss, 1962; Reilly *et al.*, 1974) and cardiovascular shock

TABLE III. Conditions Capable of Producing Reversible
Electrocerebral Silence

Intoxication	Cardiovascular shock
Sedatives	Hypothermia
Barbiturates	Metabolic states[a]
Benzodiazepines	Hepatic encephalopathy
Meprobramate	Hyperosmolar coma
Mecloqualone	Preterminal uremia
Methaqualone	Severe electrolyte imbalance
Trichloroethylene	Acid–base imbalance
Other	
Anesthesia	

[a]The role of these conditions as primary causative agents of ECS has not been clearly established.

(Jørgensen, 1974). The suppressive effect of all EEG activities by both hypothermia and hypotension resulted in the recommendation that a minimal body temperature of 37°C and minimal arterial blood pressure of 80 mm Hg be required for the accurate interpretation of ECS (President's Commission, 1981; Walker, 1985). Some metabolic/toxic states have also been implicated in the reversible suppression of EEG activities (Bennett, 1980; Plum and Posner, 1980). However, their role as primary causative agents has not been established (Chatrian, 1980). Transient ECS, usually lasting 2–3 hr, can also be found immediately after a major cerebral accident, especially if it produces significant hypoxia and hypotension (Chatrian, 1980; Jørgensen, 1974).

3.3. Interpretation of ECS in Children with Probable Brain Death

The guidelines of the AEEGS (1979) included a warning that the significance of ECS in infants and children under 3 years of age is not clearly established. Similar warnings, but with a cutoff age of 1 year, are also given by the International Federation guidelines (Walker, 1985).

A detailed review of the literature indicates that there are very few studies exploring the role of EEG in the diagnosis of brain death in the young. There were 43 children (8.5%) among the 503 patients who comprised the population of the American National Collaborative Study (Walker, 1985). At the time of the original publication, the authors of the report did not separate in their analysis this group as deviant from any other age group. However, they do not offer a breakdown of the ages of the children within the first decade. Furthermore, it is unclear how many children satisfied the combination of the basic factors, i.e., cerebral unresponsiveness, apnea, and ECS. In fact, the EEGs of children under 1 year of age were not entered in the analysis of the data (Bennett, 1980; see also Chapter 17, this volume).

Studies of mixed populations that included some children indicate that a flat isoelectric EEG is diagnostic of brain death in the appropriate clinical setting (McGinty et al., 1985). Pampiglione and Harden (1968) reported that all seven children who had isoelectric EEGs following cardiocirculatory arrest died within 4 days; however, these investigators did not report either the exact ages of the patients or the clinical status and examination at the time of the EEG. This relative paucity of data raises concerns about the value of the EEG in the diagnosis of brain death in children. Furthermore, there are three reports involving three patients beyond the immediate newborn period in which the investigators claimed that there was a return of EEG activity after a period of ECS that varied in duration from 31 hr to almost 2 weeks. The evidence for the return of EEG activity in the first patient reported by Green and Lauber (1972) was inconclusive. An extracephalic reference was not used simultaneously with the EEG, and therefore an artifactual source for the recorded activity could not be excluded. The patients described by De Oliviera *et al.* (1984) and by Juguilon and Reilly (1982) did not fulfill the clinical criteria depicted in Table I. These patients had isoelectric EEGs while they responded to painful stimuli. In fact, the patient of Juguilon and Reilly (1982) had essentially flat EEGs for at least 2 weeks, while brainstem, somatic, and primitive reflexes persisted. A subsequent computed tomography (CT) scan showed marked hydranencephaly. This clinical picture is compatible with the diagnosis of neocortical death described by Mizrahi *et al.* (1985) rather than of brain death.

In order to evaluate the role of the EEG as a confirmatory test in the diagnosis of brain death in children, we organized a multi-institutional retrospective study (Alvarez *et al.*, 1988) involving the affiliated hospitals of the Albert Einstein College of Medicine, Bronx, New York; the Hospital of the State University of New York at Stony Brook, Stony Brook, New York; Miami Children's Hospital, Miami, Florida; and Maimonides Hospital, Brooklyn, New York. The study population was obtained by reviewing the EEGs of children under 5 years of age that showed the presence of ECS. All EEGs were obtained using the guidelines of the AEEGS. Once an isoelectric EEG was identified, the patient's chart was reviewed to ascertain that the patient met the adult clinical criteria for brain death (see Table I) and had been in that state for at least 6 hr prior to the EEG. Patients with conditions that could mimic brain death or produce ECS (see Section 3.2) were excluded. The results of other ancillary tests, the clinical course, and the eventual outcome of all patients were also recorded and analyzed. A total of 52 such patients were seen during the period between January 1982 and December 1986.

Table IV depicts patients according to chronological age. The etiology of coma was known in all children. Of the 52 children, 31 (60%) died spontaneously, and 21 (40%) were disconnected from the respirator after satisfying the criteria for the determination of brain death of their particular hospital. Of the 31 patients who died spontaneously, 14 (45%) had 2 EEGs with ECS (24 hr apart). Seventeen patients (55%) with ECS in their EEG died before a second one was obtained. Six children had autopsies, and all showed the characteristic pathological changes of brain death (Black, 1978*b;* Walker, 1985). Twenty-one children were disconnected from the ventilator after satisfying the particular hospital criteria for the determination of brain death. In this group, all patients were over 3 months of age. Fourteen patients (67%) had two EEGs with ECS (24 hr apart) before being disconnected from life-support systems, while 7 (33%) had only one EEG. CBF study obtained in two patients demonstrated absence of cerebral blood flow (CBF). In three other patients, neuropathological postmortem examination confirmed brain death. Ten of the patients were organ donors, all of whom had two EEGs with ECS (24 hr apart) before being disconnected from the life-support system. ECS persisted in all patients who had a second EEG.

The results of this study suggest that an isoelectric EEG can accurately confirm the diagnosis of brain death in children under 5 years of age, provided that the clinical criteria (Table I) are satisfied. A second EEG 24 hr later does not add to the verification process and may not be necessary.

TABLE IV.   Age Distribution

Age	No. of patients
<3 mo	3
3 mo to 1 yr	7
1–2 yr	14
2–3 yr	8
3–4 yr	8
4–5 yr	12
Total:	52

The only other study on brain-death determination that included a significant number of children below the age of 5 years was performed by Drake *et al.* (1986). It involved 61 children from newborn to 18 years, 53 of whom satisfied the criteria for brain death. The latter subpopulation was not broken down into age groups. In their study, once ECS was present in patients who satisfied the clinical criteria for brain death, somatic death eventually followed. Repeat EEGs did not alter the prognosis or diagnosis, corroborating the conclusion of our study.

Our results may need to be reproduced in a larger cohort of patients including more neonates under 3 months of age (52 weeks conceptual age), since our study contained only three such infants. Infants below the age of 3 months may share many of the EEG characteristics of the newborn and in this aspect should probably be treated as such (see Section 3.4).

3.4. EEG and Brain Death in Newborn Infants

In newborn infants and especially in premature babies, the role of the EEG in the determination of brain death remains unclear. The newborn brain appears to be very sensitive to insults and can show complete absence of electrocerebral activity in response to numerous intrinsic or extrinsic factors. There are two reports in which the EEG of newborn infants showed ECS and then later normalized. One of the neonates was a premature infant who did not meet the clinical criteria for brain death because he had decorticate and decerebrate movements (Engel, 1975). The other was a 6-week-old infant with seizures prior to the clinical diagnosis of brain death (Green and Lauber, 1972). We have observed transient ECS in the EEG of an infant after a relatively small bolus of diazepam and in another after a prolonged seizure. In this setting, the EEG should therefore be cautiously used for the confirmation of cerebral death. Unfortunately, in this particular age group, the other ancillary test normally used in the diagnosis of cerebral death, CBF determination, may also be inaccurate.

The presence of open fontanelles and sutures makes the skull of the newborn an expandable chamber. In the absence of a closed nonexpandable skull, it is possible that the edema caused by brain death may not be sufficient to increase the intracranial pressure (ICP) above the mean arterial pressure (MAP) and impede CBF. In support of this possibility is the report of an infant who met the clinical criteria for brain death but who had demonstrable CBF on positron emission tomography (PET) scan (Altman *et al.*, 1986). We are also aware of an adult with persistent CBF to the side of a large cranial defect, even though he met all other criteria for brain death. Postmortem studies verified brain death (Alvarez *et al.*, 1988). These observations suggest that a hemodynamically closed system may be necessary for the occurrence of the physiological changes responsible for the absence of CBF in brain death and that such a system may not be present in the newborn.

The Task Force of Pediatric Neurologists (see Chapter 14, this volume) proposed criteria that may be useful in the diagnosis of brain death in the newborn period. These criteria may be applied 7 days after the insult. The guidelines require two examinations documenting the clinical criteria shown in Table I as well as two EEGs separated by at least 48 hr. To date, data to support these recommendations are not available.

3.5. EEG and CBF Studies

The diagnostic value of EEG and CBF studies in diagnosing brain death is frequently compared. There are reports demonstrating no detectable flow to the brain in clinically brain-dead patients whose EEGs show some electrocerebral activity (Ashwal *et al.*, 1979; Drake *et al.*, 1986). In all cases, ECS eventually developed and somatic death soon followed. This observation should not be construed as evidence that the EEG cannot reliably confirm brain death in the appropriate clinical setting; rather, this may be evidence that the EEG is more specific than, although not as sensitive as, CBF determination. The presence of discernible EEG activity indicates that there are still some viable neurons despite the occurrence of massive brain edema that has raised the ICP above the MAP and resulted in the absence of CBF. Nevertheless, in spite of the presence of some EEG activity, the eventual outcome in all these cases is somatic death. The CBF at levels not detected by angiography is insufficient to meet the metabolic requirements of the brain and, because of the no-reflow phenomenon (Fisher *et al.*, 1977), once CBF is absent, ECS and brain death will inevitably follow.

While the EEG can be altered by certain factors, such as intoxication, hypothermia, or shock, CBF studies can be affected by conditions that alter the MAP/ICP ratio. After demonstrable brain death, the presence of open sutures and fontanelles (in the newborn) (Altman *et al.*, 1986), cranial defects (craniotomy) (Avarez *et al.*, 1988), and even severe brain atrophy (Blend *et al.*, 1986; Alvarez *et al.* 1987a) can result in ICPs below MAPs and permit CBF, producing false-negative results. Furthermore, in the absence of brain death, conditions that momentarily increase the ICP above the MAP, such as head trauma and Reye syndrome, can also result in transient absence of CBF producing false-positive results for brain death (Mitchell *et al.*, 1962; Rosenklint and Joorgensen, 1974). Thus, both EEG and CBF studies have their specific limitations; once physicians are aware of these limitations, they can choose the appropriate test for each particular setting.

4. EPILOGUE

The development and adoption of brain-death standards serve multiple goals. Such standards allow for the establishment of uniform determination and pronouncement of death. They help the decedent's family understand the hopeless situation and reduce the painful and demonstrably futile waiting period preceding somatic death. They transfer medical resources from people who are dead to others who will benefit from them. Finally, under appropriate circumstances, they increase the availability of scarce organs for donation.

In our experience, there are not many children who become organ donors. At Bronx Municipal Hospital in New York, 95 children under 15 years of age died over a 5-year span (1982–1986). This figure represents 0.6% of a total of 14,880 admissions during the same period (newborn infants excluded). Of 52 patients declared brain dead (Fig. 2), 56% were considered medically unacceptable as donors. The parents refused to give consent in 17 cases (74%). Thus, only 6 children, 26% of all suitable patients, became donors.

The low mortality of children is a major reason as to why so few potential donors are available. Another reason may be the cause of death. Infectious diseases and metabolic disorders are common causes of death in this age group. These patients are not medically suitable donors.

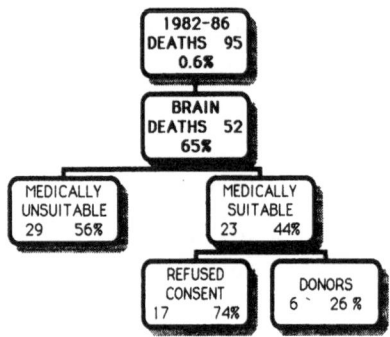

FIGURE 2. Tree chart depicting the incidence of children beyond the neonatal period until the age of 15 years who became donors over a 5-year period. Total deaths are depicted as percentage of all admissions (newborn infants excluded).

Furthermore, it may be extremely difficult for parents to give consent because of the great emotional stress they are under. Consequently, doctors are frequently hesitant even to approach the parents.

The need to increase organ and tissue donations from suitable candidates has led to the development of new legislative procedures affecting hospital organ procedurement. In New York State, a new law became effective on January 1, 1986. This new law mandates that for all deaths either

1. A note must be placed in the chart by the physician stating that the patient is not a suitable candidate because of medical exclusionary criteria (e.g., sepsis, transmissible disease, chronic disease) or because the family has expressed contrary intentions or there is reason to believe that an anatomical gift is contrary to the decedent's beliefs.
2. Consent for an anatomical gift must be pursued.

To increase potential organ transplant candidates requires the development of standard guidelines for the determination of brain death in young children. On the basis of the available data, the notion that the criteria for the determination of brain death used in adults should not be used in children between the ages of 3 months and 5 years is not justified. Indeed, in this age group, once the uniform clinical criteria have been satisfied, a single EEG with ECS is sufficient to confirm brain death. Unfortunately, there is a paucity of data concerning children below the age of 3 months, especially premature newborn infants; further studies may be necessary in order to develop separate brain-death criteria for this particular age group. The suggestions of the Task Force of Pediatric Neurologists are a promising beginning.

ACKNOWLEDGMENTS. This work was supported in part by Grant NS 20253 from the National Institute of Neurological and Communicative Diseases and Stroke. We wish to thank Ms. Donna Platyan for her help in typing this manuscript.

REFERENCES

Allen, N., Burkholdor J., Molinari G., and Comiscioni J., 1980, Clinical criteria of brain death, *NINCDS Monog. No. 24*, NIH PUbl. No. 81-2286, 77-147.

Altman, D. I., Perlman, J. M., Powers, W. J., Herscovitch, P., Dodson, W. E., Raichle, M. E., and Volpe, J. J., 1986, Exuberant brainstem blood flow and intact cerebral blood flow despite clinical and pathological evidence for brainstem and cerebral necrosis in an asphyxiated newborn infant, *Ann. Neurol.* **20**:409.

Alvarez, L. A., Lipton, R. B., and Moshé, S. L., 1987, Normal cerebral radionuclide angiogram and electrocerebral silence in the presence of severe cerebral atrophy, *Neuropediatrics* **18**:112.

Alvarez, L. A., Moshé, S. L., Belman, A. L., Maytal, J., Resnick, T. J., and Kielson, M., 1988, EEG and brain death determination in children, *Neurology (NY)* **38**:227–230.

Alvarez, L. A., Lipton, R. B., Hirschfeld, A., Salamon, O., and Lantos, G., 1988, Angiography and brain death determination in the setting of a skull defect, *Arch. Neurol.* **45**:225–227.

American EEG Society, 1979, Minimum technical standards for EEG recording in suspected cerebral death, in: *Current Practice of Clinical Electroencephalography* (D. W. Klass and D. D. Daly, eds.), pp. 492–496, Raven, New York.

Arfel, G., and Weiss, J., 1962, Electroencephalogramme et hypothermie profonde, *Ann. Chir. Thorac. Cardiovasc.* **1**:666–674.

Ashwal, S., and Schneider, S., 1979, Failure of electroencephalography to diagnose brain death in comatose children, *Ann. Neurol.* **6**:512–517.

Bennett, D. R., 1980, A review of the electroencephalographic data from the cerebral survival study, *NINCDS Monogr. No. 24*, NIH Publ. No. 81-2286, 148–180.

Bennett, D. R., Hughes, J. R., Korein, J., and Merlis, J. K., 1976, *Atlas of Electroencephalography in Coma and Cerebral Death*, Raven, New York.

Beresford, H. R., 1984, Severe neurological impairment: legal aspects of decision to reduce care, *Ann. Neurol.* **15:**409–414.

Black, P. M., 1978*a*, Brain death. I. *N. Engl. J. Med.* **299:**338–344.

Black, P. M., 1978*b*, Brain death. II *N. Engl. J. Med.* **299:**393–401.

Blend, M. J., Pavel, D. G., Hughes, J. R., Tan, W. S., Lansky, L. L., and Toffol, G. J., 1986, Normal cerebral radionuclide angiogram in a child with electrocerebral silence, *Neuropediatrics.* **17:**168–170.

Chatrian, G. E., 1980, Electrophysiologic evaluation of brain death: A critical appraisal, in: *Electrodiagnosis in Clinical Neurology* (M. J. Aminoff, ed.), pp. 525–588, Churchill Livingstone, New York.

De Oliviiera, W. M., De Oliviiera, M. L. J., Pereira, I. E., Epiphanio, E. B., and Valadao, G. C., 1984, Reavaliacao dos criterios clinicos e electrencefalotgraficos de determinacao da morte cerebral na crianca, *Arq. Neuropsiquiatr.* **42:**25–31.

Drake, B., Ashwal, S., and Schneider, S., 1986, Determination of cerebral death in the pediatric intensive care unit, *Pediatrics,* **78:**107–112.

Drury, I., Westmoreland, B. F., and Sharbrough, F. W., 1985, EEG studies in a locked in and locked out state due to severe acute inflammatory polyradiculopathy, in: *Proceedings of American EEG Society Meeting, Atlanta: AEEGS, 1985.*

Engel, R. C. H., 1975, *Abnormal Electroencephalograms in the Neonatal Period* Charles C. Thomas, Springfield, Illinois.

Fischgold, H., and Mathis, P., 1959, Obnubilations, comas et stupeurs, *Electroencephalogr. Clin. Neurophysiol.* suppl 11.

Fisher, E. G., Ames, A., Hedley-White, E. T., and O'Gorman, S., 1977, Reassessment of cerebral capillary changes in acute global ischemica and their relationship to the "no-reflow phenomenon," *Stroke* **8:**36–39.

Green, J. B., and Lauber, A., 1972, Return of EEG activity after electrocerebral silence: Two case reports, *J. Neurol. Neurosurg. Psychiatry* **35:**103–137.

Harvard Medical School, 1968, A definition of irreversible coma: report of the Ad Hoc Committee of the Harvard Medical School to examine the definition of brain death, *JAMA* **205:**337–340.

Jørgensen, E. O., 1974, EEG without detectable cortical activity and cranial nerve areflexia as parameters of brain death, *Electroencephalogr. Clin. Neurophysiol.* **36:**70–75.

Juguilon, A. C. C., and Reilly, E. L., 1982, Development of EEG activity after ten days of electrocerebral inactivity: A case report in a premature neonate-hydranencephaly or massive ventricular enlargement, *Clin. Electroencephalogr.* **13:**233–239.

Langendorf, F. G., Mallin, J. F., Masdeu, J. C., Moshé, S. L., and Lipton R. B., 1986, Fulminant Guillain-Barré syndrome simulating brain death, *Electroencephalogr. Clin. Neurophysiol.* **64:**74 (abst.).

Margolick, D., 1984, New York's highest court rules life ends when the brain dies, *New York Times,* (October 31, 1984), p. A1.

McGinty, L. K., Valderzant, C. W., Aldrich, M. S., and Sackellares, J. C., 1985, Single EEG in brain death determination, in: *Proceedings of American EEG Society Meeting, Atlanta, AEEGS, 1985.*

Mitchell, O. C., Torre, E., Alexander, E., and Davis, C. H., 1962, The non-filling phenomenon during angiography in acute intracranial hypertension, *J. Neurosurg.* **19:**766–774.

Mizrahi, E. M., Pollack, M. A., and Kellaway, P., 1985, Neocortical death in infants: Behavioral, neurologic, and electroencephalographic characteristics, *Pediatr. Neurol.* **1:**302–305.

Moshé, S. L., and Alvarez, L. A., 1986, Diagnosis of brain death in children, *J. Clin. Neurophysiol.* **3:**239–249.

National Collaborative Study, 1977, An appraisal of the criteria of cerebral death: A summary statement, *JAMA* **237:**982–986.

New York State Task Force on Life and the Law, 1986, The determination of death, 1-48.

Pampiglione, G., and Harden, A., 1968, Resuscitation after cardiorespiratory arrest, *Lancet* **1:**1261–1265.

Plum, F., and Posner, J. B., 1980, *The Diagnosis of Stupor and Coma*, FA Davis, Philadelphia.

Powner, D. J., 1976, Drug-associated isoelectric EEGs: A hazard in brain death certification, *JAMA* **236:**1123.

President's Commission, 1981, Guidelines for the determination of death: report of the medical consultants on the diagnosis of death to the President's Commission for the Study of Ethical Problems in Medicine and Biomedical and Behavioral Research, *JAMA* **246:**2184–2186.

Reilly, E. L., Brunberg, J. A., and Doty, D. B., 1974, The effect of deep hypothermia and total circulatory arrest on the electroencephalogram in children, *Electroencephalogr. Clin. Neurophysiol.* **36**:661–667.

Rosenklint, A., and Joorgensen, P. B., 1974, Evaluation of angiographic methods in the diagnosis of brain death. Correlation with local and systemic arterial pressure and intracranial pressure, *Neuroradiology* **7**:215–219.

Schwartz, J. A., Baxter, J., and Brill, D. R., 1984, Diagnosis of brain death in children by radionuclide cerebral imaging, *Pediatrics* **73**:14–18.

Setzer, N., 1985, Brain death: Physiologic definitions, *Crit. Care Clin.* **1**:375–396.

Tharp, B. R., 1980, Neonatal and pediatric electroencephalography, in: *Electrodiagnosis in Clinical Neurology* (M. J. Aminoff, ed.), pp. 67–117, Churchill Livingstone, New York.

Ventura, M. G., and Masser, P. G., 1985, Defining death: Developments in recent law. *Crit. Care Clin.* **1**:397–425.

Vernon, D. D., and Holzman, B. H., 1986, Brain death: Considerations for pediatrics, *J. Clin. Neurophysiol.* **3**:251–265.

Walker, A. E., 1985, *Cerebral Death*, Urban & Schwazenber, Baltimore.

III

ISSUES IN BRAIN DEATH RELATED TO ORGAN DONATION

19

ESTIMATION OF ORGAN AND TISSUE DONOR POOL FROM MULTIPLE CAUSE OF DEATH STATISTICS

R. JOHN C. PEARSON and STEPHANIE G. PRATT

1. INTRODUCTION

There is considerable uncertainty as to the size of the potential pool of donors for transplantation of organs and tissues, and the need to review the size of the pool is predicated on three factors: (1) the current shortage of kidney donors, (2) the growth in number of other transplants being performed in the United States, and (3) the low proportion of potential donors actually harvested.

In 1979, dialysis facilities reported that 6311 of their patients were on registries awaiting a cadaveric kidney transplant (Health Care Financing Administration, 1980), and, by 1986, the number was reported to be 9000 (American Council on Transplantation, 1987), despite a growth in the number of kidney cadaveric transplants from 4885 in 1981 to 7695 in 1985 (American Council on Transplantation, 1987). Rapaport and Cortesini developed the scenario, from multiple sources, that the incidence of end-stage renal disease (ESRD) in the United States was 24,000 per year, that the prevalence in 1984 was 75,000, and that the prevalence would double in 10 years and redouble in 10 years after that.

Transplantation of the other organs is a more recent development, and estimates of the recipient pool are not well developed. However, the urgency is less for such estimates as the number of patients with failing hearts, cirrhotic livers, and type 1 diabetes would appear to greatly outnumber the current potential for transplantation, both in terms of the organs and the teams available to perform the procedures. As of 1985, about 500 pancreata had been transplanted in the world (Pisano, 1985), 300 of which had been transplanted in the United States (American Council on Transplantation, 1987). By June 1984, 568 livers had been transplanted in the United States and 424 in Europe (Starzl *et al.*, 1985). In the United States in 1985, 731 hearts and 30 heart–lungs were transplanted (American Council on Transplantation, 1987). In 1985 26,000 corneal transplants were performed (American Council on Transplantation, 1987), but it has been esti-

R. JOHN C. PEARSON • Department of Community Medicine, West Virginia University Medical Center, Morgantown, West Virginia 26506. STEPHANIE G. PRATT • Office of Health Services Research, West Virginia University Medical Center, Morgantown, West Virginia 26506.

mated that 250,000 Americans could benefit from the procedure (American Council on Transplantation Statistics, 1985); worldwide, however, especially where trachoma is endemic, the numbers needed are in the tens of millions. Between 100,000 and 200,000 bone grafts are currently being performed each year in the United States (Friedlaender, 1985). Skin grafts are needed by many of the 130,000 burn victims each year in the United States, of whom 70,000 have stays in intensive care units (ICUs) and 10,000 die (Montgomery, 1979).

Two large studies have been conducted to review the potential for kidney donations and the actual numbers of donors. The first, conducted by the Centers for Disease Control (CDC) (Bart et al., 1981a), reviewed the medical records of 10,420 deaths in 67 large short stay hospitals in 1975 in Georgia, Kansas, and Missouri. Selecting patients on the basis of the same medical criteria as in Table I and II, the investigators used a narrow and a broad definition of potential donation, the difference between them being largely that of age: the narrow definition being 5–55 and the broader one newborn to 65. The broader definition doubled the potential donor pool from 1.7% to 3.5% of hospital deaths. Using the narrower definition, at that time standard in the hospitals, only 19.3% of the potentially available kidneys were actually retrieved.

The follow-up study in 34 of the 37 hospitals in this study located in Georgia was conducted from 1976 to 1979 to determine more closely the factors related to failure to achieve organ procurement and to see whether a higher proportion of retrievals could be achieved by professional education (Bart et al., 1981b). Factors associated with higher procurement included age between 7 months and 15 years, white race, death in the ICU, and hospital stays of 2 or 3 days. With broadening of the criteria for donation, three times as many kidneys were procured as had been during the prior 3 years; nevertheless, the retrieval rate was only 15% overall.

The second study was conducted in Ontario on deaths in hospital during 1981 and 1982 (Robinette et al., 1985). Of the 71,323 deaths, 2562 (3.6%) were considered suitable for kidney donation, but only 233 decedents became donors (9%). A large number of factors were found to impede the translation from potential into actuality: lack of interest of hospital personnel or lack of preparedness or organization; concerns by families about death really having occurred, about mutilation, or about their religious or fatalistic attitudes; families' lack of time to become prepared; and problems with logistics and transportation both within and between hospitals. The causes of death considered suitable for donation included only brain tumor; head trauma, brain

TABLE I. Guidelines for Transplantable Organs

Circulatory status	Organs (beating heart donor required)			
	Kidney	Heart	Liver	Pancreas
Physiological age limits	1–65 yr	1–45 yr	2 mo–45 yr	1–65 yr
Timing of procurement	Donor must have *intact* cardiovascular system; must have adequate perfusion of all vital organs			
Consent	Consent of legal next-of-kin required; consent of medical examiner/coroner if applicable			
Location/designation of procurement	Performed in hospital operating room by transplant team or local surgeon, with heart, liver, and pancreas teams retrieving their respective organs			
Potential recipients	End-stage renal disease	Terminal heart failure	End-stage liver failure	Juvenile diabetes with complications
Medical criteria	Present or imminent brain death; no systemic infection or extracranial malignancy except skin; no pre-existing renal disease; negative hepatitis, HTLV-3, VDRL			

TABLE II. Guidelines for Transplantable Tissues

Circulatory status	Tissues (beating heart not required)			
	Skin	Bone	Heart valves	Eyes
Physiological age limits	15–75+ yr	Over 15 yr	2 mo–55 yr	No limit
Timing of procurement	<24 hr cool; <6 hr warm	<24 hr cool; <12 hr warm		
Consent	Consent of legal next-of-kin required; consent of medical examiner/ coroner, if applicable			
Location/designation of procurement	Performed in hospital operating room by tissue recovery team			
Potential recipients	Burns	Bone defects, trauma	Heart valve replacement	Corneal damage
Medical criteria	No systemic infection or malignancy; no CNS degenerative disease; no diseases of unknown etiology; negative serology; no heart trauma or valvular disease			No exclusion

injury, aneurysms, etc.; asphyxia; and poisoning. Divided by age groups, 6% were aged 12 or less, 32% aged 13–40, and 62% aged 41–65.

The aim of this study is to review causes of death in children aged 4 months through 19 years in the United States, to assess the upper limit of potential donors, and to discuss by how much these numbers need to be reduced to reach a more realistic level. This is the first time the multiple cause-of-death file has been used for this purpose (Israel *et al.*, 1986).

2. METHODS

In this study the age groups assigned for consideration were 4 months to 19 years, 4 months being the youngest age for transplantation of any organ at West Virginia University (WVU) at the time of assignment (later lowered to 2 months, as shown in Table I) and 19 years as the upper limit for childhood.

At WVU Medical Center, guidelines exist for the harvesting of kidneys, hearts, livers, pancreases, skin, bone, heart valves, and eyes. These guidelines include physiological age limits, the timing of procurement, the consent needed, the location of procurement, the potential recipients, and the medical criteria (West Virginia University Hospital guidelines). These medical criteria govern who may not be a donor (see Tables I and II). These guidelines were followed for this study.

A computer tape was obtained from the Division of Vital Statistics, National Center for Health Statistics (NCHS), which contained the public file on all deaths in children of these ages for the latest available year, 1984. The information included not only the single cause of death usually used in vital statistics but also a recoding that used all the causes of death listed on the death certificate and rationalized them according to predetermined criteria (Transax, 1984).

Up to 20 coded causes of death can be taken from the death certificate for each patient. Accident cases included not only the external cause of death [e.g., fall, motor vehicle accident (MVA), suicide] but also the body organs affected. Also on the tape was all the other information coded from the death certificate, including age, sex, and race and location of death. The tape includes 37,484 deaths.

Three samples were drawn for in-depth analysis before the whole file was used to produce the major findings in this study. The first sample was all deaths on the third and eighteenth days of the month (these days were chosen randomly by coin toss), and each individual death was listed on a separate line by age, in months, 4–11, and in years, 1–19. For each individual, all recoded multiple causes of death, up to 20, were listed in ascending order of International Classification of Disease (ICD) code (Manual of the International Statistical Classification of Diseases, Injuries and Causes of Death). Separate listings were made in this way for deaths as inpatients (IP), deaths in the emergency room or outpatient department (ER/OPD), inhospital deaths not specified as to where (Hospital NOS), deaths on arrival (DOA), deaths out of hospital (i.e., at home, in other institutions, or in other locations), and deaths not specified as to location (NK). Of the 2601 patients who died, 618 were inpatients, 306 were DOA, 299 died in ER/OPD, 517 died in Hosp NOS, 857 died out of hospital, and 4 deaths were NK.

Each individual death in the first sample was reviewed according to the criteria for transplantation listed by organ in Tables I and II. This was done separately for liver, kidney, and heart. Consultation with the professor of pediatrics was conducted when there were diagnoses that might or might not qualify for consideration as a donor. From this review, a listing of ICD numbers was compiled separately for each organ and tissue, as listed in Table I, that would disqualify decedents from being considered as a donor.*

Accordingly, for the major analysis, computer programs were written for each organ and tissue separately in order to enumerate the number of decedents by age that could be considered as donors. For both the organs and the tissues, the locations of death were analyzed separately. These programs were used for all deaths in the file.

The second sample was drawn to confirm that the first sample was a representative one. It consisted of deaths on the eighth and twenty-third days of the month. This sample included 2457 deaths and had a similar distribution by location of death. The age distribution of the two samples was also comparable: under 1 year, 394 and 390; 1–4 years, 488 and 498; 5–9 years, 280 and 266; 10–14 years, 383 and 316; and 15–19 years, 1056 and 987.

The third sample, also from the NCHS tape file, comprised all deaths to West Virginia residents. It was analyzed to determine whether the use of multiple causes of death improved the determination of transplantability as compared with the single cause of death used in the regular reporting in vital statistics documents. It was found that there was useful information predicating organ retrieval, or not, in two areas: for accident cases, there was added precision in terms of multiple parts of the body injured, or in terms of no mention of multiple injuries. For all cases, but predominantly for the nonaccident deaths, there was information on complications, usually septic, but less often in terms of postoperative complications. Among infants, the predictability of organ transplant was affected in five of 23 deaths. Among the older children, it was affected in 32 of 72 deaths, of which 19 were MVA fatalities and three other accidents. In all, 35% of deaths were more accurately assessible.

In addition to the analysis of the multiple causes of death file, two small pilot studies were conducted to get a feel for the circumstances of death and the factors, other than medical criteria, that could affect the proportion of potential donors that would become actual. Case records of deaths in children at WVU Hospital during 1986 were reviewed. Medical examiner records were examined for deaths in children in 51 of the 55 counties of West Virginia for 1986.

*Listing available from authors.

3. FINDINGS

3.1. Analysis of Multiple Causes of Death File

The number of inpatient decedents who were potential donors of the organs and tissues within the age range 4 months to 19 years, once exclusions have been made on medical criteria, is presented in Tables III and IV. However, it is likely that the numbers of organs shown in Table III will be increased by the deaths recorded as hospital NOS, some at least of whom will have died as inpatients, and by deaths in the ER/OPD, some of whom will be there some hours in a

TABLE III.   Age Distribution of Inpatient Potential Donors of Organs;
United States, 1984[a]

Age	Kidney	Heart	Liver	Pancreas
4–11 months				
4	—	—	171	—
5	—	—	145	—
6	—	—	117	—
7	—	—	110	—
8	—	—	84	—
9	—	—	79	—
10	—	—	46	—
11	—	—	59	—
			811	
1–19 years				
1	393	182	426	450
2	244	123	238	253
3	153	75	152	164
4	92	49	89	100
5	90	55	89	94
6	69	38	65	75
7	60	31	58	67
8	63	32	64	68
9	54	30	53	57
10	62	28	65	69
11	70	38	70	73
12	58	31	55	61
13	86	53	84	90
14	56	32	54	62
15	86	52	81	92
16	107	67	99	113
17	105	68	98	114
18	125	94	119	131
19	115	73	108	129
	2088	1151	2067	2262
<1 year	—	—	811	—
	2088	1151	2878	2262

[a]Exclusions on the basis of medical criteria only.

TABLE IV.   Age Distribution of Potential Donors of Tissues: United States, 1984[a]

Age	Skin	Bone	Heart valves[b]	Eyes
4–11 months				
4	—	—	243	1436
5	—	—	231	1106
6	—	—	206	797
7	—	—	154	592
8	—	—	120	517
9	—	—	133	455
10	—	—	107	336
11	—	—	107	348
			1301	5587
1–19 years				
1	—	—	658	2876
2	—	—	446	1920
3	—	—	311	1391
4	—	—	238	1124
5	—	—	200	955
6	—	—	167	880
7	—	—	173	832
8	—	—	168	769
9	—	—	142	701
10	—	—	170	757
11	—	—	167	758
12	—	—	194	923
13	—	—	257	1148
14	—	—	254	1355
15	552	541	372	1809
16	725	700	486	2449
17	848	856	550	3006
18	1022	1036	685	3738
19	1192	1229	805	4269
	4339	4362	6443	31660
<1 year	—	—	1301	5587
	4339	4362	7744	37247

[a]Exclusions on basis of medical criteria only.
[b]Data exclude cases in which hearts would be transplantable intact.

brain-dead status. The total number of decendents in the ER/OPD and in the Hospital NOS is presented in Table V.

The upper limit of potential organs that may be retrievable, therefore, ranges from 2088 (IP only) to 5342 (IP + ER/OPD + NOS) kidney donors, 1151 to 3545 hearts, 2878 to 7316 livers, and 2262 to 5722 pancreases. The percentages of all children's deaths that these numbers represent, together with the percentages for the tissues, are presented in Table VI. The percentages range from a low of 3.1% for inpatient hearts to 84.5% for eyes. It must be clearly understood that these numbers and percentages represent the upper limit and are not realistic in terms of actual retrieval, for a variety of attitudinal and logistic reasons that will be explained.

TABLE V. Age Distribution of Potential Donors of Organs[a]

Age	Kidney	Heart	Liver	Pancreas
4–11 months				
4	—	—	337	—
5	—	—	227	—
6	—	—	178	—
7	—	—	134	—
8	—	—	95	—
9	—	—	90	—
10	—	—	84	—
11	—	—	80	—
			1209	
1–19 years				
1	450	275	486	499
2	299	203	298	317
3	209	146	206	220
4	155	104	144	159
5	110	81	102	114
6	113	75	106	116
7	94	55	94	94
8	88	67	89	90
9	71	53	71	74
10	85	50	86	87
11	87	62	82	91
12	110	66	107	113
13	111	76	110	117
14	120	88	116	128
15	132	102	131	142
16	174	131	166	187
17	235	208	230	245
18	280	236	271	289
19	331	292	325	350
	3254	2370	3220	3432
<1 year	—	—	1209	—
	3254	2370	4429	3432

[a]Deaths in ER/OPD plus hospital NOS (United States, 1984). Exclusions on basis of medical criteria only.

3.2. Deaths of Children in WVU Hospital, 1986

There were 32 children whose death certificates were completed at WVU Hospital in 1986, including deaths as inpatients, in the ER and DOA. Of the 32, 13 were certainly unsuitable for transplantation because of the medical criteria, e.g., malignancies and sepsis. Of the remaining 19, four had organs taken for transplantation (Table VII). An additional five children were suitable for transplantation, and of these the parents of one refused transplantation. Of the remaining 10, four cases were uncertain on medical grounds and six on social grounds.

The actual transplantation rate of four of nine (44%) is higher than that generally cited in the

TABLE VI.   Numbers and Percentages of All Deaths in Children Aged
4 Months to 19 Years Who May Have Organs and Tissue Retrieved
for Transplantation: United States, 1984

	IP only	IP + ER/OPD + NOS
Kidneys	2,088 (5.6%)	5,342 (14.3%)
Heart	1,151 (3.1%)	3,521 (9.4%)
Liver	2,878 (7.7%)	7,307 (19.5%)
Pancreas	2,262 (6.0%)	5,694 (15.2%)
Skin	4,339 (11.6%)	
Bone	4,362 (11.6%)	
Heart valves[a]	5,368 (14.1%)	7,744 (20.7%)
Eyes	31,660 (84.5%)	

[a]Varies by potential retrieval of whole hearts.

TABLE VII.   Deaths in Children Aged 4 Months to 19 Years: WVU Hospital, 1986

Age	Total	Transplanted	Suitable	Maybe	Unlikely	No
4–11 mo	7	—	—	1	1	5
1–4 yr	9	1[a]	2[b,d]	2	1	3
5–9 yr	6	1[a]	1[b]	1	2	1
10–14 yr	3	—	1[c]	—	—	2
15–19 yr	7	2[a,c]	1[c]	—	2	2
	32	4	5[e]	4[f]	6[g]	13

[a]Heart only.
[b]Liver only.
[c]Heart, lungs, kidneys.
[d]Liver, pancreas, kidneys.
[e]Suitable: 14-month with CHD; liver, pancreas, and kidney; 3-year-old with CHD; liver only; 9-year-old with CHD; died
postoperatively; liver only; 10-year-old head injury; transplant refused, all organs; 18-year-old head injury; all organs.
[f]Maybe: 3 with CHD died postoperatively with poor renal output; 1 6-month-old died weighing 4.4 kg; athrepsia, CHD.
[g]Unlikely: no parent present at death; very short histories of conditions (MVA, myocarditis) and very short hospital stay.

literature; however, only one pair of kidneys was harvested and, for this organ, the proportion is
in line with other studies (Montgomery, 1979; Pisano, 1985; Robinette et al., 1985).

3.3.   Medical Examiner's Cases, West Virginia, 1986

There were 118 deaths. All five cases harvested were accident cases, aged 2, 5, 17, 17, and
17 years, each of whom had had a period of days in coma—time for the family to come to terms
with their grief (Table VIII).

Of the 13 probably suitable, two were drownings, seven MVAs, two head injuries, and two
gunshot wounds. These cases were judged probably suitable in that they were not so disfigured
as to preclude donation, death inhospital, and family present before death. Six were comatose in
hospital for a period of 2 or more days, for one of whom donation was refused, and the remainder
had cardiopulmonary resuscitation (CPR) maintained in the emergency room for some hours. For
two, the gunshot wound to the abdomen and the teenager run over by a truck, only the contents
of the chest could have been harvested.

Of the six possibly suitable cases, five died after a brief spell of CPR in the emergency room

TABLE VIII.   Medical Examiner Data for
Children Aged 4 Months to 19 Years:
West Virginia, 1986

119 cases
5 harvested
13 probably suitable (1 refused)
6 possibly suitable
95 not suitable for organ donation
Up to 80 suitable for tissues

and one died after a spell of coma in hospital. These cases were judged possibly suitable on medical grounds but had no family available to give consent for donation. One, aged 10, was being treated for *Hemophilus influenzae* infection. Three of the other five had trauma to the chest but had abdomens that appeared intact. Of the remaining two cases, one had a head injury and one had multiple injuries, but neither had such trauma to chest or abdomen as to preclude donation.

Of the 95 unsuitable for organ transplant because of death out of hospital or DOA, 15 had been dead for too long for the tissues to be usable. Of the 80 remaining, 21 required autopsy because the cause of death needed explication, and for many of the 15 homicides and suicides, there would probably have been delays while the police conducted investigations. For only 5 of the 95 was there a likelihood that grief over the death could have been worked over beforehand. These five had longstanding congenital conditions, hydrocephalus, cerebral palsy, and Down syndrome. The remaining 90 were all sudden and unexpected deaths, so the potential even for tissue transplantation would be low, especially as many came from deprived neighborhoods and many did not have relatives present at death or at arrival at the medical examiner's office or hospital, factors found in the Ontario study to be poor predictors of transplantation (Robinette *et al.*, 1985). This review demonstrated that 5 of 118 (4%) patients became donors, and an additional 18 of 118 (15%) might have been suitable.

4.   DISCUSSION

4.1.   Comparison with Other Studies

Compared with the CDC study (Bart *et al.*, 1981*a, b*), this study is national in scope rather than regional, considers all deaths rather than inpatient deaths only, uses the same medical criteria as far as can be determined from the published information, and includes all organs and tissues that may be transplanted except for the rare heart–lung combination instead of only the kidneys. However, this study uses death certificates instead of an extensive review of hospital charts, with the result that there is no information on duration of hospital stay for the inpatients nor any information on whether the patient was in the ICU, both of which were predictors of organ retrieval. Nor is there any information in this study, except in the small trace studies, on whether organ donation was requested or on whether parents were present at or before death and to be available for a request for donation.

Compared with the Ontario study (Robinette *et al.*, 1985), this study is American national rather than Canadian provincial, includes all organs and tissues rather than kidneys alone, and includes a wide range of diagnoses of death among potential donors. Both studies use death certificates, but this study uses multiple causes of death. Only one hospital had chart review in this study, as compared with eight in the Canadian study. This study included all deaths, rather than only inpatient deaths.

Compared with both of the other studies, this study uses a narrower age range. None of the age groups used in the other studies could be compared easily with the ages in this study, even though the data presented here were analyzed separately for each month in infancy and each year thereafter, as their data on available kidneys covered a broader age group. The CDC proportion of 1.7% of hospital deaths that were potential donors referred to the age range 5–55 years.

Compared with the other studies, this study has no breakdown by the size or type of hospital in which the child died. However, their data may be indicative of what would be found nationally in that there was considerable agreement in the other two studies. In the CDC study, 62% of inpatient deaths occurred in the 7% of hospitals that were large. In Ontario, 62% of the potential donors, according to their (unspecified) criteria, died in teaching hospitals, and 80% died in hospitals with 400 or more beds.

Two caveats on the upper limit of potential donation may have lowered the limit by a small fraction. Not all infections would necessarily limit donation, depending on the success and duration of therapy; however, it is probable that the mention of sepsis on the death certificate would indicate that it contributed directly to the death or was a contributory factor. Also, it is more likely that physicians would commit sins of omission rather than of commission when undertaking the chore of completing the death certificate. The second caveat is that death certificates are in error, to differing extent, with different conditions (Stehbens, 1987). No assessment can be made on the significance of this to this study.

4.2.   Approaching a More Realistic Level of a Potential Donor Pool

Estimating what proportion of the upper limit of potential donors would be a realistic level of expectation for organ and tissue retrieval is an imprecise art, not a science at all, as there are very few indicators to work with.

The CDC studies were able to show 19.3% (Bart et al., 1981a) and 15% (Bart et al., 1981b) retrieval of kidneys from potential donors, with 21% from 7- to 11-month-olds, 26% from 1- to 4-year olds, and 22% from 5- to 14-year olds; the retrieval rate below 7 months was minimal, and in the age range 15–39 was 12% (Bart et al., 1981b). The Ontario study found a 9% retrieval of kidneys from potential donors. At WVU Hospital, the retrieval rate of any organ was 4 of 9,

TABLE IX.   Realistic Estimate as to Likely
Donor Pool of Organs and Tissues in Children
Aged 4 Months to 19 Years:
United States, 1984

Tissue	N
Kidneys[a]	450
Heart	280
Liver	610
Pancreas	480
Skin	350
Bone	350
Heart valves	260
Eyes[a]	2500

[a]Number of donors; double the number for number of kidneys
and eyes.

but only 1 of 9 for kidneys. In the medical examiner's case series, 5 of 18 were harvested (28%), but there was no information as to which organs were retrieved.

This study has the additional difficulty in deciding what proportion of the ER/OPD deaths and of the hospital NOS deaths should be added to the inpatient deaths to form the potential pool. In addition, there is the problem of estimating the proportion of hospitals in which the deaths occurred that would be ready, willing, and able to enlist donors.

A rough guess would be that, for organ retrieval, 60% of deaths would occur in hospitals that would participate, and 20% of inpatients and 10% of the ER/OPD and hospital NOS deaths would become donors. On this basis, the number of organs that are realistically retrievable would be as shown in Table IX.

As regards tissues, it may be realistic to suggest that skin, bone, and eyes could be retrieved from 80% of the hospital deaths and from 10% of all patients dying there or DOA. For heart valves, the proportion of hospitals may be 60%, as with the organs, and the retrieval rate 10% of those heart patients whose whole organ is not retrieved. These guesses are shown in Table IX as well.

ACKNOWLEDGMENTS. We would like to thank William A. Neal, professor and chairman of pediatrics, West Virginia University Hospital, for his review of uncommon diseases and their potential for transplantation; Daniel Thistlethwaite, fourth-year medical student, for collaboration in reviewing the literature and discussing the project; the Division of Vital Statistics, National Center for Health Statistics, for willing, warm, and timely collaboration; and Naomi J. Cassi, secretary, for the many times she had to retype this manuscript.

REFERENCES

American Council on Transplantation Statistics, 1985, cited by Graham, C. R. Jr., 1985, Eye banking: A growth story, *Transplant. Proc.* **17**(suppl 4):105–111.

Bart, K. J., Macon, E. J., Whittier, F. C., Baldwin, R. J., and Blount, J. H., 1981*a*, Cadaveric kidneys for transplantation: A paradox of shortage in the face of plenty, *Transplantation* **31**(5):379–383.

Bart, K. J., Macon, E. J., Humphries, A. L., Jr., Baldwin, R. J., Fitch, T., Pope, R. S., Rich, M. J., Langford, D., Teutsch, S. M., and Blount, J. H., 1981*b*, Increasing the supply of cadaveric kidneys for transplantation, *Transplantation* **31**:383–387.

Friedlaender, G. E., Bone banking and clinical applications, *Transplant. Proc.* **17**(suppl 4):99–104.

Health Care Financing Administration, 1980, End Stage Renal Disease Program, Second Annual Report to Congress.

Israel, R. A., Rosenberg, H. M., and Curtin, L. R., 1986, Analytic potential for multiple cause-of-death data, *Am. J. Epidemiol.* **124**(2):161–179.

Manual of the International Statistical Classification of Diseases, 1977, *Injuries and Causes of Death*, 9th rev. WHO, Geneva.

Montgomery, B. J., 1979, Consensus for treatment of "the sickest patients you'll ever see," *JAMA* **241**(4):345–346.

Pisano, L., 1985, Critical comments on present and future possibilities and advantages of pancreas transplantation in insulin-dependent diabetes mellitus, *Transplant. Proc.* **17**(suppl 2):135–140.

Rapaport, F. T., and Cortesini, R., 1987, The past present and future of organ transplantation, with special reference to current needs in kidney procurement and donation, *Transplant. Proc.* **17**(2):3–10.

Robinette, M. A., Marshall, W. J. S., Arbus, G. S., Beal, K., Bennett, R. C., Brady, W., Harris, D. M., Rimstead, D., Morrin, P., Seaver, R., and Stiller, C. R., 1985, The donation process, *Transplant. Proc.* **17**(suppl 3):45–65.

Starzl, T. E., Iwatsuki, S., Shaw, B. W., Jr., and Gordon, R. D., 1985, Orthotopic liver transplantation in 1984, *Transplant. Proc.* **17**(1):250–258.

Stehbens, W. E., 1987, An appraisal of the epidemic rise of coronary heart disease and its decline, *Lancet* **1**:606–610.

Transax, 1984, The NCHS System for Producing Multiple Cause-of-Death Statistics. Vital and Health Statistics, Series 1, No. 20, USDHHS (PHS) 86-1322.

West Virginia University Hospital, 1987, Guidelines for transplantable organs and tissues.

20

Use of Anencephalic Infants as Organ Donors

Crossing a Threshold

RONALD E. CRANFORD and JOHN C. ROBERTS

1. CURRENT PRACTICE

My interest in this area began in June 1986, when I received a call from a pediatric neurologist on the east coast. She called me in my capacity as chairman of the Ethics and Humanities Committee of the American Academy of Neurology because she had become quite concerned when she had heard of professionals involved in the transplant movement discuss the increasingly common practice of using anencephalics as organ donors.

Because of this call and the concerns she raised, I started to do a literature search and began calling professionals around the country involved in the care of newborns and the transplant movement. I was astonished to find that there were at least 15 cases reported in the medical literature on the use of anencephalics as organ donors (Martin *et al.*, 1969; Potter *et al.*, 1970; Fine *et al.*, 1970; LaPlant *et al.*, 1970; King *et al.*, 1971; Lawson *et al.*, 1973; Salvatierra and Belzer, 1975; Iitaka *et al.*, 1978; Schneider *et al.*, 1983; Ohshima *et al.*, 1984). I was even more astonished to discover that, in these case reports, there was essentially no discussion of the moral-legal implications of this practice. In my conversations, I also learned that using anencephalics as organ donors had occurred in the past and was occurring now, but only uncommonly. I was a little surprised, but not a great deal, to learn how strongly some parents felt in these individual cases and how disappointed and frustrated parents and health-care providers were when they learned that the organs of the anencephalic infants could not be used because of moral or legal concerns. I was also surprised, and disappointed, at the narrow views of some health-care professionals concerning their enthusiasm to remove organs in these children coupled with their seeming unawareness of the major moral-legal problems that this practice presented.

RONALD E. CRANFORD • Department of Neurology, Hennepin County Medical Center, Minneapolis, Minnesota 55415. JOHN C. ROBERTS • Department of Internal Medicine, Abbott-Northwestern Hospital, Minneapolis, Minnesota 55404. Dr. Cranford gave the original conference presentation. However, Dr. Roberts contributed substantially to the original research and thinking on this subject and agrees with the opinions expressed in this chapter. Thus, it was decided to coauthor the paper but to retain the first-person narrative.

I found only a few articles in the literature directly addressing the moral–legal issues, one by Fletcher *et al.* (1986) and another by Caplan (1987). I was disturbed by statements made by Harrison, which I believed were categorically false (e.g., his description of anencephalics as "brain absent") (Harrison, 1986*a, b*). Anencephalics have minimal and poorly functioning brainstem and cerebellum, but they do not fit under the category of whole-brain death, nor is it medically accurate to call them brain absent. I was also concerned about proposals for the specific medical management of anencephalics designed to permit retrieval of organs, which I found particularly objectionable and medically unfeasible. Some of these included (1) letting the infant "die," then resuscitating the infant and removing the organs; (2) letting the infant deteriorate to the point of whole-brain death and then removing organs; and (3) cooling the patient not only to preserve the organs and minimize warm ischemia time but also to allow the infant to develop whole-brain death, and then removing the organs.

My initial reaction to this preliminary review was the following. If using anencephalics as organ donors is a justifiable medical practice, and I think that it probably is under appropriate circumstances, then we should be up front about what we are doing, clarify the medical facts as much as possible, and raise the important moral–legal issues this practice presents. To continue to advocate a policy of using anencephalics as organ donors without a full-scale public debate is, in my opinion, simply wrong, as well as counterproductive. It undermines the trust and confidence of the public in the medical profession and the transplant movement at a time when trust and confidence are so critical.

2. ANENCEPHALY

Anencephaly is an uncommon birth defect, occurring in approximately 0.5–2 of every 1000 live births in the United States (Nakano, 1973). Thus, it is estimated that there may be 1000–5000 born each year; probably a realistic number would be 2000–3000. Prevalence rates, however, vary considerably with some factors: environmental, maternal, sex, ethnic groups, and location. For example, the prevalence rate in Great Britain is about 1–5 times higher than in the United States.

These patients have a devastating and observable neurological malformation. The cerebral hemispheres are usually completely absent, as is most of the cranial vault. A variable amount of brainstem and cerebellum is present. The eyes are usually present, but the face is severely malformed. This congenital malformation is so severe that it can readily be distinguished from other birth defects. A few other, extremely rare, neurological syndromes can be confused with anencephaly, such as amniotic band syndrome and mosaic forms of trisomy 13 and 18. This defect can be diagnosed with an extremely high degree of certainty, both *in utero* by measuring levels of serum α-fetoprotein (AFP) and ultrasonography, and after birth by clinical examination of the child.

Because of the major defect in the cranial vault, exposing the infant's primitive nervous system, and because of the poorly developed brainstem, these infants will die soon after birth from infection or respiratory insufficiency. Thus, these children, in addition to having no cerebral hemispheres and thus being completely unconscious, are truly dying; only 10% or less live more than 1 week, and the longest reported, well-documented, survivor in the medical literature is 4½ months.

3. ARGUMENTS FAVORING ANENCEPHALICS AS ORGAN DONORS

The strong arguments in favor of using anencephalics as organ donors focus on five major points:

1. Anencephalic infants have an utterly hopeless prognosis. They are permanently unconscious and terminally ill, and the diagnosis can be easily established both *in utero* and at birth with an extraordinarily high degree of certainty. Regardless of the degree of therapeutic efforts, most will die within days, and only a few may live for weeks. Because these infants are permanently unconscious and can experience no pain or suffering, hence can never be aware of what happens to them, a strong argument can be made that, like other permanently unconscious patients, they have no interest in treatment, i.e., treatment can neither benefit nor harm them. Given the traditional laws in this area, however, specifically on homicide, and our traditional moral and medical norms, any lethal action such as the removal of vital organs would be construed as killing, i.e., homicide. Thus, it may be reasonable to say that, from a medical–moral standpoint in terms of a developing consensus on permanently unconscious patients, anencephalic patients cannot be harmed by the removal of vital organs but, given the current laws on homicide, they can be considered to have been killed. It should be noted that anencephaly is one of the few conditions, if not the only one, in which many would argue that it is justifiable to do a third-trimester abortion (Chervenak *et al.,* 1984). Even among physicians who would never do an abortion in any other situation, anencephaly may be considered a justifiable reason for performing an abortion.

2. Organ donation is of great value to the recipients—the hundreds or thousands of newborns and infants who now, because of refinements in operative techniques and the ability to control the immunosuppressive response, can benefit from receiving the organs from the anencephalic infants. In recent years, there has been an extraordinary demand for small organs. A large number of infants who may have died otherwise of major organ malformations or failure can now be restored to potentially normal health by transplantation of vital organs from infants and small children. These include liver, heart, kidneys, lungs, bone marrow, and pancreatic islet cells. The number of young children in whom brain death develops is not enough to cope with the increasing demand for small organs, and it is unlikely, even with more extensive educational programs, that this pool of brain-dead children will satisfy the demand.

3. There is great benefit for the parents of anencephalics, knowing that some good can come of an otherwise tragic situation. Part of the benefit for parents is recognizing that the neurological damage is so overwhelmingly severe and readily apparent by merely looking at the infant that they can justify organ donation and thus receive solace and consolation.

4. There is value for health-care professionals in knowing that recipients and also parents of the donors can benefit, bringing some meaning to a hopeless condition.

5. Organ donation in these situations is good for society in terms of saving lives and decreasing costs—although one could argue that society cannot afford to pay for unlimited organ donation and that money and time spent on transplantation could be more wisely allocated elsewhere.

4. PERSPECTIVE, CONCERNS, QUESTIONS

Even in the face of these overwhelmingly persuasive pragmatic reasons justifying the practice of organ donation in anencephalic infants, however, it is important to place this practice in a broader perspective. What is disturbing to note, for example, is that, in the cases reported in the medical literature and in my conversations with numerous physicians involved in the care of these infants, there seems to be little discussion and very little apparent awareness, until recently, of the substantial moral–legal issues raised by this practice.

The use of anencephalics as organ donors is a major leap forward, crossing a line that has not been crossed before—the removal of vital organs from living persons for purposes of transplantation. This practice, even though it may be permissible, is medically, morally, and legally unprecedented. It will have significant impact on the active euthanasia debate and on fetal therapy and experimentation as well as on other major controversial issues. The moral significance of this step forward (or backward, in the minds of many) should not be taken lightly, even by those in favor of the practice.

The moral and legal status of anencephalics is closely linked to the status of permanently unconscious patients in general. There needs to be a major medical and public policy debate over the rights and interests of permanently unconscious patients in general. As part of this broad debate, we should address the similarities and differences between anencephalics and persistent vegetative state patients (Cranford, 1984).

Three major medical distinctions exist between anencephalics and patients in a persistent vegetative state:

1. In anencephalics, the damage to the brain is not only disastrous, but easily recognizable and diagnosable by clinicians, and readily observable to parents and laypersons.
2. The diagnosis of anencephaly by AFP and ultrasound *in utero,* and by clinical observation at birth is essentially 100% accurate.
3. Anencephalics, unlike persistent vegetative state patients, are truly dying. Most die within a matter of minutes, hours, or days.

To argue that anencephalic infants or other forms of permanently unconscious patients are dead in the same sense as cardiorespiratory or whole-brain-dead patients is a radical departure from our traditional understanding of death, as noted by Capron and others (Blakeslee, 1986).

Furthermore, removing vital organs such as heart, lungs, liver, or both kidneys from anencephalic infants is the proximate cause of death—even though these infants are permanently unconscious and truly dying. To justify a policy that stopping treatment in these patients is permissible is one thing; to remove vital organs or to give a lethal injection, both inherently lethal, is a horse of a different moral color. There is no medical–moral consensus concerning the morality of using anencephalics as organ donors, but the traditional case and statutory law seems clear—such an action would currently be construed as homicide. It may be that, as we begin to develop a consensus, and as these cases are challenged in court, judges and juries will find this is a form of justifiable homicide or, if anencephalic infants are classified as dead or in some other category of neither alive or dead, it will not be possible to kill something that is already dead, or not living, or not a person. But the fact remains that by any reasonable interpretation, removing vital organs from living persons—even those who are permanently unconscious and dying—can only be construed as directly causing death.

The medical practice and public policy situation here is roughly analogous to the medical practice of active euthanasia. In both situations, there is no consensus as to what is medically or morally justifiable, but the laws are clear (at least in theory) that physicians performing these practices will run the risk of criminal prosecution and public censure. There is no guarantee whatsoever, or reasonable probability, as to what either prosecuting attorneys will do or judges and juries will decide when these cases are brought to their attention—and rightly so, as no reasonable medical or societal consensus exists in either circumstance. Also, the idea of removing vital organs from anencephalic infants while these children are still alive (even though permanently unconscious and unable to suffer) may offend our moral and emotional sensibilities.

In my opinion, the only way to handle this dilemma is to be up front about what we are doing, even if we run the chance of temporarily offending moral and emotional sensibilities. In the short run there will, and perhaps should, be a strong public reaction to this practice. To achieve the greatest possible good by minimizing warm ischemia time, hence the possibility of irreparable damage to organs, and to be honest about what we are doing, the only morally permissible and medically feasible way of managing these infants when removing organs is to continue maximal treatment and transfer the infants to the operating room, where they are given muscle relaxants. After organs are removed, treatment is stopped. From a purely objective standpoint, it would not be necessary to give anesthesia, since the infant is not capable of pain and suffering, but often it is emotionally disturbing to health-care providers and others not to give anesthesia in this context, even though it is medically irrational to do so. Handling cases in this manner would make it fairly obvious what we are doing; that is, causing the death of the infant by the removal of vital organs. Apparently many, not ready to face this fact and the moral dilemmas it presents, continue to manage these cases in a more surreptitious manner, such as devising new and "creative" ways of diagnosing brain death; these practices are to be condemned. If the most appropriate way of medically managing the removal of organs from these infants cannot be explained to the public and satisfactorily defended, it should not be done at all.

What will be the impact of the newer *in utero* diagnostic studies, such as AFP and ultrasound, when the diagnosis can be made sooner and more often and when ultrasound becomes routine? What will be the frequency of live anencephalic births if ultrasound is made a routine procedure during pregnancy in the United States (as it appears to be headed in that direction), and if there is more education of the public concerning the severity of the deficit in the anencephalic infant? If this is a situation in which most parents would opt for abortion when they find out their infant is anencephalic, this would markedly decrease the number of anencephalics born alive and could make the whole issue of anencephalics as organ donors relatively moot.

5. RECOMMENDATIONS AND COMMENTS

After my review of the medical literature, consideration of the facts and of the moral and legal issues, discussions with numerous professionals involved in this area, and further reflection, here are some of my preliminary recommendations:

1. The continued use of anencephalics as organ donors cannot be justified unless there is a commitment by the medical profession to a full-fledged debate on the relevant medical–moral–legal issues and unless physicians are willing to conduct this practice in a more open and consistent manner. If this practice is eventually accepted, the medical profession and society have crossed a new threshold. The practice of using anencephalics as organ donors, i.e., the removal of vital organs for purposes of transplantation, causing the death of patients, is medically, morally, and legally unprecedented.

2. The debate over the moral permissibility of the practice of anencephalics as organ donors cannot be easily distinguished and isolated from other related moral dilemmas, especially the status of permanently unconscious patients. Part of this dialogue involves showing the similarities and differences between anencephalics and other forms of permanently unconscious patients, such as those in a persistent vegetative state. Other major issues at the beginning of life include the changing views on abortion, the treatment of seriously ill newborns and the Baby Doe laws, and the much broader and probably more significant issue of fetal organ and tissue donation. Thus, the practice of anencephalics as organ donors cannot, and should not, be viewed in a narrow perspective, although some would strongly argue that anencephalics, because of the severity of the defect and the accuracy of the diagnosis, should be treated separately from all other medical syndromes, including other forms of permanently unconscious patients, such as those in a persistent vegetative state.

3. In the near future, anencephalics and other forms of permanently unconscious patients will probably be viewed as a category separate from the living and from the dead. The merits of arguments for and against this unique position should be brought forward and

publicly debated. To attempt to label anencephalics as dead and then work backward to justify and rationalize one's position retrospectively seems counterproductive; moreover, it is wrong. Attempts to include anencephalics and other permanently unconscious patients under the Uniform Determination of Death Act (UDDA) are simplistic and misguided and should be strongly discouraged (Blakeslee, 1986; Parachini, 1986; Giannelli, 1987). The only reasonable and socially justifiable way of legally sanctioning this highly controversial practice would be either to amend the Uniform Anatomical Gift Act to include anencephalics (and perhaps other permanently unconscious patients) for the purposes of organ donation or to create an entirely new moral and legal category separate from the living and the dead and then allow for organ donation in this class of patients.

4. The medical profession should take an active leadership role in this debate and not view it as a narrow debate on the use of anencephalics as organ donors. National medical societies in the neurological sciences, such as the Child Neurology Society and the American Academy of Neurology, have a compelling obligation to study these issues and begin to develop positions—in other words, to truly act as leaders. Legal norms will, and should, follow evolving reasonable standards of medical practice, not the reverse. That is what happened with the whole-brain-death issue, and it is what should happen here. Public trust and confidence are at stake here, and physicians and other health-care professionals should be willing to face (and lead the discussion of) the extremely difficult value judgments that lie ahead.

5. Health-care institutions, through institutional ethics committees or other means, should begin to develop practices and written policies to balance the rights and needs of all concerned parties and to minimize the possibility of abuses and untoward implications for other patients. These policies would include, for example, evaluation of appropriate surrogates, as well as the intentions and motivations of parents and surrogates, so as to limit the possibilities of conflicts of interest and abuses.

6. In the final analysis, the benefits of a medical and social policy supporting the practice of anencephalics as organ donors probably will, and should, prevail over the risks and implications. One can develop a plausible and strong argument that anencephalics should be used as organ donors under appropriate circumstances, notwithstanding the substantial moral implications.

7. At some point in the ongoing debate and evolution of this issue, health-care professionals and others will need to bring about changes in attitude and public policy by retrieving organs from anencephalics in an open fashion, running the risk of adverse publicity and criminal prosecution. It is hoped that, when this is accomplished, they will receive the support of medical colleagues and others who will defend this practice while raising the broader issues that need to be considered.

REFERENCES

Blakeslee, S., 1986, Law thwarts effort to donate infants' organs, *New York Times* Sept. 9, 19–20.
Caplan, A., 1987, Should fetuses or infants be utilized as organ donors?, *Bioethics* **1**(2):119–140.
Capron, A. M., 1987, Anencephalic donors: Separate the dead from the dying, *Hastings Ctr. Rep.* **17**(1): 5–9.
Chervenak, F. A., Farley, M. A., Walters, L., Hobbins, J. C., and Mahoney, M. J., 1984, When is termination of pregnancy during the third trimester morally justifiable?, *N. Engl. J. Med.* **310**:501–504.
Cranford, R. E., 1984, Termination of treatment in the persistent vegetative state, *Semin. Neurol.* **4**:36–44.
Fine, R. N., Korsch, B. M., Stiles, Q., Riddell, H., Edelbrock, H. H., Brennan, P., Grushkin, C. M., and Lieberman, E., 1970, Renal homotransplantation in children, *J. Pediatr.* **76**:347–357.

Fletcher, J. E., Robertson, J. R., and Harrison, M. R., 1986, Primates and anencephalics as sources for pediatric organ transplants: Medical, legal, and ethical issues, *Fetal Ther.* **1**:150–164.

Gianelli, D., 1987, Anencephalic infant moral dilemma, *Amer. Med. News* April 17, 2–32.

Harrison, M. R., 1986*a*, The anencephalic newborn as organ donor: Commentary, *Hastings Ctr. Rep.* **16**(2): 21–23.

Harrison, M. R., 1986*b*, Organ procurement for children: The anencephalic fetus as donor, *Lancet* pp. 1383–1385.

Iitaka, K., Martin, L. W., Cox, J. A., McEnery, P. T., and West, C. D., 1978, Transplantation of cadaver kidneys from anencephalic donors, *J. Pediatr.* **83**:216–220.

King, L. R., Gerbie, A. G., Idruss, F. S., Swenson, O., Siegel, Alan, DelGreco, F., Grayhack, J., Gross, M., Gonzales, E., and Stolpe, Y., 1971, Human renal transplantation with kidney grafts from the newborn, *Invest. Urol.* **8**:622–628.

LaPlant, M. P., Kaufman, J. J., Goldman, R., Gonick, H. C., Martin, D. C., and Goodwin, W. E., 1970, Kidney transplantation in children, *Pediatrics* **46**:665–677.

Lawson, R. K., Bennett, W. M., Campbell, R. A., Pirofsky, B., and Hodges, C. V., 1973, Hyperacute renal allograft rejection in the human neonate, *Invest. Urol.* **10**:444–449.

Martin, L. W., Gonzales, L. L., West, C. D., Swartz, R. A., and Sutorius, D. J., 1969, Homotransplantation of both kidneys from an anencephalic monster to a 17 lbs boy with Eagle–Barrett syndrome, *Surgery* **66**:603–607.

Nakano, K. K., Anencephaly: A review, *Dev. Med. Child Neurol.* **15**:383–400.

Ohshima, S., Ono, Y., Kinukawa, T., Matsuura, O., Tsuzuki, K., and Itoh, S., 1984, Kidney transplantation from an anencephalic baby: A case report, *J. Urol.* **132**:546–547.

Parachini, A., 1986, Science, ethics clash over infant organ donations bill, *L. A. Times* Dec. 2.

Potter, D., Belzer, F. O., Rames, L., Holliday, M. A., Kountz, S. L., and Najarian, J. S., 1970, The treatment of chronic uremia in childhood I transplantation, *Pediatrics* **45**:432–443.

Salvatierra, O., and Belzer, F. O., 1975, Pediatric cadaver kidneys: Their use in renal transplantation, *Arch. Surg.* **110**:181–183.

Schneider, J. R., Sutherland, D. E. R., Simmons, R. L., Fryd, D. S., and Najarian, J. S., 1983, Long-term success with double pediatric cadaver donor renal transplants, *Ann. Surg.* **197**:439–442.

21

RELAXING THE DEATH STANDARD FOR ORGAN DONATION IN PEDIATRIC SITUATIONS

JOHN A. ROBERTSON

1. INTRODUCTION

A major ethical and legal constraint in organ procurement is the requirement that organs be removed only from dead patients. Although kidneys and bone marrow are obtained from living donors, the dead donor rule controls the procurement of hearts, livers, and most kidneys. Brain-death tests of death permit the removal of these organs from heart-beating but brain-dead sources.

The shortage of pediatric organs for transplant now forces us to consider whether the dead donor rule should be strictly adhered to in all circumstances. Several situations arise in which viable organs could be obtained from persons who are irreversibly comatose and near death but who do not yet satisfy criteria of brain death. One such situation concerns pediatric patients who appear to be brain dead but, because of the uncertainty of brain death diagnosis in infants and children, have not been used as cadaveric organ sources. Similarly, anencephalic newborns cannot now be sources of organs for transplant, since they still have brainstem function.

Since our voluntary system of organ procurement depends crucially on public confidence that organ donation does not harm or slight the interests of donors, it is with much trepidation that I raise the question of altering the dead donor rule in order to facilitate organ procurement. The taboo against using nondead donors is so strong that any discussion of altering the rule could stimulate fears (reflected in novels and films such as *Coma*) that organs will be taken from vulnerable living patients and thus discourage organ donation.

Yet the needs of children with end-stage organ disease and of parents faced with near-brain-dead infants present a strong case for assessing the merits of continued adherence to the dead donor rule. The potential use of anencephalic newborns as organ sources illustrates the need for such a reassessment.

The 2000–3000 anencephalic infants born each year could be an important source of organs for a variety of perinatal and pediatric conditions, possibly saving the life of infants who would otherwise die. Parents of anencephalics are increasingly requesting that their organs be used for transplant. If anencephalic infants are to be a source of viable organs, it may be necessary to

JOHN A. ROBERTSON • School of Law, University of Texas at Austin, Austin, Texas 78705.

remove organs before brain stem function ceases. Yet since brainstem function remains, anencephalics are not yet legally brain dead and could not be used under existing law. The dead donor rule would have to be changed to permit use of anencephalic organs (Harrison et al., 1986).

Given the great value of anencephalic organs to recipients and their families, and the meaning that the parents of anencephalic newborns would derive from donation, it is appropriate to examine more closely the reasons for adherence to this rule in the case of anencephaly and other situations of near death.

2. LIMITING CONDITIONS FOR RELAXING THE DEAD DONOR RULE

To highlight the core value issues, let us consider a situation that meets the following restrictive conditions. First, the family has freely and knowingly consented to the donation and have on their own requested that their anencephalic child's organs be donated to other needy children so that some good may emerge from their own personal tragedy. Their attending physician has had no part in their discussion of donation with organ procurement and transplant personnel.

Second, organ removal before total brain death is the only way to ensure a viable heart, liver, or kidney for transplant. If waiting for the cessation of brainstem function will permit use of the organs, there is no need to violate or change the dead donor rule. In the situation envisaged, however, this alternative does not exist.

Third, the use of the anencephalic organ is essential to save the life of the prospective pediatric recipient. Sufficient research has occurred to establish that transplant of the anencephalic heart, liver, or kidney is a safe and effective therapy for the recipient, and will enable him or her to have an otherwise normal life. No other organs are available, and temporary therapies are no longer efficacious.

Fourth, the diagnosis of anencephaly is accurate to a high degree of medical certainty. The diagnosis has been made according to a consensus protocol agreed on by leading medical experts in the field. Three physicians have confirmed that the potential donor clearly fits the diagnostic category.

If these four conditions are met, should removal of the anencephalic organs before brainstem function ceases be permitted? That is, should the dead donor rule—a legal requirement that would bar use of anencephalic organs before brainstem function ceases—be relaxed in this situation to permit the desired organ donation and transplant to occur?

A change in the law to permit the use of anencephalic organs in this situation could occur in one of two ways. The law could be changed by redefining brain death to mean cortical or upper brain death rather than the total absence of brain activity, including brainstem activity, as the law now states. For example, Veatch and others have argued for a redefinition of brain death as cortical death, thereby preserving the rule that only dead persons may be an organ source (Veatch, 1975).

An alternative approach would keep brain death as total brain death and address directly the legality of relaxing or altering the dead donor rule in the situation described above. If the dead donor rule is to be altered, this approach would seem to be preferable. As Alexander Capron (1987) has pointed out, "adding anencephalics to the category of dead persons would be a radical change, both in the social and medical understanding of what it means to be dead and in the social practices surrounding death." Relaxing the dead donor rule will also have complications, but they will be fewer than would occur through reaching the same result by redefining death.

What then are the arguments against relaxing the rule in these cases? Two concerns—the interests of the donor and the interests of others and society—need analysis.

3.   THE DEAD DONOR RULE AND HARM TO THE ORGAN SOURCE

A major reason for the requirement that the organ donor be dead is to protect the donor from being harmed by organ removal. If the donor is dead, taking his organs will not harm him. By contrast, if he is alive, it is assumed that removing organs will kill or otherwise injure him.

This view of the dead donor rule, however, assumes that the live donor has interests in continued living and in not being physically injured. While this assumption is true in most instances and should thus be strictly followed, it may not apply to situations of irreversible coma, near-dead pediatric patients, and anencephalics.

Such patients, although legally still alive, may no longer have interests to be respected in living or in avoiding physical harm. Consider first the situation in which an organ or tissue is removed without causing brain death, as would occur with removal of bone marrow or a kidney for transplant from an anencephalic newborn. Such infants are not sentient and thus would not be harmed by the surgical intrusion. Indeed, even removing a kidney would not harm the source. Such patients lack interests that can be harmed by nonlethal organ or tissue removal.

A similar conclusion should follow even if organ retrieval directly caused death, as would occur if the heart or liver were taken from an anencephalic newborn to transplant to another infant. It is widely accepted that all sustaining medical treatments, including nutrition and hydration, can be withheld from anencephalic patients. (Baby Doe Regulations, 1985). Since they will not recover and while still alive have none of the experiences that make living a good for them, it may be reasonably be said that they have no further interest in living. Therefore, they may be allowed to die by having treatment withheld. Indeed, some persons would recognize a societal duty or moral obligation to withhold treatment in order that they might die.

If anencephalic infants have no interest in living and thus no right to be treated, it is unclear how actively causing their death by organ removal injures them any more than would passive killing by withholding treatment. Active killing by organ removal neither harms the anencephalic infant nor violates its right to life, since it has no further interest in living, hence would no longer have a right to life. Thus, concern for the rights and welfare of the organ source cannot justify the dead donor rule with anencephalic organ sources. In arguing against the use of anencephalic donors because they are "the most vulnerable patients," Professor Capron assumes without analysis that they have interests to protect, when that is the very issue that needs to be addressed (Capron, 1987).

Some persons might argue, however, that anencephalic infants still have an interest in being treated with dignity and with respect, and that removing their organs or tissue before death violates the dignity or respect owed all living human subjects. Indeed, the law would still treat them as legal subjects and might treat organ removal causing brain death as homicide. Yet if anencephalics lack all cognitive capacity, have no interest in further living, and are insensate, it is difficult to see how they retain an interest in being treated with dignity or retain other interests that the law should protect. Cortical death with some remaining brainstem function deprives them of all interests, including the interest in being treated with dignity.

In sum, viewing the matter from the perspective of the anencephalic patient, it is difficult to see how their interests can be harmed by tissue or organ removal before total brain death. It may be that these patients are still legally alive, but a requirement that they be dead before organ removal cannot be justified as necessary to protect their interests. Anencephalics fall into the class of living human entities who lack interests that must be protected. Protecting their interests does not justify foreclosing this source of organ donations in the situations described.

The need to treat vulnerable incompetent patients with dignity and respect is an important societal or community concern. But it is a concern of society—of other persons—and not of the irreversibly comatose or near-dead patient himself. Societal interests, rather than the interests of the cortically dead but living patient, must then be examined to understand the dead donor rule.

4. HARM TO OTHERS AND THE DEAD DONOR RULE

Surely society has an interest in how we treat near-dead but living persons, even if those persons no longer have interests that require protection. Two kinds of societal interests exist in such situations.

4.1. Slippery Slopes and Loose Categories

A major societal concern in such near-death situations is restricting the proposed practice to organ sources who clearly lack interests at the time of removal, thereby preventing the practice from spilling over to incompetent patients who retain interests in avoiding pain, death and undignified treatment.

Although often presented as a slippery slope problem, this concern is more accurately viewed as a problem of loose categorization. The danger in accepting a category of living human subjects who lack interests and thus may be used as an organ source is that this category will not be defined carefully and strictly enough to confine the practice to those for whom it is justified.

The danger here is not that we will become so inured to removing organs from live persons that anyone in the hospital will become fair game for the organ procurement team. Rather, the danger is that the category will defy strict specification and spill over to less clear cases. These cases might include persons who have real interests in avoiding pain and in staying alive, even though they have severely diminished capacities and are not competent to make choices concerning their treatment. If taking organs before death from some clear cases will inevitably lead to removal in nonjustifiable cases, the interest of those persons who are erroneously included in the category argues against it.

While the risk of loose and inaccurate categories cannot be ignored, the power of this concern depends on how likely the risk is. No program of removing organs from near-dead persons should begin until this danger has been thoroughly examined and negated, as the restrictive conditions set out above attempt to do. It may be that the categories can be defined strictly enough to dispose of this risk. For example, better tests of pediatric brain death will greatly reduce the risk that near-dead infants with valid interests will be used as organ sources. Similarly, criteria for defining anencephaly can also be tightened and diagnostic safeguards built in to ensure that it is a true case of anencephaly rather than a case of microcephaly, hydranencephaly, or other conditions that do not justify similar treatment to anencephaly. The mere risk of error and mistake should not prevent such schemes if reasonably tight safeguards and procedures for applying the criteria have been adopted any more than the risk of misdiagnosis prevents taking organs from brain-dead adults.

4.2. Use as a Mere Means: Taking Organs without Causing Death

A second major societal concern arises from the symbolic or cultural meaning of using people in this way. This concern has two components: (1) the mere use of the incompetent as means to the utility of others, which arises whether or not organ removal causes the organ source's death; and (2) that which arises when procurement itself actively causes the death of the organ source.

The first aspect of this symbolic concern is the violation of human dignity that some persons perceive in any use of a living human subject to advance the good or interest of others. Although the organ source has no interests being harmed, it appears that he or she is being used as a means to the good of others. In this instance, the good advanced is that of the recipient and his or her family and that of the family who requests that the organs be used.

Some persons would object to the use of anencephalic or other near-dead subjects in this way, since it appears to denigrate their worth and to exhibit a crass willingness to use others as a mere means. Treating near-dead subjects as organ sources, even with the consent of the family, might be perceived as a violation of community norms of respect for persons.

Such objections arise frequently in medical ethical discussions. They reflect a principle of Kantian ethics that makes some sense when applied to rational, autonomous beings, if the consent of those beings to the use is missing (Singer and Kuhse, 1987). However, it is not a compelling objection (other than in some symbolic sense) when the subject used is not harmed by the intervention in question. Indeed, established practices in a wide variety of circumstances show societal willingness to use both competent and incompetent subjects to advance the interests of others. The key ethical question in such cases is whether a competent patient has consented to such use or, if incompetent to decide, whether the use harms or benefits the subject.

The debate over the use of children who are incompetent to consent in research illustrates the issue. The policy position that emerged from the famous McCormick–Ramsey debate was that children could, with parental consent, be used in research that might benefit them or, if no therapeutic benefit was likely, research that posed minimal risk (Harrison, 1986). The mere fact of use to aid others was deemed ethically acceptable if no harm to the subject would occur and a benefit to others could be shown. Similarly, bone marrow and kidneys may be taken from children and incompetent patients if they derive a net benefit from the donation, e.g., are not harmed (Robertson, 1976).

The important question is not the use of one patient for the good of others, but the circumstances of the use. Even if we recognize some constraints on such use, we cannot and should not forbid all such uses. The question is whether the use is respectful and justified. When parents find meaning in donating organs at a time of tragedy from an infant who is not harmed by the donation and another person and family gain immeasurably, one may reasonably view the entire transaction as respectful of human needs and dignity, even though a nonconsenting subject is used as a means to the good of others. A contrary view may motivate persons not to donate or accept such organs, but it does not suffice to ban the practice in the restrictive conditions described above.

4.3. Symbolic Concerns in Actively Causing Death

The symbolic concern with actively causing death to obtain organs from near dead persons who lack interests poses a more difficult problem than merely using the near dead subject as a means for the good of others. Although they lack interests in further living and thus are not harmed by organ removal, the prohibition against active killing is violated.

The importance of this threshold is evident in developing norms and practices for withholding life-sustaining treatment. While withholding life-sustaining treatment is now medically, ethically, and legally accepted when the patient consents or, if incompetent, ceases to have further interest in living, a firm line in favor of passive and against active euthanasia exists (Robertson, 1983). Active killing is legally proscribed, even when a fully informed competent patient requests it in order to avoid severe pain.

The concerns behind maintaining the firm line against active euthanasia involve slippery slope and category spillover of the kind discussed earlier But even if those concerns could be assuaged, the symbolic costs of permitting active killing in a medical setting would remain. Legalization of active killing might symbolize a weakening of the societal commitment to respect all human life and the prohibition against taking life. The ferocity of the abortion debate illustrates the strength of such a commitment as well as the need to hold the line even more firmly in other settings. Yet once we see that when the patient lacks interests, that line is a symbolic or constitutive commitment and not a matter of rights or obligations of justice, we can ask whether the symbolic gains are always so great that the loss of benefits to persons in deviating from it is justifiable.

Despite the firmness of the norm against active killing, some breaches have been accepted in certain exceptional circumstances. For example, certain practices with dying patients that hasten death are widely accepted. Administration of opiates that depress respiration in terminally ill patients is justified by the specific intent to relieve pain, even though such drugs might actively hasten death.

Consider also the common practice in organ procurement of shifting management of a patient at a certain point from saving the donor's life to preserving his organs for transplant. The therapy designed to save life by withholding fluids to minimize brain swelling and herniation suddenly shifts when further treatment is considered hopeless and fluids are aggressively pushed to ensure perfusion of the organs to preserve their viability for use in transplantation (Pittsburgh Transplant Foundation, 1984). Such shift in management actively hastens brain death, yet it occurs in a patient who no longer has any meaningful interests. While not yet widely known or debated, it is likely that such a practice would be accepted. The symbolic loss is small, and the benefits to recipients and society are great.

Although the line against active killing should be staunchly maintained, it is not clear that it need be absolute. Situations testing this line will increasingly occur, as the present situation shows. Once we protect the interests of persons at risk, however, the symbolic costs and benefits of maintaining or deviating from the line must be addressed. In the restrictive circumstances that I have assumed, a reasonable argument for recognizing an exception to the rule against active killing (hence the dead donor rule) can be made.

Whether other pediatric and adult situations would also qualify requires further study. Each situation has to be examined on its own terms, once the symbolic barrier ceases to be absolute. The question for policymakers in each case should be whether the benefits of maintaining this symbolic line outweigh the benefits to others of breaching it. When carefully addressed in these terms, few cases may qualify for the exception, although an occasional situation, such as relaxing the dead donor rule for anencephalic organ sources, might be identified. Good ethical analysis thus may enable us to keep the rule without losing the benefits that accrue from a few narrow deviations from it.

5. CONCLUSION

We have seen that the arguments against tissue and organ retrieval from patients who are not yet brain dead cannot easily be sustained on grounds of preventing harm to the organ source. The central concern is that others will be hurt by loose categories and slippery slopes or, more likely, by the discomfort at openly recognizing that near dead persons are actively being killed to obtain organs. In the final analysis, the concern is a symbolic rather than a patient rights concern. But symbols are sources of meaning and constitute the moral nature of the community. They have a substantive weight of their own, even if the organ source's rights or welfare are not implicated and thus cannot easily be ignored.

A crucial difference between symbolic and rights concerns is that the former may be more easily traded off than the latter. The community may not override the rights of persons, but it may, if persuaded of the wisdom of doing so, alter its investment in key symbols. Without violating rules of justice or obligations to persons, the community may choose to give meaning to grieving families and life to needy transplant recipients at the price of loosening the barrier against active killing.

With organ removal from near-dead pediatric patients and anencephalics, the issue between utility and symbolic concerns is squarely posed. If the very restrictive conditions described above are satisfied, a good case for relaxing the dead donor rule exists.

However, those restrictive conditions probably cannot be satisfied, as too much is still experimental and unknown in pediatric transplantation to make the case for giving up the symbolic benefits of the dead donor rule. (Experimental use of anencephalic organs may also be premature.) Furthermore, it has not yet been clearly established that anencephalic organs would be nonviable when brain stem function ceases or that preservation options such as cooling of the dying anencephalic would not preserve organs. As with many medical–ethical dilemmas, it appears that the factual array that would make otherwise unethical actions ethical often cannot be met.

But the current difficulty in satisfying these conditions should not blind us to the nature of the conflict and the possibility of meeting the conditions in the future. Indeed, a separate issue is whether the same restrictions should be met to justify nonlethal donations of bone marrow and kidneys from anencephalics. If organ removal does not itself cause death, the symbolic costs of using anencephalic organs are lessened and may be justified in circumstances that would not justify lethal organ removal. Symbolic costs, however, will remain and will continue to require compelling justification, such as a last resort for the needy patient, even if the standard of efficacy that might justify active killing could not be met. Thus, it may be ethical to begin experimental use of anencephalic kidneys, which can be obtained without actively causing the source's death, even if removal of hearts and livers cannot now be justified.

Until more certain benefit from relaxation of the dead donor rule can be established, this important threshold—although rooted in symbolic rather than rights concerns—should be staunchly maintained. The problem of pediatric organ supply, however, will continue to focus attention on these issues and require us to compare the symbolic costs and the gains to recipients and families of a change in the dead donor rule in certain narrow circumstances. There may be a time when such a change is desirable.

REFERENCES

Baby Doe Regulations, 1985.

Capron, A. M., 1987, Anencephalic donors: Separate the dead from the dying, *Hastings Cent. Rep.* **17**(1): 5–9.

Harrison, M. R., 1986, The anencephalic as organ donor, *Hastings Cent. Rep.* **16**(2):21–3.

Harrison, M. R., Robertson, J. A., and Fletcher, J., 1986, Animals and anencephalics as pediatric organ sources, *J. Fetal Ther.* **1**:150–164.

Pittsburgh Transplant Foundation, 1984, Post Mortem Organ Procurement Protocol, Pittsburgh.

Robertson, J. A., 1976, The substituted judgment doctrine and organ donations from incompetent patients, *Col. Law Rev.* **45**:59–80.

Robertson, J. A., 1983, *The Rights of the Critically Ill,* pp. 92–94, Ballinger Press: Cambridge, MA.

Singer, P., and Kuhse, H., 1986, The ethics of embryo research, *Law Med. Health Care* **14**:137–139.

Veatch, R. W., 1975, The whole-brain oriented concept of death: An outmoded philosophical formulation, *J. Thanatol.* **3**:13–17.

22

THE DEFINITION OF DEATH
Unresolved Controversies

ROBERT M. VEATCH

1. THE CONCEPT OF DEATH

During the 1970s, as states rapidly adopted brain criteria for pronouncing death, many believed that the definition of death debate would soon be over. A few romantics would hold onto the heart as the critical organ for considering a person alive, but they would be overpowered by more reasonable people oriented to the brain as the locus for determining whether a person was dead. Eventually those committed to the respiratory and circulatory function would die off, and a wide-spread consensus would dominate public policy.

Now, 20 years after the meetings of the Harvard Ad Hoc Committee, substantial (but not total) consensus exists at the legal level. At the same time, the issue remains one of lively debate and controversy. Even more telling, just beneath the surface there appears to remain substantial confusion and ambiguity. It is measured in statements by highly educated professionals as well as laypersons about people who are simultaneously "brain dead and about to die," about physicians with patients they consider "brain-dead" who ask families for permission to turn off life supports so the patient can die, and about "brain-dead" people who retain brain stem function so that they live for years.

All these statements represent a continuing imprecision in our use of language, but also lingering doubt about exactly what it means to be dead. It should be clear, after the years of debate, that, insofar as we are engaged in public policy discourse, we are dealing with the questions of when persons should be treated the way our society normally treats the dead: when they should be treated as corpses, when the burial process should be initiated, when wills should be read, when health insurance payments should cease and life insurance payments be made, when grief should begin, when vice-presidents should succeed to the presidency, as well as when organs may be removed for transplantation.

ROBERT M. VEATCH • Kennedy Institute of Ethics, Georgetown University, Washington, D.C. 20057.

2.   DEATH OF THE PERSON AS A WHOLE

It should be clear that we are only interested in the death of the person as a whole. We are not interested in the death of body parts. This is one reason why the time has come to stop talking about "brain death" or "heart death." To be sure, individual organs do cease functioning irreversibly. Figuratively, we can say they "die," but that is both imprecise and linguistically confusing. It is imprecise because normally individual cells or tissues within organs can remain living long after the critical functions have been lost. It is imprecise also because it is really the functions that are critical, not the organs normally associated with those functions.

It is linguistically confusing because to use the now archaic term "brain death" can mean two radically different things. It can refer to the death of the person as a whole based on the irreversible loss of brain function together with the claim that that function is what is necessary for the person to function as a whole. By contrast, it can mean something quite different. It can mean the death of the organ in a person who may still be living (based on the belief that what makes the person "whole" still remains—the presence of the flowing of vital bodily fluids or, in religious frameworks, the presence of a soul). Brain death can mean both the death of the person based on brain function loss and the death of the brain in a still-living person. As such, the term is too confusing to be used any longer. It should be abandoned.

Even so, we still must answer the question of when a person should be treated as dead. Even the most conservative thinker agrees that some persons should be considered to have died even though some tissues or cells remain living. The critical question is one of philosophy and social policy. When should persons be considered dead, that is, when should they be considered to have lost whatever it is that makes them an integrated entity, a person-as-a-whole rather than a residual collection of living cells or tissues of a disintegrated being?

It should be clear that no amount of science can answer such a question. It is not a scientific question. This is not to say that there can be no objectively "right" answer to the definition of death question. Some problems in ethics may meaningfully be thought to have objectively correct answers. That genocide is wrong or that racism is wrong can usefully be thought of as being objectively true propositions. They are not true, however, because of any scientific proposition or any scientific discovery. If they are statements with truth value, it is because some ethical questions can meaningfully be thought of as being true or false, even though they are not questions lending themselves to scientific investigation.

The question "Should the patient be treated as dead?" is exactly like the question "Is it wrong to stop a life-sustaining treatment?" Changing the question to "Is the person really dead?" adds nothing more. It is analogous to asking "Is it really wrong to stop life-sustaining treatment in this patient?" A person may really be dead only in the sense that it is really wrong to stop the life-sustaining treatment or to practice genocide. Being dead, strange as it may seem, is not a biological state in any interesting policy sense. Having lost all cellular or all organ-level function is indeed a biological state about which biological scientists may have expertise, but diagnosing such conditions has virtually nothing to do with claims about persons being dead. By such formulations human life remains in isolated hair follicles, in perfused heart muscle, and in laboratory-stored frozen sperm cells.

3.   FOUR UNRESOLVED ISSUES IN PUBLIC POLICY

Even with the debate over the past two decades and the extensive legislative and judicial decision-making regarding the definition of death, several unresolved problems remain. The debate is unexpectedly intractable over at least four issues. These issues will arise invariably in decisions about declaration of death in pediatric cases. In fact, pediatric cases will often introduce special decisions to these controversies that need attention.

3.1. Values in Neurological Criteria for Loss of Brain Function

There is increasing recognition that the more technical question of how to measure the irreversible loss of function in the brain is a question that must be kept separate from the policy question of whether to treat as dead persons who have irreversibly lost brain function. This gives rise to a division of labor that is reflected in most state definition of death statutes. They generally take on only the policy task, authorizing, in fact requiring, death to be pronounced when there is irreversible loss of total brain function. In doing so, the statutes normally make clear that the determination that brain function has been irreversibly lost should be made on the basis of currently acceptable medical standards. This is because it is assumed that this is a technical neurological question that should be answered based on the most current scientific evidence and is a question that only those with neurological expertise can answer.

In fact, neurological scientists have over the years come up with several sets of criteria (Harvard Medical School, 1968; President's Commission for the Study of Ethical Problems in Medicine and Biomedical and Behavioral Research, 1981; Mohandas and Chou, 1971; Walker *et al.*, 1977). It is assumed that good scientists should, in principle, be able to construct sets of criteria such as these (as opposed to answering the broader policy question) without drawing on their personally held beliefs and values. This is a manifestation of what philosophers would call the fact/value dichotomy (Kohler, 1966; Hudson, 1969).

While this works as a simplified version of the story, unfortunately it will probably not be adequate for more subtle analysis, especially for cases involving pediatric decisions. It is increasingly recognized that the distinction between scientific judgments and value judgments cannot be rigidly maintained (Kuhn, 1962; Popper, 1968; Veatch, 1976b). It has always been recognized that, in fact, scientists attempting to answer a scientific question such as when brain function is irreversibly lost will be influenced by their personal values. Those standing in moral or religious traditions committed to the legitimacy of considering persons with irreversible loss of brain function dead will be more inclined to accept the enterprise of constructing criteria for brain function loss and to accept the conclusion that a particular set of tests measures the functional loss. Personal biases do, in fact, influence the scientific enterprise, but many standard procedures are available to minimize these influences. It is normally held that the ideal is to eliminate them completely. While that ideal cannot be achieved, we should try to get as close as possible.

Recently, however, there has been a shift in the argument. Some are claiming that the scientific enterprise and the process of reporting scientific conclusions inevitably must incorporate evaluative judgments. Out of an infinite number of observations that an observer might make, he or she should report only the important ones, and deciding which ones are important is an evaluative task. The very conceptualization of what is observed requires a use of concepts and terms that can not be independent of cultural and linguistic conventions that are in turn dependent on systems of beliefs and values. Most importantly, deciding what is worth reporting and what conclusions to draw is necessarily evaluative.

In particular, concluding that there is adequate evidence that a function is irreversibly lost will depend on the kinds of risks perceived to be at stake. Consider the various sets of neurological criteria for irreversible loss of brain function. Among the countless decisions that must be made is a determination of how often and over how long a period the tests must be repeated before concluding that someone has irreversibly lost function. The Harvard criteria called for a period of 24 hr (Harvard Medical School, 1968). The Minnesota criteria call for a 12-hr testing period (Mohandas and Chou, 1971). The more recent reports of the National Institute of Neurological and Communicative Disorders and Stroke (Walker, 1977) and of the consultants to the President's Commission (President's Commission for the Study of Ethical Problems in Medicine and Biomedical and Behavioral Research, 1981) call for testing periods of 6 hr.

Some of this difference can be accounted for by some scientific advances and additional data that have become available over the years. However, much of the difference is simply a matter of how willing various commentators are to risk different types of errors. Anyone deciding on criteria for irreversible loss of brain function must consider two types of errors: (1) erroneously concluding that brain function has been lost when it has not been, and (2) erroneously concluding it has not been lost when it has.

At first it would seem that the first kind of error is the more serious and that it should be avoided at all costs. Assuming there is legal authorization to pronounce death based on loss of brain function, that error would lead to pronouncing someone dead who really is not. The policy of avoiding error at all costs is not practical, however. Presumably, repeating the tests over a longer period will be safer. If one were literally only concerned about falsely pronouncing death, the period for repeating the tests could be made much, much longer. It could be weeks or longer.

There are also serious moral risks in treating dead people as alive, just as there are moral risks in treating living people as dead. Organs for transplant will be lost, scarce resources will be used, and, most importantly, there will be an assault on the dignity of the deceased by confusing his corpse with his living self.

Although the criteria adopted must be quite safe in avoiding the error of falsely calling someone dead, there must be a reasonable compromise. They must avoid the error of treating dead persons as alive. Otherwise, we could simply revert to heart and lung criteria and completely avoid the moral and conceptual risk of using brain criteria. However, this compromise will require deciding how to balance these two types of moral risk. Choosing the correct length of time is nothing more than deciding what confidence level we want in concluding that function loss is irreversible, which is a moral decision about how to balance off two kinds of risks.

In pediatric cases, an analogous problem arises. Criteria that have been developed for adult patients will be applied to children only by making some assumptions. At least for a while the data will not be as solid as for the adult cases. A decision will have to be made about when the criteria are adequately enough tested to be used in cases involving children. That decision, although it sounds "purely scientific," in fact will be based on the values of those making the choice. It will be based on their assessment of the risk of considering a brain-damaged child dead when he is alive with serious brain damage and their assessment of the risk of considering a child alive when he is really dead.

For some people who really believe that seriously brain-damaged children (such as those in a persistent vegetative state (PVS)) should actually be treated as dead, there is virtually no (moral) risk in too rapid an adaptation of adult criteria to children. For those who consider a permanently vegetative life infinitely precious and to be preserved at all costs, but who consider the child with irreversible loss of all function dead, this error will be much more serious, and much more rigorous testing of criteria and much more rigorous criteria will be appropriate.

To make matters more complex, it is likely that people with neurological expertise, people who are going to be choosing criteria sets, are probably atypical on the moral and philosophical positions regarding when persons ought to be treated as dead. The data are not all in, but it is reasonable to assume that people who come from a very special sociological, economic, and educational group and who give their lives to clinical work relating to brain function probably have atypical ways of valuing brain function as opposed to heart and lung function. Whether they place more or less emphasis on the value of brain function, they will be atypical and will choose criteria sets based on those atypical values. Society will be getting those values when it accepts the "medically standard" criteria for what appears to be a scientific judgment.

3.2. Higher Brain and Whole-Brain Formulations

These moral and philosophical positions that influence selection of criteria for measuring brain function loss have even more direct bearing on the policy question: whether we ought to say regarding persons who have lost brain function that the person as a whole is dead. Since functions are lost at varying times, for any person some functions will have been lost while others remain. No one holds that all bodily functions must be lost for the person as a whole to be dead. On the other hand, no one holds that the person as a whole is dead whenever any function is lost.

For a decade or so, the debate was between those who held that circulatory and respiratory functions were critical for the person to be considered alive "as a whole" and those who held that brain function was critical. No one asked precisely which brain functions were critical for the person to be alive as a whole. Increasingly, we have recognized that not even all brain functions cease at precisely the same time. The common wisdom is that there should be loss of all brain function in order for the person to be treated as dead. Certainly not just the loss of some isolated function would be sufficient. But even when there is massive irreversible brain damage, all functions may not be lost.

Much more work needs to be done to identify exactly what functions can remain when the person as a whole is considered dead. It is not even obvious that it is functional loss that is critical. Some, including persons within the medical community, hold that it is not function but anatomical structure that is critical (Byrne *et al.*, 1979). It is crucial to realize that there is no scientific argument against that position. If someone wants to hold that persons are alive as long as the anatomical structure of the brain remains intact, there is no evidence that could be mounted to the contrary.

At another level, even among those who accept the claim that function is significant, it is important to realize that cellular level function will remain when all supercellular function has been lost. That explains why some criteria permit small electrical potentials to appear on an EEG when a person is said to have lost all brain function (Walker *et al.*, 1977). Clearly, at some level, some electrical activity is still present. If it is at the cellular level, so the argument goes, it is insignificant to the functioning of the person as a whole and therefore can be ignored.

The more difficult question is whether some supercellular functions may still be present when it is concluded that the person has lost that which is necessary to function as a whole. The first level of the problem arises when we decide whether to accept spinal reflexes as indicating a presence of crucial functioning of the central nervous system (CNS). Since the days of the Harvard Committee, Henry Beecher has argued that spinal activity does not count (Beecher, 1970). The reasoning here must be that even though spinal reflexes indicate CNS activity at the supercellular level that permits bodily integration over considerable distances, this should really not be enough to count as the body functioning "as a whole," that is, as an integrated activity with all its basic essential elements present.

Once the tenuous nature of the spinal reflex exclusion is recognized, it will be more important to ask similar questions about lower brainstem reflexes. Is there really anything more essential about a cough reflex or an eye-blink reflex just because it is mediated through the brainstem rather than the top of the spinal cord? If not, could it not be possible for a person to be considered to have lost what is essential to integrated functioning while an isolated supercellular brainstem-mediated reflex remains active?

If that is the case, we need to confront more directly exactly what it is that is essential. To many of us, especially those working within the Judeo-Christian tradition, a human does not function as a whole if there is no capacity for the integration of mental and bodily function (Engelhardt, 1975; Veatch, 1975; Haring, 1973). That, of course, is a philosophical or theological conclusion, but so is the conclusion that there is adequate integration of bodily function when brainstem reflexes are present, even though the capacity for consciousness is absent. For that matter, it is also a religious or philosophical conclusion when one holds that circulatory and respiratory integration is sufficient integration of bodily activity for a person to be treated as living as a whole.

The test case involves persons who have no future capacity for consciousness or social integration but who retain brainstem activities, including respiratory regulation. Patients in truly permanent vegetative states are in such a condition (Cranford and Smith, 1979; Jennett and Plum, 1972). So are cases reported by Brierley and colleagues (1971). In fact, if it could have been confirmed that Karen Quinlan's condition was truly one of irreversible unconsciousness (which it might have been), she would also have been ''dead'' based according to this notion that death is the loss of bodily integration of mental and physiological function.

This position is often called the cerebral or cortical or neocortical definition of death because it is assumed that these tissues are essential to the presence of consciousness or other mental activity (Brierley *et al.*, 1971). This term is not a good one for several reasons. For one, the presence of capacity for consciousness cannot be exactly coterminus with the presence of cerebral or cortical activity. Some such activity might be present with no remaining capacity for consciousness. On the other hand, at least theoretically, a person might be conscious with no cerebral tissue intact, either because other brain centers have taken over some of this function or an artificial organ has been created that could replace the naturally functioning tissue (Tomlinson, 1984). We might hold that it would be immoral to hook up a person to a computer, constituting an artificial organ for consciousness, but such a person would probably still be considered alive, especially if the computer were attached to a body with sensory and motor connections.

In order to overcome the problems with terms that are overly precise in localizing consciousness, some of us have taken to referring to this position with the purposely more vague term ''higher-brain-oriented concept of death,'' implying that the function that is normally associated with the higher brain is the *sine qua non* of a person functioning as an integrated whole. No matter how much physiological activity is integrated, the person should be treated as dead, according to this view, if there is no remaining capacity for consciousness.

Insofar as Judeo-Christianity holds that the human is an integration of body and soul and that mental function is a kind of modern surrogate for the soul, then Judeo-Christianity ought to support this higher-brain-oriented concept of death. This is not an abandonment of the notion that the death of the individual as a whole occurs when there is a breakdown in integration at the organismic level. Rather, it is the position that the permanent dissociation of mental and physiological function constitutes a breakdown in integration. In fact, at least some Protestant and Catholic scholars hold this view. Secular observers also support it to the extent that they share in this view that places significance on the integration of mental and physiological function.

A number of arguments have surfaced against this position. Several appear in the President's Commission report. First, the Commission argued that accepting this view would be entering into the philosophical debate about ''personhood'' (President's Commission for the Study of Ethical Problems in Medicine and Biomedical and Behavioral Research, 1981). While some defenders of the higher brain formulation rely on specific personhood (Engelhardt, 1975) or personal identity (Green and Wikler, 1980) theories, others do not. In fact, it is possible to hold any position regarding personhood (or to hold that personhood is not a meaningless concept) and still hold that individuals should be considered dead when higher brain functions are lost. One could hold, for example, that there are some nonpersons who are nevertheless still living humans who deserve all the rights and protections of society and its laws. Deciding who is a person would, in this circumstance, be irrelevant to deciding who is dead.

Second, it was argued by the Commission that in order for a conceptual formulation of death to be incorporated into public policy, it has to be amenable to clear articulation (President's Commission, 1981). It is claimed that the higher brain formulation cannot be reduced precisely to particular measures or tests. While that is true, it is not the case that irreversible loss of higher brain function has to be measured precisely in order for this concept of death to be operationalized. As with the whole-brain-oriented formulation, we may be able to measure with adequate certainty that higher brain function has been lost in some cases, even if we cannot with certainty guarantee that all such cases. This could be done by diagnosing PVS provided the judgment can be made with adequate certainty that some group of PVS patients are truly "permanent." It is interesting that the Commission itself concluded that it was possible to know with adequate certainty that some patients have irreversible loss of consciousness (President's Commission, 1983). The Commission cannot simultaneously argue that we can never measure irreversible loss of consciousness in individuals who retain some brain function.

Third, the Commission argues that choosing a "higher brain" definition would "depart radically from the traditional standards" (President's Commission, 1981). This argument raises two problems. First, it implies that adopting a whole-brain-oriented concept of death does not depart radically from traditional standards. This is based on the dubious claim that the whole-brain-oriented definition of death has operated throughout history and that all that has happened recently is the adoption of new measures or tests or criteria for determining that individuals have died. This requires assuming that the physician who used to feel the pulse or watch for respiration was doing so only because this was an indirect way of measuring brain function. That simply is not believable. The evidence is clear that shifting to a brain-oriented definition was conceptually controversial, at least for a while. Many people once held, if they could be asked clearly, that persons with no brain function but with heart and lung function were really alive. Only by a radically conceptual shift could even these people be called dead. Both the whole-brain-oriented concept and the higher-brain-oriented concept are "radical departures from tradition." Second, the Commission's claim implies that a radical departure is wrong. Unfortunately, we are probably in a situation where a radical departure is necessary because it is conceptually superior. Even if only the higher brain formulation were a radical departure, it should still be adopted if it is right. It is odd to argue against a position on the grounds that it is a departure from an older, less accurate position.

The Commission concluded with a *non sequitur*. It says that "irreversible cessation of all brain functioning is sufficient to determine death of the organism." That position is basically beyond dispute today, but it is irrelevant. What we need to know is whether it is a necessary condition, not a sufficient one. The Commission has not made a case that individuals with spontaneous respiration and no further capacity for consciousness must be considered alive. Since many secular philosophical positions reject that view and many religious traditions seem to as well, it is hard to see why the one position, the whole brain oriented one, should be forced on dissenters, whether they be more conservative (heart and lung oriented) or more liberal (higher-brain oriented).

One of the group of cases involving moral controversies in pediatrics involves infants born without the capacity for consciousness. Anencephalics, for instance, would be conceptualized very differently if a higher-brain-oriented definition of death were adopted. Although "anencephalic" ought to refer to infants "without encephalon," in fact, such infants have brainstem function. However, they lack higher function capacity. Thus, with either a heart-and-lung-oriented concept or a whole-brain-oriented concept, such infants are alive. With a higher-brain-oriented concept, they would never have been alive. They would perhaps be morally and legally akin to living gamete cells or embryos or early term fetuses that do not have the moral and legal standing of full members of the moral community. They are living human tissue, no doubt, but they are not to be treated as members of the moral community. They would never have lived.

The practical implications are less severe than may be apparent, however. Even if anencephalic infants are treated as living based on a whole-brain-oriented definition of death, they are certainly candidates for a decision to allow them to die. Thus, regardless of a definition of death, they may be dead very soon. In one case, however, they never would have lived (just as other human tissues are now treated for public policy purposes as if they never had lived).

3.3. States without Statutes

If it is the case that several definitions of death are within reason, new problems are created. States have, over the past two decades, gradually expressed their policy choice regarding death. This has been done either by statute (in 40 jurisdictions) or by judicial case law (in 7 jurisdictions including some that also have statutes). In four states (Delaware, Minnesota, South Dakota, and Utah), there is no case law, and their legislatures have refused to adopt such legislation in spite of organized efforts to get statutory definitions passed. The question this poses is what definition of death ought to be used in jurisdictions that have not acted to adopt a new definition.

Some might have argued that the social consensus is so clear that physicians should feel free to use the new definition even without legal authorization to do so. Insofar as the traditional definition of death is a common law definition and common law evolves, it could be maintained that the common law has, in fact, changed, so that the physician can or should use a brain-oriented definition.

This could lead to chaos, however. In the first place, it seems hard (although not impossible) to conclude that a state that has had the opportunity to adopt a new statutory definition and refused to do so has had its common law evolve to the position the legislature has refused to adopt. Individual practitioners could nevertheless maintain that the law has changed. They could take it upon themselves to assume the new law and stand by to have their position tested by court review. That is risky to the clinician, however. Moreover, it is morally problematic. It is an act of hubris to assume as a private citizen that the law has changed and proceed to act as if it had. It is especially bold on a matter that will mean the death of the patient if the private citizen's guess about the status of the law happens to be wrong.

It is far more responsible to assume that the traditional common law definition remains in effect and work to get that law changed. For almost all cases, there will be little practical difference. Any patient who suffers such severe neurological deficit that he has irreversibly lost all brain function is surely a good candidate for a decision to be allowed to die. The next of kin ought to be approached to determine whether the patient has expressed treatment refusal wishes and, if not, the next of kin, functioning as the surrogate, should decide whether further life support should be foregone.

As alternative brain-oriented definitions become more plausible, permitting individual physician discretion will become even more controversial. Some physicians act as if they have discretion now under laws authorizing death pronouncement based on brain-oriented criteria. In fact, no such discretion exists. The laws state that "death shall be pronounced" when brain function is irreversibly lost. They do not permit physicians to use their own discretion to delay pronouncing death in order to permit family members to accept the patient's fate or for any other purposes. Certainly they do not permit physicians to opt for an alternative brain-oriented formulation, such as a higher-brain-based one.

It is no more permissible for a physician to use his discretion to deviate from the traditional common law definition than from a newer definition. In fact, if physicians have the right to use their own private judgments based on their own philosophical convictions to change the definition of death away from the heart-and-lung-oriented one, there is no reason why they should be limited to the whole-brain formulation. They might just as reasonably opt for the higher-brain definition. The personal views of private citizens on what they think the definition of death ought to be can not be decisive in a public practice as fundamental to the rights of persons as deciding whether they are dead.

3.4. Freedom of Conscience

While clinicians should not be able to pick their personal definition of death and impose it on patients, should they be able to pick their own definition with regard to their own deaths? Ought anyone be able to pick their own definitions of death? The idea that people could pick their own definition of death at first seems preposterous. Death is often thought to be a matter of biological fact. Such facts are not a matter of personal choice based on personal ideology.

It is now clear, however, that being dead is not a matter of biological fact. Having one's brain function or heart function irreversibly lost is a matter of fact, at least within the limits of the value choices that must be made in even these determinations. By contrast, deciding that the organism as a whole no longer exists involves some judgment calls. In particular, it requires determining how much of the organism must still be functioning in order for it to exist "as a whole."

Besides the public policy debate is not exactly over whether the organism exists "as a whole." Rather, it is over when, for public policy purposes, we should treat the organism as if it no longer exists "as a whole."

The question is precisely like that of deciding whether it is appropriate to forgo treatment in a terminally ill patient. In deciding whether to forgo treatment, an evaluative judgment must be made based on some system of beliefs and values. In pluralistic society, we have affirmed that competent persons should have the maximum freedom to make these moral choices based on their own values (President's Commission, 1983). With regard to incompetent patients, we first honor the patient's own wishes to the extent they can be determined. If they cannot be determined, there is substantial support for transferring this decision to the next of kin to act as surrogate (President's Commission, 1983; Veatch, 1984). Fifteen jurisdictions now authorize by statute next-of-kin decisions in such cases (American Association of Retired Persons, 1986). In other states, the presumption of next-of-kin surrogacy is widespread. It is endorsed by groups such as the President's Commission (1983). There must be some limit on these decisions. In particular, persons are not allowed to refuse treatment when the interests of third parties are seriously threatened (President's Commission, 1983; Veatch, 1976a). Moreover, with regard to next-of-kin and other surrogate decisions, it is clear that judgments about what the patient would have wanted or what is in the patient's best interest must be within reason (Veatch, 1984).

People in a liberal society deserve exactly the same discretion to incorporate their personal philosophical and religious beliefs and values in the case of the definition of death. Christians ought to support higher-brain death; Orthodox Jews favor the heart-and-lung definition. The judgment that the individual as a whole is to be treated as dead for public policy purposes does not require any more uniformity than the decision to let an individual die. Once it is realized that they are both essentially moral or policy questions and not questions of scientific fact, a policy permitting limited freedom of conscience in the only sensible one.

The arguments against permitting individual discretion are weak. The most often cited argument is that "Were a non-uniform standard permitted, unfortunate and mischievous results are easily imaginable" (President's Commission, 1981). The "unfortunate and mischievous results" are never spelled out. Presumably the critics have in mind such things as the fact that life insurance payments would be made at different times depending on when a person is considered dead. Likewise, health insurance payments would cease at the time the person were treated as dead. Other social impacts could include affects on homicide prosecutions. [If an early point of death is chosen, homicide prosecution may be possible when it would not be if the patient were to "live" long enough for the statutory time period to elapse (*State v. Watson*, 1983).] Additional social implications could be imagined for the allocation of scarce medical resources, grieving, and so forth.

What is important is that, while each of these implications is potentially troublesome, no one has demonstrated that they will, in fact, be disruptive. For ease of public policy administration, the most appropriate way to proceed would be for each jurisdiction to adopt one definition of death (presumably a whole-brain-oriented one) and permit individuals to deviate within a specified range (including heart and lung based definitions and possibly higher brain definitions as well). It seems likely that only the most highly motivated will actually act on conscience to opt for a secondary definition. If so, very limited economic and social impact is likely.

Moreover, whatever problems of this sort can be anticipated, they are exactly the same that would occur with much greater magnitude from a policy of permitting decisions to forgo treatment. Deciding whether to forgo treatment determines when life and health insurance policies pay off; it could affect homicide prosecutions; it could affect grieving, property transfer, and so forth. Moreover, deciding to forgo treatment, say, for a permanent vegetative state (PVS) patient, could affect the time of death much more radically. A PVS patient, if treated aggressively, may live for decades. By contrast, a patient with a dead brain will die by all definitions in a matter of a week or two. If we are concerned about social policy confusion resulting from variations in the time of death attributed to personal choice, we should be much more concerned about decisions to forgo treatment rather than decisions about when death has occurred.

The use of a new definition of death in pediatric cases poses what might be thought to be special problems if individual discretion is permitted. Children are never competent to pick their definition of death, so a surrogate would have to choose. It might be argued that the mischief that would occur if people had discretion in picking a definition of death is more serious when surrogates do the picking. In some cases malicious surrogates could arrange a death to meet their financial or emotional desires rather than the welfare of the patient. Moreover, it is not clear on what basis surrogates should have the right to opt for a special definition of death for a child.

First, it should be noted that this could arise only if the right to choose a definition of death is extended to the surrogate as well as the individual while competent. A conscience clause could be written so that it only applies to persons who pick their own definition of death at a time while they are still conscious and competent.

By contrast, there are good reasons why this right should also be extended to family surrogates. We normally give family members the right to make fundamental choices regarding the lives of incompetent members. Parents choose school systems, religious training, and so forth. These are decisions that are at least as critical as a definition of death. Yet we affirm the importance of the family as a fundamental unit entitled to and requiring great freedom (President's Commission, 1983). We place limits on familial discretion but, as long as families operate within reason, we accept such familial discretion as an important right and responsibility.

There is no reason why this same limited discretion should not apply in choosing a definition of death from among reasonable options. The fact of the matter is that when families have been given discretion in the decision to forgo treatment, a decision that has much more potential for mischief than the choice of a definition of death, there are only rare reports of mischief or seriously irresponsible decision-making. In such cases, the legal apparatus exists to override the irresponsible surrogate. That same legal authority would exist in cases involving surrogate choices of a definition of death that deviates from the state-authorized default position.

The President's Commission goes on to argue that the definition of death is "one of legal status, on which turn the rights and interests not only of the one individual but also the other people and of the state itself." It concludes, "the subject is not one for personal (or familial) self-determination" (President's Commission, 1981). That, of course, is not a real argument. While there are impacts on others, they are not nearly as great as the impact of deciding to forgo treatment. Moreover, if there are impacts on others, they could easily be corrected by public policy or statute. For example, if we discovered that Medicare encountered significant additional expenses by maintaining people with dead brains who wanted to be treated as alive, we could simply create a diagnosis-related group (DRG) for individuals with dead brains that had offered no funding for such care, beyond diagnosis and confirmation of prognosis.

Some opponents of a conscience clause imply that clinicians should use discretion in either pronouncing death or in informing families in cases where there is known to be reservation about the concept of death based on brain function. This is surely a much more offensive approach. It implies the clinician has a right to use discretion, even though the patient or family has no such discretion. In fact, the law states that the person shall be pronounced dead when brain function is lost. No discretion is or should be permitted. If the family's concerns are dealt with by deceiving them after death has been pronounced, that surely is an unacceptable assault on their dignity and a violation of the minimum requirements of honesty.

The Commission seems to go wrong when it holds that "there is no personal discretion as to the fact of death when either criteria is [sic] met" (President's Commission, 1981). It is true that, within limits, it is a fact that a brain has irreversibly ceased functioning. It is not a fact that persons who have lost brain function have lost enough bodily function that they ought to be treated as dead. That is not a factual matter, except as one holds that any ethical or evaluative choice is a "moral fact."

Two states, New York and New Jersey, have considered adopting a definition of death with a conscience clause. The New York State Task Force has endorsed a model law that states:

> A person may be pronounced dead upon suffering irreversible cessation of all circulatory and respiratory functions; or, in the case of a person whose heartbeat and respiration are maintained on the basis of mechanical means, upon a determination that the person has sustained an irreversible cessation of all functions of the brain, including the brain stem; provided that no action shall be taken in reliance upon the provisions of this section with regard to a person whose heartbeat and respiration are maintained on the basis of mechanical means if to do so would violate the sincerely held religious or moral beliefs or convictions of the individual, as earlier announced by the individual himself or as attested to by a family member or next friend, or in the case of a minor or incompetent person, if to do so would violate the sincerely held religious or moral beliefs or conviction of the person's parent or guardian.

New Jersey at the present time is considering a similar proposal. There is no good reason to force a definition of death on Jews or others for whom a brain-oriented definition violates their theological positions. Respect for the conscience of minorities requires a conscience clause, just as it requires honoring special views about treatment refusal.

4. CONCLUSION

Determining the definition of death has resulted in an intriguing controversy, in part because it is so fundamental an issue, but also because the interplay between medical science and moral choices is so complex. While the movement in favor of a whole-brain-oriented definition is substantial, we still do not have anything like a societal consensus. Some still hold out for a heart-and-lung-oriented definition. An increasing minority is becoming convinced that persons should be treated as dead when they lose higher brain function, even if brain stem reflexes remain. Given the fact that these are fundamentally unscientific issues and that even what appears to be science, measuring the irreversible loss of function, in principle has to incorporate some moral and evaluative choices of the creators of the criteria, it seems reasonable to grant personal freedom at least within limits imposed by the society's obligation to protect the interest of others. These are controversies that are not likely to be resolved soon.

REFERENCES

American Association of Retired Persons, 1986, *A Matter of Choice: Planning Ahead for Health Care Decisions*, A.A.R.P., Washington, D. C.

Beecher, H. K., 1970, The new definition of death, some opposing views, Presented at the meeting of the American Association for the Advancement of Science, December 1970.

Brierley, J. B., Adam, J. A. H., Graham, D. I., and Simpson, J. A., 1971, Neocortical death after cardiac arrest, *Lancet* **2**:560–565.

Byrne, P. A., O'Reilly, S., and Quay, P. M., 1979, Brain death—an opposing viewpoint, *JAMA* **242**:1985–1990.

Cranford, R. B., and Smith, H. L., 1979, Some critical distinctions between brain death and the persistent vegetative state, *Ethics Sci. Med.* **6**:199–209.

Engelhardt, H. T., 1975, Defining death: A philosophical problem for medicine and law. *Annu. Rev. Respir. Dis.* **1975**:587–90.

Green, M. B., and Wikler, D., 1980, Brain death and personal identity, *J. Philos. Public Affairs* **9**(2):105–133.

Haring, B., 1973, *Medical Ethics*, Fides, Notre Dame, Indiana.

Harvard Medical School, 1968, A Definition of Irreversible Coma, Report of the Ad Hoc Committee of the Harvard Medical School to Examine the Definition of Brain Death, *JAMA* **205**:337–340.

Hudson, W. D., 1969, *The Is/Ought Question*, Macmillan, London.

Jennett, B., and Plum, F., 1972, Persistent vegetative state after brain damage, *Lancet* **1**:734–737.

Kohler, W., 1966, *The Place of Value in a World of Facts*, Mentor, New York.

Kuhn, T. S., 1962, *The Structure of Scientific Revolutions*, University of Chicago Press, Chicago.

Mohandas, A., and Chou, S. N., 1971, Brain death: A clinical and pathological study, *J. Neurosurg.* **35**:211–218.

New York State Task Force on Life and Law, July, 1986, *The Determination of Death*.

Popper, K. R., 1968, *The Logic of Scientific Discovery*, Harper Torchbooks, New York.

President's Commission for the Study of Ethical Problems in Medicine and Biomedical and Behavioral Research, 1981, *Defining Death: Medical, Legal and Ethical Issues in the Definition of Death*, U. S. Government Printing Office, Washington, D.C.

President's Commission for the Study of Ethical Problems in Medicine and Biomedical and Behavioral Research, 1983, *Deciding to Forego Life-Sustaining Treatment: Ethical, Medical, and Legal Issues in Treatment Decisions*, U. S. Government Printing Office, Washington, D. C.

State v. Watson 191 N.J. Super. 464 (1983).

Tomlinson, T., 1984, The conservative use of the brain-death criterion—A critique, *J. Med. Philos.* **9**:377–393.

Veatch, R. M., 1975, The whole-brain-oriented concept of death: An outmoded philosophical formulation, *J. Thanatol.* **3**:13–30.

Veatch, R. M., 1976a, *Death, Dying, and the Biological Revolution*, Yale University Press, New Haven, Connecticut.

Veatch, R. M., 1976b, *Value-Freedom in Science and Technology*, Scholars Press, Missoula, Montana.

Veatch, R. M., 1984, Limits of guardian treatment refusal: A reasonableness standard, *Am. J. Law Med.* **9**:427–468.

Walker, A. E., Diamond, E. L., Moseley, J. I., 1977, An appraisal of the criteria of cerebral death—A summary statement, *JAMA* **237**:982–986.

IV

NEEDS AND POSSIBILITIES IN TRANSPLANTATION

23

Developments in Immunosuppression
The Secret to the Success of Organ Transplantation

Charles T. Van Buren

1. INTRODUCTION

For centuries, surgeons have operated on patients in order to remove diseased tissues or to manage traumatic injuries. The objectives of practitioners of such an extirpative discipline became to minimize the surgical tissue loss or to adapt the patient to a regrettable but necessary disability. Only during the twentieth century has the focus of surgery expanded from ablation of disease and shifted toward the restoration of lost function by transplanting living and normally functioning tissues and organs from one individual to another. The success of clinical transplantation has been limited by the transplant surgeon's understanding of the body's immune response to transplanted tissues and by effective modulation of this response through suppression of the immune system. An understanding of the history of clinical immunosuppression enables one to understand both the limitations and the future of clinical organ transplantation.

The surgical techniques for performing solid organ transplants were initially described by Alexis Carrel (1910). He reported the successful transplantation of a functioning kidney from one dog to another. Carrel also described the inevitable biological consequence of such a transfer of a solid organ from one host to another—increasing swelling, inflammation, and eventual thrombosis of the transplanted organ. Although Carrel received the Nobel prize for his pioneering work, it remained for another group of investigators to elucidate the mechanism for the rejection response. Billingham *et al.* (1953) demonstrated that successful transplantation of skin grafts from one mouse strain to another could be accomplished if fetal mice were injected with spleen cells from the donor mouse strain prior to the skin engraftment. This tolerance to foreign tissue was specific to the tissue of the donor mouse and could not be established following maturation of the host mouse's immune system. These experiments led to the concept that the immune system actively surveys the body to destroy foreign tissue; acceptance of transplanted tissue is dependent

CHARLES T. VAN BUREN • Division of Immunology/Organ Transplantation, University of Texas Medical School at Houston, Houston, Texas 77030.

221

on suppression of this response or permits the immune system to recognize the tissue as self, and not foreign.

The first successful renal transplant attempted to thwart the normal cellular and antibody response to foreign tissue by eliminating the stimulus for such a response. This experiment, performed in 1954, was the first in a unique series of living related transplants between identical twins—individuals who were genetically identical and consequently incapable of rejecting one anothers' tissues (Merrill *et al.*, 1956). The initial patient in this remarkable series, was R.H., a 24-year-old man who presented with chronic renal failure presumed secondary to glomerulonephritis. Following identification of a brother who by history was an identical twin to the patient, both the patient and his potential donor underwent blood typing and further testing to confirm identity. Skin grafts were exchanged between host and donor, and the lack of rejection confirmed that the twins were identical. R.H. received a kidney from his twin donor, had prompt onset of function of the newly transplanted organ, and quickly excreted the fluid and wastes that had accumulated due to his chronic kidney failure. The only concern was the development of proteinuria, which persisted even after removal of the patient's diseased native kidneys. Although these transplants documented that functional organs could successfully be transferred between identical twins, the rarity of individuals with renal failure who had the good fortune to have such a donor limited the impact transplantation would have on the population. Moreover, identical twin renal transplant recipients who had initially had renal failure due to glomerulonephritis demonstrated a disturbingly high incidence of recurrent disease in the transplanted kidney; more than 60% of patients developed recurrence of the autoimmune disease, and a large number of the identical twin population lost their isografts due to recurrent disease (Glassock *et al.*, 1968). Thus, even in biologically favored matches, some sort of suppression of the immune system would be required to treat the original disease.

Approaches to suppression of the immune response can be divided into three broad categories: physical factors, which include the use of radiation therapy and lymphoid-depletion treatments, such as thoracic duct drainage; chemical immunosuppression, including the use of corticosteroids, antiproliferative agents, and most recently, cyclosporin; and biologic immunosuppression, which includes the use of antilymphocyte serums, either polyclonal or monoclonal, donor-specific blood transfusions, and, most recent, therapy directed against those proteins synthesized as messengers of the immune response system. Progress in each of these areas over the past three decades has been marked by the narrowing in the spectrum of the populations of cells targeted by the immunosuppressive regimen.

2. NORMAL IMMUNE RESPONSE

Before analyzing the benefits and limitations of each of these modes of therapy, it is appropriate to review the normal immune response to an organ transplanted between nonidentical members of the same species, in a very general fashion. Following transplantation, foreign proteins presented by the transplanted organ are engulfed and processed by circulating macrophages. These proteins that evoke the most vigorous immune response are coded for by the major histocompatibility complex (MHC), a series of genes located on the short arm of the sixth chromosome in man. Processing these foreign proteins (antigens) both focuses these products for response by other elements of the immune system and stimulates production of interleukin-1 (IL-1) from the activated macrophage. This protein acts on the next group of immunoreactive cells to be involved in the immune response to an antigen, the lymphocytes. Lymphocytes are categorized into two populations: T lymphocytes, which are primarily involved in direct cell–cell killing of incompatible cells and in mounting a cellular rejection response; and B lymphocytes, which, following activation, mature into plasma cells capable of producing a specific antibody to neutralize a corresponding antigen. Finally, T lymphocytes are further subcategorized into T-helper lymphocytes (T_H), which are vital to expansion and propagation of an immune response; T-suppressor lymphocytes (T_s), which can suppress an ongoing or incipient immune response; and T-cytotoxic lymphocytes (T_c), those mature differentiated lymphocytes capable of destroying a specific target cell based on its unique surface antigens.

Following antigen processing, production of Macrophages focus antigen to which T lymphocytes may respond. IL-1 leads to activation of lymphocytes and production by the T_H cell of interleukin-2 (IL-2), a signal vital for expansion of the number of specific T_c cell lines directed against the processed antigen. The T_H cell is also required to focus the antigen for the B lymphocyte and to provide growth factors essential to expansion of plasma cell lines. The final result of this immune activation by foreign antigen is the generation of T_c lymphocytes, which are directly injurious to the transplanted tissue, and plasma cells producing specific antibodies, which lead to cellular destruction and thrombosis of the transplanted organ.

3. SUPPRESSION OF THE IMMUNE RESPONSE

3.1. Physical Treatment

Ionizing radiation was the first physical treatment used to modify the immune defenses of the body. Gamma radiation leads to irreversible crosslinking of DNA and destruction of cells. Rapidly dividing cells, such as T and B lymphocytes, are especially sensitive to such effects. Although sublethal total-body irradiation facilitated transplantation in animal species, unacceptable toxicity due to bone marrow suppression limited its usefulness in clinical study (Murray et al., 1962).

Serendipitous observation that therapeutic radiation of lymph node bearing regions of the body to treat Hodgkin lymphoma resulted in suppression of cellular immune responses and selective reduction of T_H subpopulations of lymphocytes raised the possibility that similar total lymphoid irradiation (TLI) protocols could be used to precondition patients prior to transplantation (Fuks et al., 1976). Myburgh et al. (1980) reported the use of TLI to confer tolerance to subhuman primates bearing kidney allografts from another host. Sampson et al. (1985) demonstrated that TLI, at a dose of approximately 2000 rads and in conjunction with pharmacological immunosuppression, can lead to successful transplantation of cadaveric renal allografts in more than 70% of cases. Concerns regarding the logistics of delivering radiation dose and of securing a kidney transplant while the effects of the TLI were optimal, nonspecific bone marrow suppression, and reports of high morbidity and mortality associated with TLI have limited widespread application of this mode of therapy (Najarian et al., 1982).

Another physical approach, focused on depletion of lymphocytes from the body, was employed by Franksson et al. (1976). This technique, thoracic duct drainage (TDD), required placement of a catheter in the thoracic duct, drainage of the lymphocyte-rich fluid from the duct, centrifugation of cellular elements, and reinfusion of the cell-free lymph into the patient. The technique appeared to enhance cadaveric renal allograft survival. However, difficulties in coordinating maximal immunosuppression with availability of a suitable cadaveric kidney, the tremendous amount of labor in the separation of lymphocytes from large volumes of thoracic duct lymph, and the sepsis associated with maintenance of the thoracic duct cannula or from infusion of contaminated lymph supernatant limited the appeal of TDD as immunosuppressive therapy.

3.2. Chemical Immune Suppression

During the first decade of the clinical expansion of transplantation, investigators experimented with a number of chemical agents in an attempt to suppress the vigorous response to a renal allograft from a nonidentical donor. Actinomycin C, a crystalline antibiotic agent isolated from a culture broth of *Streptomyces,* is a compound that binds avidly to the guanine base of DNA. The drug inhibits rapidly proliferating cells of normal or neoplastic origin and, by blocking the transcription of RNA, leads to suppression of immune responsiveness. Unfortunately, toxicities such as mucositis with gastrointestinal (GI) disturbances and myelosuppression leading to pancytopenia limited successful use of this agent to manage renal transplant patients (Murray *et al.,* 1962).

Schwartz and Dameshek (1959) heralded the first promising immunosuppressive agent with the introduction of 6-mercaptopurine. This analogue of the purine bases inhibited purine biosynthetic pathways and proved effective in limiting lymphoproliferative responses by interfering with DNA synthesis. Since the drug was not specifically targeted for lymphoid cells, toxicities included myelosuppression and damage to GI epithelium due to the rapid turnover of these cellular elements. Calne *et al.* (1962) reported the use of an imidizole derivation of 6-mercaptopurine (azathioprine) to suppress renal allograft rejection in the mongrel dog. The combination of this purine antimetabolite with the nonspecific anti-inflammatory effects of corticosteroids represented the first clinically effective immunosuppressive regimen for use in clinical organ transplantation.

During the ensuing decade, clinical programs in cardiac, liver, kidney, and, to a lesser extent, small bowel and pancreas transplantation developed at selected academic centers. The mainstay of immunosuppression was the azathioprine–prednisone regimen. The narrow window between therapeutic immunosuppression and myelosuppression often limited its efficacy, and mortality of cadaveric allograft recipients due to sepsis approached 25% at many academic centers (Tilney *et al.,* 1978).

Substitution for azathioprine by other nonspecific immunosuppressive agents, such as cyclophosphamide, replaced one set of complications with another. Cyclophosphamide is an alkylating agent that binds covalently to the nucleobases of DNA and RNA. When timed to coincide with immunostimulation, administration of cyclophosphamide can result in effective immunosuppression (Starzl *et al.,* 1973). Toxicities such as myelosuppression and hemorrhagic cystitis can prove limiting, and the drug has been used most extensively to replace azathioprine when the latter agent has led to drug induced hepatitis and jaundice.

Using combinations of these nonspecific immunosuppressive drugs, centers have reported 1-year graft success rates ranging from 25% to 40% for vital organs (liver, cardiac) to 50% for cadaveric renal allograft survival (Starzl *et al.,* 1981; Watson *et al.,* 1980; Tilney *et al.,* 1978). Inadequate induction of immunosuppression, resulting in allograft rejection, or overimmunosuppression, usually as a consequence of treatment for rejection, limited widespread application of organ transplantation to treat end organ disease. In this area of nonspecific antiproliferative immunosuppressive agents, high-dose corticosteroids were often a mainstay of antirejection therapy. The anti-inflammatory effects of corticosteroids has long been recognized, and these agents were used early as antirejection therapy (Zukoski *et al.,* 1965). More recent investigations have demonstrated that steroids interfere with production of lymphokines vital to the propagation of a rejection response (Dupont *et al.,* 1984; Cupps and Fauci, 1982). However, steroid-induced peptic ulcer disease, aseptic hip necrosis, cataract formation, and steroid-induced diabetes mellitus impaired the quality of life of those patients who were able to weather the assaults of rejection or infection. Clearly, therapy directed against more specific elements of the immune response was required for widespread application of the technical successes of transplantation.

3.3. Biological Immunosuppression

The next group of immunosuppressive reagents to be clinically tested were antibodies raised in mammals against human lymphocytes. Najarian and colleagues reported the use of an equine serum directed against Epstein–Barr transferred human lymphoid cells to improve results in cadaveric renal transplantation (Najarian *et al.*, 1976). The preparation, antilymphoblast globulin (ALG), when combined with azathiaprine–prednisone therapy, reduced the incidence of rejection and improved graft survival. Other groups reported the use of polyclonal globulin preparations directed against human thymocytes (ATG) to enhance results in liver, cardiac, and heart lung transplantation (Starzl *et al.*, 1967; English *et al.*, 1982; Reitz *et al.*, 1982). Although the products clearly improved immunosuppressive efficacy, these immunosuppressive regimens still often resulted in overimmunosuppression and overwhelming viral infection (Simmons *et al.*, 1977). In addition, neoplasms such as lymphoma and Kaposi sarcoma developed in ALG- or ATG-treated transplant patients at rates much higher than expected in the general population (Cleary *et al.*, 1984; Penn, 1981). These neoplasms, associated with cytomegalovirus (CMV) infections, underscored the necessity to limit the target of treatment both to improve suppression of rejection and to maintain host defenses against infection.

The difficulty in manufacture of polyclonal antilymphocyte preparation, the variability of biological activity from lot to lot, and the heterogeneous mixtures of immunoglobulins present have at times limited production or efficacy of these biologic immunosuppressives. Monoclonal antibody preparations, derived from a single-cell immunized against human T lymphocytes, obviate many of the problems posed by ALG or ATG. OKT$_3$ is a murine-derived monoclonal antibody product directed against the T$_3$ antigen present on all mature human lymphocytes. Clinical trials with this agent have demonstrated increased efficacy in the treatment of rejection episodes refractory to steroid therapy (Thistlethwaite *et al.*, 1987). The drug is predictably effective, can be administered by peripheral venous infusion, and causes few side effects after the administration of the first dose. Few studies exist, however, comparing the benefit of monoclonal with polyclonal antilymphocyte preparations. The logistics of administration and previous familiarity with the product seem to dictate which product is used at a given center.

The latest monoclonal antibody directed against cellular elements of the immune response focuses on the IL-2 receptor. This protein, present on the cell surface of lymphocytes, appears soon after the cell is activated by antigen. Cells bearing IL-2 receptors appear to be dependent on binding of IL-2 to this receptor in order to proliferate. In a murine cardiac transplant model, the use of antibody directed against the IL-2 receptor effectively blocked rejection of the allograft (Kirkman *et al.*, 1985). Clinical studies to test this new specific weapon against rejection in human allograft recipients are eagerly awaited.

4. BIOCOMPATIBILITY

During the 1970s, much of the progress in transplantation was directed toward minimizing toxicity of immunosuppressive therapy and tailoring the immunosuppressive regimen to the needs of individual groups of patients. Tissue typing became refined as a means of maximizing the compatibility between donor and recipient. In the living related donor renal allograft recipient, outcome depended on the compatibility between donor and recipient. Individuals who shared, with the donor, the same two chromosomes that carried the major histocompatibility complex (MHC) could expect up to 95% 1-year renal graft survival from such a well-matched kidney (Salvatierra *et al.*, 1980). On the other hand, individuals who shared only one chromosome bearing the MHC genes and who demonstrated a strong immune response to donor cells in tissue culture could anticipate a 50% chance of success, no better than that anticipated if that patient had received a graft from an unrelated cadaver donor. To increase the frequency of successes, transplant centers depended increasingly on tissue typing to identify the most compatible donor. Application of this search to cadaveric organs led to the establishment of organ-sharing systems to optimize the tissue match on a regional or national basis (Report of the Task Force on Organ Transplantation, 1986).

Kerman *et al.* (1981) reported that another testable factor, the strength of the immune response of the recipient, could predict graft outcome. A panel of nonspecific immunological assays—skin-test responses to microbial antigens, panel mixed lymphocyte culture (MLC), active T-rosetting cells, and spontaneous blastogenesis—were used to designate individuals as strong or weak immune responders. For the patients who were strong responders, 1-year cadaveric renal allograft survival under azathioprine–prednisone therapy was only 35%, while weak immune responders had a 1-year allograft survival approaching 65% (Kerman *et al.*, 1980). More aggressive immunosuppressive therapy could alter the outcome; ATG therapy improved 1-year renal allograft survival to 65% in strong immune responders, while the survival in weak immune responders could not be improved. These data demonstrated that the biological responsiveness of the host as well as the tissue compatibility of the donor could affect the outcome of the transplant. Modulation of immunosuppressive therapy based on these variables could improve the chance of a successful transplant.

In 1973, another factor was identified that appeared to affect clinical results in renal transplantation. Opelz *et al.* (1973) reported that untransfused cadaveric renal allograft recipients had a significantly worse outcome than did recipients who had been transfused with at least one unit of blood prior to transplantation. This beneficial effect of blood transfusions was confirmed by others in both animal and clinical studies (Okazaki *et al.*, 1980; Spees *et al.*, 1980). The basis of this beneficial effect seemed to be twofold: first, as a screening test, to sensitize and eliminate from the potential recipient pool strong immune responders, who would make antibodies directed against the human leukocyte antigens (HLA) present on the white cells in the unit of blood; and second, as a form of immunosuppression, resulting in the generation of suppressor T cells to dampen the rejection response to the kidney transplant (Smith *et al.*, 1981). Thus, blood transfusion prior to transplantation emerged as a adjunct to immunosuppressive drugs.

Salvatierra *et al.* (1980) extended the benefits of blood transfusion to the living related renal transplant setting. The group previously described to be at high risk of rejection—recipients with a high MLC response to haploidentical living related donors—were purposely transfused with 3 units of blood from the potential kidney donor. If the patient did not develop antibodies directed against the donor due to these transfusions, a living related transplant was performed; 95% of these kidneys were functioning 1 year following transplant—a marked improvement from the 50–60% success rate anticipated with conventional (azathioprine–prednisone) immunosuppression. The disadvantage of this approach was that up to 30% of prospective donors were eliminated for use by development of donor-specific antibody responses in the transfused patient. Although this disadvantage was diminished by treatment with azathioprine before transfusion, the loss of a potential living related donor has proved a major disadvantage of donor-specific transfusion therapy (Anderson *et al.*, 1982). This form of therapy also results in a high number of reversible rejection episodes, necessitating high-dose steroid therapy. Thus, the high rate of successful transplants comes at the expense of morbidity due to antirejection therapy.

5. CYCLOSPORIN

Progress in clinical transplantation has not developed incrementally, but with quantum leaps. The development of azathioprine heralded the era of clinical transplantation with acceptable success rates. In 1976, a new drug was described that appeared to have potent immunosuppressive properties (Borel *et al.*, 1976). This fungus-derived peptide, cyclosporin, was initially used clinically for kidney transplant recipients by Calne, one of the pioneers of the azathioprine era of transplantation (Calne *et al.*, 1979). Although the drug appeared to have formidable side effects, with both kidney and liver toxicity, the agent reduced the incidence of rejection and improved the 1-year success rate in cadaveric renal allograft recipients to 80% (Kahan *et al.*, 1985). Cyclosporin therapy also improved the success of living related transplants, with 92% 1-year success of haploidentical high-responder recipients of living related donor renal allografts, without the use of donor-specific transfusion (Flechner *et al.*, 1984*a*). The incidence of rejection was lower in cyclosporin-treated recipients than that observed with donor-specific transfused patients. Moreover, up to 30% of living related renal allograft recipients could be weaned off corticosteroid therapy, further improving the post-transplantation quality of life (Flechner *et al.*, 1984*b*). Thus, the cyclosporin era of transplantation has both ushered in improved graft outcome and decreased drug-induced morbidity.

The improved results observed in cyclosporin-treated kidney transplant recipients has been paralleled by a marked improvement in results in liver, pancreas, heart, and lung transplantation (Sherlock, 1983; Sollinger *et al.*, 1987; Schroeder and Hunt, 1986; Toronto Lung Transplant Group, 1986). Not only has the overall success rate improved, but mortality due to infection has markedly decreased. This decrease in mortality has occurred despite the expansion of recipient criteria to include older and sicker patients. Frazier *et al.* (1988) recently reported an 83% 1-year heart transplant success rate in patients over the age of 60. The use of mechanical hearts as temporary support measures to bridge the gap between end-stage cardiac function and transplantation has become an accepted mode of medical therapy (Renlund *et al.*, 1987). Herein lies the crux of the current dilemma in transplantation: The gains in availability of organs by the more efficient use with better immunosuppressive therapy have been offset by a dramatic expansion of the potential recipient pool, because of increased interest in this increasingly safe model of therapy and because of more lenient screening procedures. Demand for transplantable organs currently outstrips the supply. An orderly system for the distribution of these limited resources has been mandated by recent federal legislation in order to avoid concerns regarding the fairness of organ allocation (Report of Task Force, 1986).

A major problem observed with cyclosporin therapy in human transplant patients has been development of significant renal and hepatic toxicity. The Stanford group has reported onset of chronic renal failure in a cardiac transplant patient treated with cyclosporin (Myers *et al.*, 1984), while all centers have experienced the difficulty in distinguishing cyclosporin nephrotoxicity from rejection (Flechner *et al.*, 1983). Hepatotoxicity is common, appears to be largely dose related, and can be associated with development of gallstones *de novo* (Lorber *et al.*, 1987). To avoid these problems, especially in cadaveric renal transplants vulnerable to acute tubular necrosis, some centers have advocated induction of immunosuppression with corticosteroids, ALG, and azathioprine (Matas *et al.*, 1988). Once the patient's renal allograft has commenced to diurese, azathioprine is replaced by cyclosporin therapy. Graft survivals up to 85% at 1 year are reported with such a strategy. While some groups have advocated the conversion of cyclosporin-treated patients to azathioprine, clinical studies of conversion therapy have resulted in frequent rejection episodes and a high incidence of graft loss (Lorber *et al.*, 1985).

Recent studies have suggested dietary manipulation of the immune response as a potent means of immunosuppressing potential transplant recipients. Studies at the University of Texas at Houston have demonstrated that a normocaloric isonitrogenous diet that is nucleotide free can enhance cardiac allograft survival in both murine and rat hosts (Van Buren *et al.*, 1983*a*, 1987). The nucleotide-free diet suppresses primary mixed lymphocyte culture responses *in vitro* and *in vivo*, delays experimental graft-versus-host disease, and suppresses sensitization to microbial or xenoantigens injected subcutaneously (Van Buren *et al.*, 1983*a;* Kulkarni *et al.*, 1984, 1987). The principal cell requiring dietary nucelotides for optimal function appears to be the helper lymphocyte; both the number of phenotypic T_H cells and the function of IL-2 production are depressed in sensitized mice maintained on a nucleotide-free diet (Van Buren *et al.*, 1985). The nucleotide free diet not only suppresses allograft rejection but also enhances the efficacy of cyclosporin. The nucleotide-free diet and low-dose CyA synergistically prolong graft survival beyond that seen with diet or the subtherapeutic dose of CyA alone (Van Buren *et al.*, 1983*b*).

Thus, provision of a nucleotide-free diet may, by lowering the required dose of cyclosporin, be able to minimize the problem with cyclosporin toxicity. In a similar fashion, Kirkman *et al.* (1985) demonstrated that provision of fish oil with cyclosporin enhances the immunosuppression seen with cyclosporin alone in a rat heart allograft model. This beneficial effect of fish oil is hypothesized to be due to provision of omega-3 fatty acids as precursors for prostagladin synthesis. Elzinga *et al.* (1987) used omega-3 fatty acid supplements to improve renal function in CyA-treated rats. The prospect for a nucleotide-free diet or fish oil, either alone or with cyclosporin, to improve clinical results in transplantation awaits further clinical trials.

The dramatic improvement in the outcome of cyclosporin-treated transplant recipients has also complicated defining the criteria on which organ allocation is based. While HLA matching between donor and recipient, immune-responder status, and blood transfusion had a significant effect on the outcome of cadaveric renal allografts managed by conventional immunosuppression, this has not been true in cyclosporin-treated patients. Individual center studies at the University of Minnesota, the University of Texas at Houston, as well as the Canadian Trial and the European Multicentre Trial fail to demonstrate any benefit of HLA matching in cyclosporin-treated renal allograft recipients (Kerman *et al.*, 1988*a;* Najarian *et al.*, 1985; Canadian Multicentre Transplant Study, 1983; European Multicentre Trial, 1983). Studies by Terasaki and the Southeastern Organ Procurement Foundation (SEOPF) appear to conflict with these conclusions (Cecka *et al.*, 1988; Sanfilippo *et al.*, 1984). Unlike SEOPF or Terasaki multicenter aggregate studies, all the previously mentioned studies demonstrating HLA typing to be irrelevant have in common the use of a standard cyclosporin based regimen which is effective in preventing rejection. SEOPF also reported that poorly matched locally distributed kidney grafts fared as well as well-matched kidney grafts shipped from outside centers (Alexander *et al.*, 1987). The above-cited studies failed to demonstrate a beneficial effect of blood transfusion on renal allograft outcome. These observations are confirmed by Opelz's analysis of pooled data from many centers, revealing the disappearance of the beneficial transfusion effect in *either* conventionally treated or cyclosporin-treated patients. Finally, immune-responder status no longer is a good predictor of outcome in the cyclosporin-treated renal transplant patients (Kerman *et al.*, 1988*b*). More effective immunosuppression negates the influence of these other factors. These findings underscore the danger in basing public policy decisions on outdated scientific data.

In contrast with these findings in renal transplant recipients, both HLA matching and blood transfusions appear to have a beneficial effect on graft outcome in cyclosporin-treated cardiac transplant recipients (Kerman *et al.*, 1988*b*). The reasons for this difference between groups of patients is unclear. A potential explanation may be that heart allografts evoke a more potent immune response, that induction of immunosuppression with cyclosporin is less efficient in cardiac allograft recipients compared with renal recipients, or that the diagnosis of rejection is more sensitive in heart transplant patients. Regardless of the explanation, the irony remains that current organ allocation policy dictates kidney distribution largely based on HLA match, for which there is little scientific support, while cardiac distribution is not based on tissue typing, despite evidence that this may lead to a higher rate of rejection and less efficient utilization of this resource. Until the scientific basis for optimal organ utilization can be defined, public policy may need to err on the utilization of these organs regionally, in order to minimize the time the organs are preserved without blood flow.

6. CONCLUSION

Organ transplantation has developed rapidly during the past three decades, passing swiftly from a technical feat that could be applied successfully only in identical twins to an almost routine method of treatment for patients with irreversible organ system disease. The current vanguard of progress focuses on increasingly complex procedures, with multiple organ or tissue replacement, and immunosuppressive regimens that are more focused and less toxic. While these medical advances are being made, public policy on organ distribution must be formulated to ensure that as many patients as possible can realize the restoration of life and function that a successful transplant can provide.

REFERENCES

Alexander, J. W., Vaughn, W. K., and Pfaff, W. W., 1987, Local use of kidneys with poor HLA matches is as good as shared use with good matches in the cyclosporine era: An analysis of one and two years, *Transplant. Proc.* **19**:672–674.

Anderson, C. B., Sicardo, G. A., and Etheredge, E. E., 1982, Pretreatment of renal allograft recipients with azathioprine and donor-specific blood products, *Surgery* **92**:315–321.

Billingham, R. E., Brent, L., and Medawar, P. B., 1953, Actively acquired tolerance of foreign cells, *Nature (Lond.)* **172**:603–606.

Borel, J. F., Feurer, C., Gubler, H. V., and Stahelin, H., 1976, Biological effects of cyclosporin A; a new antilymphocytic agent, *Agents Actions* **6**:468–475.

Calne, R. Y., Alexandre, G. P. J., and Murray, J. E., 1962, A study of the effects of drugs in prolonging survival of homologous renal transplants in dogs, *NY Acad. Sci.* **99**:743–761.

Calne, R. Y., Rolles, K., White, D. J., Thiru, S., Evans, D. B., McMaster, P., Dunn, D. C., Craddock, G. N., Henderson, R. G., Aziz, S., and Lewis, P., 1979, Cyclosporin A initially as the only immunosuppressant in 34 recipients of cadaveric organs: 32 kidneys, 2 pancreases, and 2 livers, *Lancet* **2**:1033–1039.

Canadian Multicentre Transplant Study Group, 1983, A randomized clinical trial of cyclosporin in cadaveric renal transplantation, *N. Engl. J. Med.* **309**:809–815.

Carrel, A., 1910, Remote results of the replantation of the kidney and the spleen, *J. Exp. Med.* **12**:146–150.

Cecka, J. M., Cicciarelli, J., Mickey, M. R., and Terasaki, P. I., 1988, Blood transfusions and HLA matching—an either/or situation in cadaveric renal transplantation, *Transplantation* **45**:81–86.

Cleary, M. L., Warnke, R., and Sklar, J., 1984, Monoclonality of lymphoproliferative in cardiac transplant recipients, *N. Engl. J. Med.* **310**:477–482.

Cupps, T. R., and Fauci, A. S., 1982, Corticosteroid-mediated immunoregulation in man, *Immunolog. Rev.* **65**:133–155.

Dupont, E., Wybran, J., and Toussaint, C., 1984, Glucocorticoids and organ transplantation, *Transplantation* **37**:331–335.

Elzinga, L., Kelley, V. E., Houghton, D. C., and Bennett, W. M., 1987, Modification of experimental nephrotoxicity with fish oil as the vehicle for cyclosporine, *Transplantation* **43**:271–274.

English, T. A., McGregor, C., Wallwork, J., and Cory-Pearce, R., 1982, Aspects of immunosuppression for cardiac transplantation, *Heart Transplant.* **1**:280–284.

European Multicentre Trial Group, 1983, Cyclosporin in cadaveric renal transplantation: One year followup of a Multicentre Trial, *Lancet* **2**:986–989.

Flechner, S. M., Kerman, R. H., Van Buren, C. T., and Kahan, B. D., 1984*a*, Successful transplantation of cyclosporine treated haploidentical living related renal recipients without blood transfusions, *Transplantation* **37**:73–76.

Flechner, S. M., Van Buren, C. T., Kerman, R. H., and Kahan, B. D., 1984*b*, The nephrotoxicity of cyclosporine in renal transplant recipients, *Transplant. Proc.* **15**:2689–2694.

Franksson, C., Lundgren, G., Magnusson, G., and Rigden, O., 1976, Drainage of thoracic duct lymph in renal transplant patients, *Transplantation* **21**:133–140.

Frazier, O. H., Macris, M. P., Duncan, J. M., Van Buren, C. T., and Cooley, D. A., 1988, Cardiac transplantation in patients over 60 years of age, *Ann. Thorac. Surg.* **45**:129–132.

Fuks, Z., Strober, S., Bobrove, A. M., Sasazuki, T., McMichael, A., and Kaplan, H. S., 1976, Long term effects of radiation on T and B lymphocytes in peripheral blood of patients with Hodgkin's disease, *J. Clin. Invest.* **58**:803–814.

Glassock, R. J., Feldman, D., Reynolds, E. S., Dammin, G. J., and Merrill, J. P., 1968, Human renal isografts: A clinical and pathologic analysis, *Medicine (Baltimore)* **47**:411–454.

Kahan, B. D., Kerman, R. H., Wideman, C. A., Flechner, S. M., Jarwenko, M., and Van Buren, C. T., 1985, Impact of cyclosporine on renal transplant practice at the University of Texas Medical School at Houston, *Am. J. Kidney Dis.* **5**:288–295.

Kerman, R. H., Floyd, M., Van Buren, C. T., and Kahan, B. D., 1980, Improved allograft survival of strong immune responder-high risk recipients with adjuvant ATG therapy, *Transplantation* **30**:450–454.

Kerman, R. H., Floyd, M., Van Buren, C. T., McConnell, R., McConnell, B. J., and Kahan, B. D., 1981, Correlation of non-specific immune monitoring with rejection or impaired function of renal allografts, *Transplantation* **32**:16–23.

Kerman, R. H., Van Buren, C. T., Lewis, R. M., and Kahan, B. D., 1988a, Successful transplantation of 100 untransfused cyclosporine-treated primary recipients of cadaveric renal allografts, *Transplantation* **45**:37–40.

Kerman, R. H., Van Buren, C. T., Lewis, R. M., Frazier, O. H., Cooley, D., and Kahan, B. D., 1988b, The impact of HLA A,B, and D_R, blood transfusions, and immune responder status on cardiac allograft recipients treated with cyclosporine, *Transplantation* **45**:333–337.

Kirkman, R. L., Barrett, L. V., Gaulton, G. N., Kelley, V. E., Ythier, A., and Strom, T., 1985, Administration of an anti-interleukin 2 receptor monoclonal antibody prolongs cardiac allograft survival in mice, *J. Exp. Med.* **162**:358–362.

Kulkarni, S. S., Bhateley, D. C., Zander, A. P., Van Buren, C. T., Rudolph, F. B., Dicke, K. A., and Kulkarni, A. D., 1984, Functional impairment of T-lymphocytes in mouse radiation chimeras by a nucleotide free diet, *Exp. Hematol.* **12**:629–699.

Kulkarni, A. D., Fanslow, W. C., Rudolph, F. B., and Van Buren, C. T., 1987, Modulation of delayed hypersensitivity in mice by dietary nucleotide restriction, *Transplantation* **44**:847–849.

Lorber, M. I., Flechner, S. M., Van Buren, C. T., Kerman, R. H., Bartosh, J., and Kahan, B. D., 1985, Cyclosporine toxicity: The effect of combined therapy using cyclosporine, azathioprine, and prednisone, *Hum. Immunol.* **13**:59–60.

Lorber, M. I., Van Buren, C. T., Flechner, S. M., Williams, C., and Kahan, B. D., 1987, Hepatobiliary and pancreatic complications of cyclosporin therapy in 466 renal transplant patients, *Transplantation* **43**:35–40.

Matas, A. J., Tellis, V. A., Quinn, T. A., Glicklich, D., Soberman, R., and Veith, F. J., 1988, Individualization of immediate posttransplant immunosuppression, *Transplantation* **45**:406–409.

Merrill, J. P., Murray, J. E., Harrison, J. H., and Guild, W. R., 1956, Successful homotransplantation of the human kidney between identical twins, *JAMA* **160**:277–282.

Murray, J. E., Merrill, J. P., Dammin, G. J., Dealy, J. B., Alexandre, G. W., and Harrison, J. H., 1962, Kidney transplantation in modified recipients, *Ann. Surg.* **156**:337–355.

Myers, B. D., Ross, J., Newton, L., Luetscher, J., and Perlroth, M. 1984, Cyclosporine-associated chronic nephropathy, *N. Engl. J. Med.* **311**:699–705.

Myburgh, J. A., Smith, J. A., Hill, R. R. H., and Browde, S., 1980, Transplantation tolerance in primates following total lymphoid irradiation and allogeneic bone marrow injection. II. Renal allograft, *Transplantation* **29**:405–408.

Najarian, J. S., Simmons, R. L., Condie, R. M., Thompson, E. J., Fryd, D. S., Howard, R. J., Matas, A. J., Sutherland, D. E., Ferguson, R. M., and Schmidtke, J. R., 1976, Seven years experience with antilymphoblast globulin for renal transplantation, *Ann. Surg.* **184**:352–368.

Najarian, J. S., Ferguson, R. M., Sutherland, D. E., Slavin, S., Kim, T., Kersey, J., and Simmons, R. L., 1982, Fractionated total lymphoid irradiation as preparative immunosuppression in high risk renal transplantation, *Ann. Surg.* **196**:442–452.

Najarian, J. S., Fryd, G. S., Strand, M., Canafax, D. M., Ascher, N. L., Dayne, W. D., Simmons, R. L., and Sutherland, D. E., 1985, A single-institution, randomized, prospective trial of cyclosporine versus azathioprine–antilymphocyte globulin for immunosuppression in renal allograft recipients, *Ann. Surg.* **201**:142–157.

Okazaki, H., Maki, T., Wood, M., and Monoco, A. P., 1980, Effect of a single transfusion of donor specific and nonspecific blood on skin allograft survival in mice, *Transplantation* **30**:421–428.

Opelz, G., Sengar, D. P., Mickey, M. R., and Terasaki, P. I., 1973, Effect of blood transfusions on subsequent kidney transplants, *Transplant. Proc.* **5:**253–259.

Opelz, G., 1987, Improved kidney graft survival in nontransfused recipients, *Transplant. Proc.* **19:**149–152.

Penn, I., 1981, Depressed immunity and the development of cancer, *Clin. Exp. Immunol.* **46:**459–474.

Renlund, O. G., Bristow, M. R., Lybbert, M. R., O'Connell, J. B., and Gay, W. A., 1987, Medicare designated centers for cardiac transplantation, *N. Engl. J. Med.* **316:**873–876.

Reitz, B. A., Wallwork, J. L., Hunt, S. A., Pennock, J. L., Billingham, M. E., Oyer, P. E., Stinson, E. B., and Shumway, M. E., 1982, Heart lung transplantation: Successful therapy for patients with pulmonary vascular disease, *N. Engl. J. Med.* **306:**557–564.

Report of the Task Force on Organ Transplantation, 1986, Organ Transplantation: Issues and Recommendations, U. S. Department of Health and Human Services, Public Health Service, Health Resources and Services Administration, Office of Organ Transplantation, April, 1986.

Salvatierra, O., Vincenti, F., Amend, W., Potter, D., Iwaki, Y., Opelz, G., Terasaki, P., Duca, R., Cochrum, K., Hanes, D., Stoney, R., and Feduska, N., 1980, Deliberate donor-specific blood transfusions prior to living related renal transplantation, *Ann. Surg.* **192:**543–552.

Sampson, O., Levin, B. S., Hoppe, R. T., Bierber, C. P., Miller, E., Waer, M., Kaplan, H. S., Collins, G., and Strober, S., 1985, Preliminary observations on the use of total lymphoid irradiation, rabbit antithymocyte globulin, and low dose prednisone in human cadaver renal transplantation, *Transplant. Proc.* **17:**1299–1303.

Sanfilippo, F., Vaughn, W. K., Spees, E. K., Light, J., and LeFor, W. M., 1984, Benefits of HLA-A and HLA-B matching on graft and patients. Outcome after cadaver–donor renal transplantation, *N. Engl. J. Med.* **311:**358–364.

Schroeder, J. S., and Hunt, S. A., 1986, Cardiac transplantation: Where are we? *N. Engl. J. Med.* **315:**961–963.

Schwartz, R., and Dameshek, W., 1959, Drug-induced immunological tolerance, *Nature (Lond.)* **183:**1682–1683.

Sherlock, S., 1983, Hepatic transplantation: The state of play, *Lancet* **2:**778–779.

Simmons, R. L., Matas, A. J., Rattazzi, L. C., Balfour, H. H., Howard, R. J., and Najarian, J. S., 1977, Clinical characteristics of the lethal cytomegalovirus infection following renal transplantation, *Surgery* **82:**537–546.

Smith, M. D., Williams, J. D., Coles, G. A., and Salaman, J.R., 1981, The effect of blood transfusion on T suppressor cells in renal dialysis patients, *Transplant. Proc.* **13:**181–183.

Sollinger, H. W., Stratta, R. J., Kalayoglu, M., Pirsch, J. D., and Belzer, F. O., 1987, Pancreas transplantation with pancreaticocystostomy and quadruple immunosuppression, *Surgery* **102:**674–679.

Spees, E. K., Vaughn, W. K., Williams, G. M., Filo, R. S., MacDonald, J. C., Mendez-Picon, G., and Niblack, G., 1980, Effects of blood transfusion on cadaver renal transplantation, *Transplantation* **30:**455–463.

Starzl, T. E., Marchioro, T. L., Porter, K. A., and Brettschneider, L., 1967, The liver: Homotransplantation of the liver, *Transplantation* **5:**790–803.

Starzl, T. E., Groth, C.G., Putnam, C. W., Corman, J., Halgrimson, C. G., Penn, I., Husberg, B., Gustafsson, A., Cascardo, S., Geis, P., and Iwatsuki, S., 1973, Cyclophosphamide for clinical renal and hepatic transplantation, *Transplant. Proc.* **5:**511–516.

Starzl, T. E., Iwatsuki, S., Klintmalm, G., Schroter, G. P., Weil, R., Koep, L. T., and Porter, K. A., 1981, Liver transplantation 1980, with particular reference to cyclosporin A, *Transplant. Proc.* **18:**281–285.

Thistlethwaite, J. R., Gaber, A. O., Haag, B. W., Aronson, A. J., Broelsch, C. E., Stuart, J. K., and Stuart, F. P., 1987, OKT$_3$ treatment of steroid-resistant renal allograft rejection, *Transplantation* **43:**176–184.

Tilney, N. L., Strom, T. B., Vineyard, G. C., and Merrill, J. P., 1978, Factors contributing to the declining mortality rate in renal transplantation, *N. Engl. J. Med.* **299:**1321–1325.

Toronto Lung Transplant Group, 1986, Unilateral lung transplantation for pulmonary fibrosis, *N. Engl. J. Med.* **314:**1140–1145.

Van Buren, C. T., Kulkarni, A. D., and Rudolph, F. B., 1983a, Synergistic effect of a nucleotide-free diet and cyclosporine on allograft survival, *Transplant. Proc.* **15**(suppl 2):2967–2968.

Van Buren, C. T., Kulkarni, A., Schandle, B. V., and Rudolph, F. B., 1983b, The influence of dietary nucleotides on cell mediated immunity, *Transplantation* **36:**350–352.

Van Buren, C. T., Kulkarni, A. D., Fanslow, W. C., and Rudolph, F. B., 1985, Dietary nucleotides: A requirement for helper/inducer T lymphocytes, *Transplantation* **40:**694–697.

Van Buren, C. T., Kim, E. E., Kulkarni, A. D., Fanslow, W. L., and Rudolph, F B., 1987, Nucleotide free diet and suppression of the immune response, *Transplant. Proc.* **19:**57–59.

Watson, D. C., Reitz, B. A., Oyer, P. E., Stinson, E. B., and Shumway, N. E., 1980, Sequential orthotopic heart transplantation in man, *Transplantation* **30:**401–403.

Zukoski, C. F., Callaway, J. M., and Rhea, W. G., 1965, Prolonged acceptance of canine renal allograft achieved with prednisolone, *Transplantation* **3:**380–386.

24

Pediatric Transplantation
Needs and Potential Donors

NANCY ASCHER

1. INTRODUCTION

Interest in pediatric organ donation and organ retrieval has been focused in part because of a perception that there are not enough pediatric organs for needy pediatric recipients. This chapter discusses the number of patients waiting for various organs and the number of pediatric donors available. It will be shown that there are more individuals of all ages waiting for organs than there are organs available. This is currently easily demonstrable for patients waiting for kidney transplants. It also appears true for other organ transplants. The problem is particularly severe for pediatric patients, and it is going to get worse.

Data assembled by the American Council on Transplantation demonstrate the growth of activity in transplantation over the past few years. There have been increased numbers of kidney transplants from 1981 to 1984, as well as increased numbers of heart, liver, pancreas, and other transplants. Approximately 10,000 kidney transplants, 800 liver transplants, and more than 400 heart transplants were performed in 1986. The number of transplant centers also continues to increase.

But many patients are waiting for various organs. Approximately 10,000 individuals in the United States are waiting for kidney transplants, but the pool of individuals who could benefit from kidney transplants probably is in the range of 80,000–90,000, the number of people who are presently on some kind of dialysis. In terms of hearts and livers, although few people are waiting currently on these transplant lists, there are many more people who could benefit from these transplants. As in kidney transplantation, it may be expected that more of these individuals will try to avail themselves of this therapy. This is probably one of the reasons that the federal government, currently funding $2 billion a year for patients with end-stage renal disease, has been reluctant to underwrite the cost of end-stage heart disease and end-stage liver disease.

NANCY ASCHER • Department of Surgery, University of California at San Francisco, San Francisco, California 94143-0780.

2. NEEDS

2.1. Kidneys

There are a number of ways to look at pediatric patients as a separate subgroup. One way is to examine the number of patients who present themselves for care. Data assembled from a group of pediatric kidney programs show the distribution according to disease of about 350 patients aged 1–18 years with end-stage renal disease. Males constitute 57%. There are many more white patients than blacks or any other ethnic group. Most interesting is that the mean age of the pediatric patients is 15 years. Two thirds of patients received cadaver grafts, but long-functioning grafts are more common in patients receiving organs from living relations. The mean age at first transplant is 12 years, 7 months. But there are disturbing problems when one compares this information with death data. That is, there are a large number of patients who die with a primary diagnosis of one form or another of kidney failure who are under 1 year of age. There are thus about 500 children under 1 year of age who might benefit from kidney transplants, indicating the need for donors. Yet these patients are not given transplants, and many centers have policies against transplanting patients this small. By contrast, relatively few patients in the mean age of those receiving transplants actually die with end-stage kidney disease.

2.2. Hearts

Data from the Battelle Institute National Heart Transplantation Study categorize individuals who would benefit from a heart transplant. As of 1984, no one was even looking at patients under 10 years of age because no one was doing transplants in patients that small (although they had been done unsuccessfully earlier). Indeed, no patients under 18 years of age had received a heart transplant. However, the field is evolving quickly because of improved immunosuppression.

The number of patients who could benefit from heart transplants is easy to determine by noting how many die of heart disease, because one of the indications for heart transplant is a high likelihood of dying without the transplant. Among patients under 1 year of age, there are 1300 children dying. These children are clearly those who could benefit from a heart transplant. A total of 2800 children die by 18 years of age. So the pool is surprisingly large.

2.3. Livers

The most common cause for which liver transplant is performed is biliary atresia. The incidence of biliary atresia is 1 per 10,000 live births in the United States. Thus, about 300 children are born every year with biliary atresia. One third of them will be cured with the Kasai operation, which leaves a minimum of 200 children who would benefit from a liver transplant, if they could live long enough. Other diseases are less frequent. Nonetheless, when added together, they amount to about the same number as children with biliary atresia. Thus there are about 400 new children every year who could benefit from a liver transplant. Roger Evans, from the Battelle Institute, accumulated data on children who died in 1979 indicating that 300 children aged 0–15 years of age versus 9500 adults aged 15–54 years die every year with end-stage liver disease. Data from 1983 indicate approximately the same numbers (with 80 patients under 1 year of age dying). Since it is estimated that about one third of children on liver transplant lists die waiting, those who die represent about one third of the patients under 1 year of age who might benefit from a liver transplant. This again suggests the possible 300 patients mentioned above.

3. DONORS

3.1. All Donors

The Centers for Disease Control (CDC) conducted several studies investigating potential donors. They examined charts of patients who died in the hospital to determine which of those patients met medical criteria for organ donation; it was determined that 1 to 3 of every 100 inhospital deaths met the medical criteria for renal donors. Since of two million people who die each year, 60% die in the hospital, and 2 of every 100 inhospital fatalities are suitable renal donors, there are 24,000 potential donors.

3.2. Pediatric Donors

Other studies of the actual numbers of donors by age demonstratated that there is a marked variation according to age distribution. Retrieval is much lower in the 2- to 6-month-old donor group or in the older donor group compared with the 5- to 14-year-old donor group, indicating that even if there were 25,000 donors, there would not be enough organs for all the possible pediatric recipients. Thus, the group less likely to receive organs are very young recipients.

In addition, infant mortality has been decreasing steadily over the years. Although there are 40,000 deaths under 1 year of age annually in the United States, a relatively small percentage fall into the category that might be considered potential donors—possibly 956 deaths. The rest of these, such as congenital anomalies, sudden infant death syndrome (SIDS), or respiratory distress syndrome (RDS), contraindicate against their use as suitable donors. These 900+ potential donors have to provide for those infants who need kidneys, livers, and hearts. But CDC studies also indicate that only 10–20% of this age group become donors, which means perhaps there will be 100–200 donors under 1 year of age to meet the needs of 1300 potential recipients for transplantation.

3.3. Alternative Solutions

There are some potential alternatives to this permanent donor shortage, and there are alternatives for the kidney transplant recipient. Living related and living unrelated donors can be used, as well as xenografts. Among heart transplant recipients, the mechanical heart is a treatment modality for the future if we are going to pursue treatment of heart disease, as are xenografts. And for livers, living unrelated partial grafts are a possibility. Hepatic dialysis is currently being tried in a number of animal models, as are gene transplants and xenografts.

25

DEVELOPMENTS IN TISSUE TRANSPLANTATION

KELVIN G. M. BROCKBANK and ROBERT T. McNALLY

1. INTRODUCTION

Shortfalls in organ donation result in prolonged waiting periods for transplant recipients. Such shortfalls could be significantly reduced through the efforts of health professionals who attend to, and are involved with, brain dead patients. The purpose of this chapter is to present some current and future developments in the field of tissue transplantation, with the aim of clarifying the importance and potential of transplantable tissues. Since large organs such as heart, liver, and kidneys are the subjects of other chapters in this volume, this chapter is restricted to small, less complex tissues, such as heart valves, veins, and islets of Langerhans. The importance of these tissues is clarified when it is realized that approximately 400,000 transplantation procedures have been performed in 1987 (Table I).

The major advances in transplantation of tissues are occurring because of efficient sterile procurement techniques, recognition of a group of immunologically privileged tissues, development of techniques for the avoidance of the transplant recipient's immune surveillance system, and improvements in tissue-preservation methods. Cryopreservation is discussed at length, while other methods of preservation are dealt with in later sections on transplantation of specific tissues. Procurement is discussed in the section on heart valves.

2. CRYOPRESERVATION

Historically, several approaches for tissue storage have been used. The most commonly used and promising method has been cryopreservation. Some alternative methods have been freeze drying, chemical treatment, tissue culture prior to transplantation, and storage at refrigeration temperatures.

The field of cryopreservation dates from 1949, when Polge et al. (1949) discovered the protective property of glycerol for bull sperm. Subsequently, Lovelock and Bishop (1959) re-

KELVIN G. M. BROCKBANK and ROBERT T. McNALLY • Research and Development, CryoLife, Inc., Marietta, Georgia 30067; Department of Pathology, Medical University of South Carolina, Charleston, South Carolina 29425.

TABLE I.   Tissue Transplant and Prosthetic
Implant Estimates for 1987

Tissue	Procedures
Heart valves	40,000[a]
Corneas	30,000[b]
Pancreas	130[c]
Skin	>100,000[a]
Blood vessels	70,000[a]
Tendons/ligaments	>100,000[c]
Bone	50,000[c]
Bone marrow	1,000[b]

[a] CryoLife estimates.
[b] American Council on Transplantation, U.S. transplant stat.
sheet (Jan. 1987).
[c] In Vivo: The Business & Medicine Report, 42–45 (1985).

ported the protective activities of dimethylsulfoxide (DMSO) in preventing freezing injury to living cells. DMSO has since become the most widely used cryoprotectant. In addition to DMSO and glycerol, both of which penetrate cells and are known as permeating cryoprotective agents, there are a variety of so-called nonpermeating cryoprotective agents. These agents include such compounds as polyvinylpyrolidone, hydroxyethyl starch, sugars, and sugar alcohols. The permeating cryoprotective agents reduce the intracellular water concentration and therefore reduce the amount of ice formed at any temperature. In addition, both permeating and nonpermeating cryoprotectants act directly on cell membranes. The mechanism of the latter interaction is not clear, but it may involve changes in colloidal osmotic pressure and modifications of the behavior of membrane-associated water by ionic interaction. For some cells, combinations of these two classes of cryoprotective agents may give optimal viability.

During the past 30 years, two major mechanisms for freezing injury to cells and tissues have been emphasized. First, there are the obvious mechanical injuries that can occur due to either extra- or intracellular ice crystal formation. Second is the danger of osmotic dehydration. Current cryopreservation technology consists of trying to maintain a balance between these two forms of injury. Basically, when freezing is performed at a rapid rate, there is a tendency for ice crystals to form both intracellularly and extracellularly. However, when cryopreservation is performed at slower rates, there is a tendency for ice crystal formation to occur first in the extracellular medium. As the extracellular ice forms, the cells are exposed to an increasingly hyperosmotic environment. This is due to water sequestration as the ice crystals grow. The cells shrink due to transport of water out of the cell in response to the osmotic imbalance caused by the increasing extracellular solute concentrations. The net result of combining optimal cooling rates and cryoprotective agents is that less of the freezable intracellular water will be converted to ice and osmotic cellular dehydration is limited.

There are several steps in developing cryopreservation procedures (Bank and Brockbank, 1987). For many tissues, especially if the desired cryoprotectant concentration exceeds 1 M, the cryoprotectant should be added in a stepwise manner in order to minimize cellular osmotic damage. It is usual to perform the cryoprotectant addition steps at a low temperature (4°C or lower). This is because cryoprotectants at the concentrations employed for cryopreservation are often toxic to tissues. Once the optimum cryopreservation conditions have been selected for a tissue, and the tissue has been cooled to liquid nitrogen temperatures, the tissue may be stored indefinitely. It is believed that the only events that occur at liquid nitrogen temperatures are interactions with subatomic particles, which give the theoretical life expectancy of cryopreserved tissues in thousands of years.

Thawing of tissues is usually performed in a 37–42°C waterbath. This is in order to thaw as rapidly as possible without achieving temperatures lethal to the tissue. The rationale for rapid warming is that it limits the growth of ice crystals that were formed during cooling. Some tissues may be sensitive to rapid warming. This is due to transient osmotic shock, because the cells are exposed to an extracellular hypertonic solution as the ice melts and are forced to rehydrate in order to maintain their osmotic equilibrium. Upon completion of the thawing procedure, the cryoprotectant solution must be removed. This is usually done gradually at 4°C in order to reduce the effects of both osmotic shock and cryoprotectant toxicity.

At this point, the importance of selection of assays for viability of tissue (Brockbank and Bank, 1987) should be emphasized. Viability may be defined as the ability of a cell or tissue to maintain itself and interact in a normal manner with its environment. The appropriate viability assays for a specific tissue are dependent on both the cell types present in the tissue and the functions of the tissue being evaluated. Cellular and tissue viability assays usually fall into either proliferative, metabolic, and/or mechanical assays. Morphological procedures, such as routine histology, surface antigen localization, transmission electron microscopy (TEM), or scanning electron microscopy (SEM), are often used as preliminary tests for identification of promising cryopreservation procedures.

Cryopreservation technology has applications for many of the tissues to be discussed. By contrast, the alternative procedures listed previously have more limited applications, usually for one or two tissues only. Therefore, these procedures will be mentioned where appropriate during the discussion of specific tissues.

3.   IMMUNOLOGICALLY PRIVILEGED TISSUES

There are three transplantable tissues that have little or no immunological reaction when transplanted in mismatched allogeneic recipients. The mechanism by which this immunological privilege is conferred is believed in all three cases to be due to isolation of the tissue from the vascular system. The three tissues to be considered here are (1) heart valves, both aortic and pulmonary; (2) corneas; and (3) cartilage. Heart valves have not yet been reported to induce the immune response in mismatched donor–recipient combinations. This could be because of two factors: (1) the endothelium lining the valve, which would be a major source of class II antigens, is largely removed during procurement, cryopreservation, and surgical implantation of the valve; or (2) the connective tissue of heart valves is very poorly vascularized, leading to very little contact between host lymphocytes and donor fibroblasts. In spite of this lack of immunological responsiveness, some investigators are currently matching for blood groups prior to transplantation of heart valves. By contrast, the situation with corneas is not quite as good. Allogeneic transplantation with corneas results in mild immunological problems in approximately 30% of patients. These problems can usually be overcome by mild short-term immunosuppression. Sanfilippo *et al.* (1986) showed that there can be a significant reduction of graft rejection in the small group of high-risk patients by tissue matching. In mature cartilage, the chondrocytes are isolated from the vascular system by a matrix consisting of fibers and fibrils embedded in an amorphous intercellular substance. Lymphocytes, the primary cells responsible for immune reactions, are unable to migrate through this cartilage matrix.

3.1.   Heart Valve Transplantation

Aortic allografts have been used for more than three decades (Murray, 1956). More recently, pulmonary homograft valve external conduits have also been employed. The earliest allograft valves were preserved by refrigeration at 4°C for days and weeks (Barratt-Boyes *et al.*, 1969). Because of difficulties with long-term storage and because of increasing demand during the 1960s, a number of alternative valve treatment procedures were employed (O'Brien *et al.*, 1987). Valves were sterilized chemically or by irradiation after nonsterile procurement. These alternative treatments resulted in nonviable heart valves. The chemical methods of sterilization attempted included formaldehyde fixation, chlorhexidine, β-propiolactone, and ethylene oxide. Freeze drying was also attempted. Freeze drying consists of freezing tissues to approximately −70°C and then drying the tissue by sublimation in a vacuum. The resulting grafts developed leaflet calcification and tissue failure within a few years after transplantation.

Most heart valves have been antibiotic sterilized and stored by varying periods at 4°C. The experience of Ross (1987) indicates that degeneration of such heart valves becomes clinically manifest at about 7 years. However, the incidence of degeneration is uncertain. Because of the slow process of degeneration, valve-related deaths are rare. Thus, patient survival is much better than valve survival, and Ross has become increasingly aware that function or survival of allografts in children is considerably better than is the case with xenografts. Valve xenografts are usually chemically fixed porcine valves. These valves have been reported to undergo rather rapid degenerative changes due to calcium deposition. This calcium deposition results in loss of leaflet flexibility. In valve allografts, some surface calcium deposition may occur, but it does not impede leaflet function. Because of these differences in calcium manifestation, allografts are frequently used in children. The allograft also has advantages over mechanical valves, and the advantages include relative freedom from danger of embolism and anticoagulant hemorrhage, freedom from hematological abnormalities associated with mechanical valves, freedom from restriction of pregnancy, and absence of danger of death due to sudden valve failure.

Mermet *et al.* (1970) reported on valve cryopreservation. Since that time, there have been several reports of valve cryopreservation. The most recent, by O'Brien *et al.* (1986) reported on a 16-year follow-up for refrigerated valves and 11-year follow-up of cryopreserved valves. Valves refrigerated for periods longer than 2 weeks may be considered nonviable (Mochtar *et al.*, 1984), in contrast with the high level of cell viability observed in cryopreserved valves (Kamp *et al.*, 1981). Within the above time frame, 23 patients receiving nonviable refrigerated valves were reoperated for leaflet perforation or rupture; by contrast, in no patient receiving viable cryopreserved valves did this complication develop. The actuarial freedom at 10 years post-transplanta-

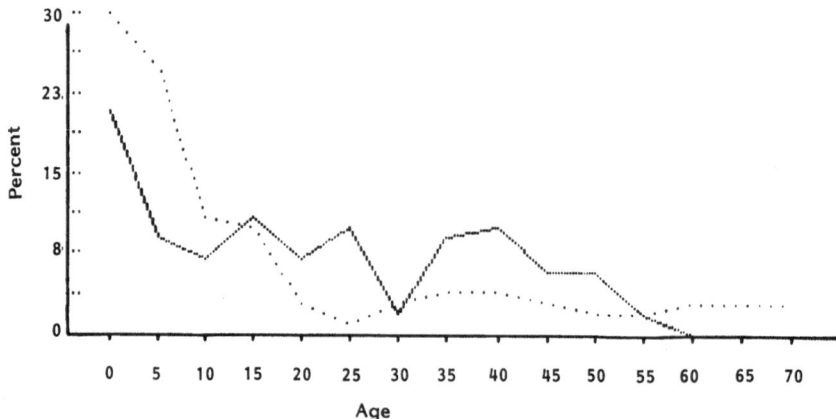

FIGURE 1. Comparison of valve donor (----) and recipient (···) age distributions.

TABLE II.   Etiology of Right-Sided Heart
Disease in Pediatric Valve Recipients

Disease	%
Pulmonary atresia	24
Tetralogy of Fallot	18
Truncus arteriosus	15
Pulmonary stenosis	15
Transplantation of great arteries	12
Miscellaneous	15

tion from all valve-related complications, including reoperation, embolism, and endocarditis, was 92% for viable cryopreserved allografts and 73% for nonviable 4°C refrigerated allografts.

CryoLife is a tissue-processing laboratory which will process tissue sent to it at the request of transplanting surgeons throughout the North American continent with the aid of various organ-retrieval services. The CryoLife allograft valve program was initiated with the arrival of the first heart in August 1984. The hearts received by CryoLife are those for which no suitable whole-heart recipient could be found. The heart donor and valve recipient age distributions of patients involved in this clinical program are indicated in Fig. 1. The donor data are based on all donors ($N = 90$) during February 1987. The recipient data are drawn from physician responses to our inquiries over a longer period in 1985 and 1986 ($N = 116$). It is obvious from a cursory examination of these curves that there are fewer pediatric donations, whereas most valves were actually placed in pediatric patients with congenital diseases of the right side of the heart (Table II). Most of the donors died in accidents; specific causes of death are indicated in Fig. 2. The donors averaged 2.5 days on a respirator (range 0–18 days). Following procurement, the hearts reached

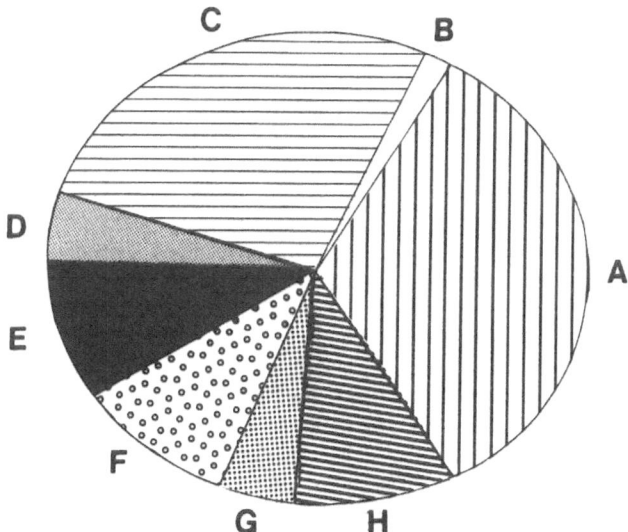

FIGURE 2. Cause of valve donor death. A, closed-head injury (34%); B, sudden infant death syndrome (2%); C, cerebrovascular accident (26%); D, transplantation (4%); E, gunshot wound (10%); F, multiple trauma (10%); G, drowning (4%); H, miscellaneous (10%).

TABLE III.   Frequency
of Procurement of Other
Organs from Donors of
Heart Valves

Organ	Frequency (%)
Kidney	86
Liver	31
Eye	14
Pancreas	13
Bone	13
Lung	3
Skin	1

the CryoLife service laboratory within the mandatory 24-hr time limit (mean 16 hr). In 98% of donations (Table III), at least one other organ (e.g., kidney, pancreas) was procured. During procurement of organs and tissues, care should be taken not to traumatize the tissues in any way, either by excessive handling, instrument contact, or dehydration. Tissues vary considerably in their ability to survive in the donor after cessation of heartbeat. This is because some tissues have limited tolerance for warm ischemia. Other tissues, such as skin, bone, and cartilage, may remain viable for several hours in the donor following cessation of heartbeat. Therefore, it is most important during the development of any specific transplant-preservation procedure to determine the requirements for prevention of cell damage due to variables during procurement and shipping.

Our efforts to increase the availability of cryopreserved heart valves have permitted surgeons to maintain valve banks. This enables the surgeons to select valves of the correct size for each individual patient. However, there is still a great need for increased tissue procurement, especially from pediatric donors for pediatric recipients.

3.2.   Corneal Transplantation

During corneal transplantation, a procedure known as penetrating keratoplasty, the central two thirds of a cornea is removed with a trephine and replaced with a similar sized donor cornea. Approximately 30,000 procedures are performed in the United States each year, and there were 3500–5000 people in the United States waiting for a donor cornea as of January 1, 1986 (Eye Bank Association of America, 1986). Therefore, as long as the supply keeps up with demands for tissues, there is very little requirement for long-term preservation. This has led to the use of short-term cold (4°C) and tissue culture (37°C) preservation techniques in corneal transplantation. Storage of cornea at low temperatures (4–6°C) was introduced by Filatov during the 1930s (Filatov, 1935). The first eye bank was founded in the United States by Paton (1945). Corneas are still, in general, stored at refrigerator temperatures. It is possible to culture corneas at 37°C in defined media for extended periods of time, but this method has not gained wide popularity because of problems with contamination of the tissue. Corneal storage became widely accepted with the introduction in 1974 of the McCarey–Kaufman (M–K) medium. This medium permits storage at refrigeration temperatures for 2–4 days. More recently, Kaufman et al. (1985) described a new cornea-preserving solution called K-Sol. K-Sol permits storage at refrigeration temperatures for 10–14 days and distribution of corneas on both a national and an international basis. The important component in K-Sol appears to be chondroitin sulfate. Chondroitin sulfate is a glycose aminoglycan. Glycose aminoglycans are long unbranched polysaccharide chains composed of repeating disaccharide units. The precise mechanism by which chondroitin sulfate confers on K-Sol the ability to store corneas is unknown.

3.3. Cartilage Transplantation

Cartilage has long been considered an immunologically privileged tissue, since it survives longer after transplantation than most other tissues, the exceptions being corneas and valves. Since cartilage has been clearly shown to be antigenic (Langer and Gross, 1974), it is believed that the matrix of cartilage acts as a barrier to protect the chondrocyte from the immune response. In long bone transplants, the calcified bone, which is below the cartilage proliferation plate, appears to function as an efficient barrier to lymphocyte invasion. However, in articular cartilage transplants, there is no physical barrier, and the immunological response that occurs at the surface of the graft results in destruction. It is crucial for a cartilage-bearing allograft that the cartilage, which does not replace or restore itself in adult life, remain biologically and metabolically functional in order to maintain its unique and essential biomechanical properties. Tomford and Mankin (1983) make it very clear in their review on investigational approaches to articular cartilage preservation that viable cartilage fares better than nonviable cartilage after transplantation. Preservation procedures for cartilage are still being developed. The best results so far have been obtained using cryopreservation (Tomford and Mankin, 1983, 1986). Cartilage is usually transplanted in cartilage-bearing allogeneic bonegrafts for reconstruction of joints damaged by trauma, degenerative diseases, and tumors. Since transplants suitable for a variety of anatomical sites, and in various sizes, are required, a large supply of tissue is necessary. Unfortunately, an inadequate supply of donor allogeneic tissue is resulting in curtailed growth of cartilage-bearing allogeneic bone transplantation.

4. BONE TRANSPLANTATION

Allogeneic bone is used for transplantation only when autogenous bone is not available. Transplantation of viable allogeneic bone will result in graft rejection. Antigens in bone grafts include those present on osteogenic cells, hemopoietic cells, vascular endothelium, nerve tissue, and connective tissue. It should be noted that under experimental conditions, all allografts, both viable and nonviable, evoke an immune response in recipients (Brown and Cruess, 1982). Results with frozen, demineralized, and freeze-dried bone have been favorable. The bone allograft produced by these techniques is nonviable; it is dead, but it is able to exert a biological function known as osteoinduction. For instance, the osteoinductive properties of demineralized bone have been used to encourage the growth of new bone in the craniofacial area of patients, principally children, with birth defects (Glowacki et al., 1981). The active component in osteoinduction is a substance known as bone morphogenic protein. This protein was isolated by Urist and collaborators (1979). The function of this protein is to induce cells of host origin to migrate into the dead bone and to form cartilage and new bone. Thus, the bone transplant acts as a stimulator for new bone formation and as a scaffold upon which the body forms new bone. It is likely that the bone morphogenic protein will soon be produced by recombinant DNA methods. Osteoinductive bone matrix powder, or recombinant bone morphogenic protein, has clinical potential in repairing fractures, deteriorating bone in aged persons, and damage due to periodontal diseases or bone cancer, in addition to use in surgery for congenital craniofacial defects.

A major problem that remains in the transplantation of cartilage-bearing bone allografts is the necessity to have both viable cartilage and nonviable bone. An approach to resolution of this problem could be to sterilize the bone with radiation while shielding the cartilage with lead. Thus, a nonviable osteoinductive bone scaffold with viable cartilage could be transplanted across immunological barriers.

5. BONE MARROW TRANSPLANTATION

The majority of diseases which have historically reduced man's average life expectancy are now prevented or cured. The result is that people now live longer and die from other diseases. Most people alive today will die of either heart disease or cancer. The aggressive therapy (irradiation and chemotherapy) for the majority of cancers destroys the bone marrow (blood-forming tissues), and if a suitable bone marrow transplant is not available, the patient will die. The methods for collection, manipulation, and cryopreservation of bone marrow are well defined (Gorin, 1986). In allogeneic bone marrow transplantation, it is extremely important to match the donor tissue to the recipient's tissues. This is done by comparison of the blood group antigens and the human leukocyte antigen (HLA) system. In excess of 50 antigens are believed to be of some significance. The level of significance of many of these antigens is still the subject of clinical investigation, and it is likely that other important antigens will be recognized in the future. The probability for problems after allogeneic bone marrow transplantation depends on the degree of match of the donor tissue to the recipient. The recipient may reject the donor bone marrow cells or, more likely, the graft's immune competent cells may reject the host. This phenomenon, known as graft versus host disease, can reduce the quality of life and be life-threatening. These problems can be overcome if it is possible to give the patients their own cells, i.e., an autologous bone marrow transplant. In the situation in which the patient is being treated for a solid tumor that does not metastasize to hematopoietic tissues, it is possible to withdraw bone marrow by aspiration prior to therapy and store the bone marrow at liquid nitrogen temperatures. However, some cancers metastasize specifically to bone marrow, and other cancers will be leukemias and lymphomas, cancers of the blood-forming tissues. In these situations, a process called bone marrow purging may be performed (Kaizer *et al.*, 1983). Bone marrow is taken from the patient prior to therapy and is treated *in vitro* with chemotherapeutic agents, which, it is hoped, will have a greater specificity for the cancer cells than for the bone marrow cells. Then, at a later time, following therapy, the patient will be infused with his own bone marrow cells, which were cryopreserved during therapy. Unfortunately, in spite of significant long-term survivals in some patients using this approach, if one cancer cell remains after purging the bone marrow, the cancer will probably recur. There are several acquired hematological diseases, e.g., aplastic anemia, which can be cured if autologous bone marrow is available for transplantation.

In addition, persons with acquired immune deficiency syndrome (AIDS) and those receiving sublethal doses of nuclear radiation would benefit from having their own bone marrow in storage. The questions therefore arises, Why are bone marrow banks not popular? The reason is that the risks of death from anesthesia during bone marrow aspiration are greater than the chances of developing a blood cell cancer or of being involved in a nuclear accident. General anesthesia is required for bone marrow collection for transplantation because 0.75–1.5 liters of bone marrow aspirate will be withdrawn. This necessitates 100 or more individual aspirations of marrow an extremely painful process.

The goal of many investigators in hematology is to develop techniques to expand small volumes of bone marrow for transplantation purposes. The rationale for this line of investigation is that for donation of small samples of bone marrow, local anesthesia is adequate. The donor can leave shortly after the procedure. Currently, it is not possible to expand human bone marrow *in vitro*, but there has been major success using mouse marrow (Dexter *et al.*, 1977), and advances in this field may occur at any moment. Success in this endeavor would make available, from small samples of bone marrow, tissue for autologous transplantation of the donor or for allogeneic transplantation of close relatives of the donor, if the level of HLA compatability permits. The future situation that is envisaged is that children would routinely donate in a single aspiration a few milliliters of bone marrow, a procedure similar to that performed routinely for diagnostic bone marrow biopsies. The bone marrow would then be expanded *in vitro* using culture conditions that are currently the subject of intensive investigation. When adequate bone marrow has been grown, the bone marrow sample would be cryopreserved and stored at approximately $-196°C$. Bone marrow has been successfully cryopreserved for several years, and it is generally believed that indefinite storage is possible, because no detectable biological deterioration should occur at these ultralow temperatures. Care would have to be taken that tissues did not warm past $-100°C$. Such temperature fluctuations cause loss of tissue viability. Bone marrow quality can be ensured both before and after cryopreservation by checking the bone marrow samples for microbial contamination and for viability of the cells required for successful bone marrow transplantation.

6. LIGAMENT AND TENDON TRANSPLANTATION

The biomechanical role of ligaments and tendons has long been appreciated, and there are many commercially available prosthetic implants. Unfortunately, for some sites, especially those that undergo flexion, these implants do not achieve satisfactory function. An example is the anterior cruciate ligament (Jackson and Drez, 1987); prosthetic materials have been unable to simulate the major histological zones that reduce stress concentrations at the ligament–bone insertion sites. Prosthetic materials developed to date are either too elastic, fail to provide adequate knee stability, or are too rigid. There have been a few studies in which cryopreservation has been attempted. These studies show that the mechanical properties of ligaments can be preserved by cryopreservation. Little is known about the viability of the cells in cryopreserved ligaments using methods that permit retention of mechanical properties. Viable cryopreservation of ligaments is complicated by the fact that there are different cell types present in this tissue: endothelial cells, chondrocytes, fibrous cartilage cells, and connective tissue fibroblasts. Cryopreserved ligaments, processed by CryoLife, are currently being transplanted experimentally in dogs, and the first clinical trials should be initiated in 1989. One of the requirements for use of allogeneic ligaments and tendons is to have available a bank of material suitable for surgical procedures. Therefore, large-scale procurement of different-sized ligaments and tendons from a variety of anatomical sites will be required in the future.

7. PANCREATIC CELL TRANSPLANTATION

The problems of immune rejection continue to be the major obstacle for transplantation of endocrine cells. The term ''endocrine'' implies that the secretions of the cell are released directly into blood vessels, rather than into ducts, as is the case with exocrine glands. Some examples of endocrine glands are the adrenal glands, the parathyroid glands, the anterior lobe of the pituitary, the thyroid gland, and the B cells of the pancreas. Because of the great significance of pancreatic B-cells for the cure of diabetes, comments are restricted to pancreatic B-cell transplantation. However, it should be noted that all the techniques mentioned here for B cells are appropriate for other endocrine glands as well. The pancreatic B cells are found scattered throughout the exocrine portion of the pancreas in richly vascularized, small masses of endocrine cells. The B cell is one type of endocrine cell found in these small masses, and the masses are known as islets of Langerhans. The B cells produce insulin in response to hyperglycemia. Therefore, it has long been the objective of many scientists to transplant the islets of Langerhans, containing B cells, into patients with diabetes who require regulated production of insulin. Immune rejection is the major obstacle to transplantation of the islets of Langerhans as a treatment for diabetes. Three methods are being developed to circumvent the tissue recipient's immune system.

Pancreatic islets have been treated with ultraviolet (uv) irradiation in the 280- to 320-nm wavelength (Hardy *et al.*, 1986). In rodents, this treatment resulted in marked prolongation of pancreatic islet allograft survival. Experiments in primates have been unsuccessful, even when transplantation has been combined with immunosuppressive cyclosporin therapy. However, it appears that primate islets are more sensitive to uv irradiation than are rodent islets and that the islets discussed in published studies were probably dead. Therefore, we must await the results of future studies employing lower doses of uv irradiation before coming to any conclusions about this approach to islet transplantation.

A second approach to islet transplantation has been advanced by Lafferty *et al.* (1986). Lafferty's method involves a short period of organ culture. Aggregates of approximately 50 islets of Langerhans are formed and cultured in an oxygen-rich solution. Following organ culture, islet allografts have reversed chemically induced diabetes in mice. Clinical studies using cultured fetal islet cells are currently in progress.

The approach to islet transplantation that is currently most promising is the technique of microencapsulation. Microencapsulation consists of enclosing islets in a membrane that is impermeable to the large host immunoregulatory molecules (antibodies) but that permits glucose from the host's circulation to diffuse freely into the islets of Langerhans. Insulin produced by the islets in response to the glucose will diffuse out. The encapsulation process, described by Lim (1983), consists of forming a suspension of islets in approximately 0.5-mm spheres of sodium alginate gel. The spheres are then coated with poly-L-lysine. By varying the molecular weight of the poly-L-lysine and the thickness of the coat of poly-L-lysine on the alginate sphere, it is possible to produce a sieve with defined molecular size restriction properties. Encapsulated islets have successfully cured chemically induced diabetic rodents across major immunological barriers. This technique holds the exciting promised of permitting use of xenografts, grafts between species, to rescue diabetic patients. In preliminary studies, we have successfully reduced the blood glucose levels of diabetic mice with transplants of cryopreserved encapsulated rat and pig islets of Langerhans. The ability to cryopreserve encapsulated tissue permits the accumulation of cells from several donors. It also facilitates shipping to surgeries, and it is not susceptible to the contamination hazards of long-term maintenance in tissue culture.

The above methods offer promise for transplantation of islets in diabetics. It should be noted that there are other approaches that we have not touched on involving manipulation of the recipient. For instance, the use of donor-specific uv light-irradiated blood transfusions or of brief pretransplant immunosuppression. Rather, we have limited ourselves to techniques for modification of the transplant in such a way that the recipient no longer recognizes the transplant as foreign.

8. BLOOD VESSEL TRANSPLANTATION

There will probably be approximately 150,000 procedures involving blood vessels this year in the United States. For procedures involving blood vessels greater than 10 mm in diameter, several prosthetic vessels are available. Prosthetic materials do not do well when used to replace vessels smaller than 10 mm in diameter. The field of small vessel research is a very active one, since there will be at least 70,000 procedures during 1987 in this vessel size range. Some approaches to solving the problem of small vessel transplantation are (1) to coat prosthetic vessels with endothelial cells (Graham *et al.*, 1980; Watkins *et al.*, 1984), (2) to grow blood vessels in tissue culture (Weinberg and Bell, 1986), and (3) to cryopreserve human saphenous veins. It should be noted that in all these approaches, the presence of vascular endothelium is considered important. The endothelium produces fibrinolytic substances and plasminogen activators, which protect against thrombogenesis (Loskutoff and Edgington, 1977), and prostaglandins, which play a role in maintaining small vessel patency (Weksler *et al.*, 1977). Both experimental and clinical reports have indicated that endothelial damage in vessels promotes both thrombosis and intimal thickening. Analysis of cryopreserved saphenous vein has previously shown extensive endothelial damage (Balderman *et al.* 1984; Sachs *et al.*, 1982). We have been actively involved in perfecting saphenous vein cryopreservation for the past 2 years. We have developed a method for cryopreservation of saphenous vein that results in a morphologically intact endothelium. In addition, we have found, using an *in vitro* clonogenic assay, that endothelial viability after cryopreservation is not significantly different from that of control unfrozen veins. Cryopreserved saphenous veins have successfully undergone preclinical trials in dogs, and a limited clinical study has been initiated in patients for whom there is no other suitable alternative. Preliminary vein post-transplant observations are extremely encouraging, but adequate data for statistical analysis will not be available until the end of 1988.

9. CONCLUSION

We have discussed some current developments and future possibilities in tissue transplantation at a time of increased tissue requirements for transplantation and medical research. Increased donation is required to ensure an adequate tissue supply. In addition to the tissues previously mentioned, there are many other tissues that could be procured as the medical incentive develops. These include lengths of gastrointestinal tract, uterus, larynx, ureter, peripheral nerves, muscles, and many glandular tissues. A major problem in building tissue banks is limited donation of tissues, which results in inadequate inventory of immunologically and size-matched transplants. The problem of limited donation is largely attributable to failure of medical personnel to identify potential donors and the reluctance of the next of kin to authorize procurement of tissue. This problem should eventually be overcome by education of both the public and the medical profession on the potential benefits of tissue and organ donation to society.

REFERENCES

Balderman, S. C., Montes, M., Schwartz, K., Hart, T., Bhayana, J. N., and Gage, A. A., 1984, Preparation of venous allografts, *Ann. Surg.* **200:**117–130.

Bank, H. L., and Brockbank, K. G. M., 1987, Basic principles of cryobiology, *J. Cardiac Surg.* **2**(suppl):137–143.

Barratt-Boyes, B. G., Roches, A. H. G., Brandt, P. W. T., Smith, J. C., and Lowe, J. B., 1969, Aortic homograft valve replacement: A long-term follow-up of an initial series of 101 patients, *Circulation* **40:**763–775.

Brockbank, K. G. M., and Bank, H. L., 1987, Measurement of post cryopreservation viability, *J. Cardiac Surg.* **2** (suppl):145–151.

Brown, K. L. B., and Cruess, R. L., 1982, Bone and cartilage transplantation in orthopaedic surgery, *J. Bone Joint Surg.* **64A:**270–279.

Dexter, T. M., Allen, T. D., and Lajtha, L. G., 1977, Conditions controlling the proliferation of haemopoietic stem cells in vitro, *J. Cell. Physiol.* **91:**335–344.

Eye Bank Association of America, 1986, *Eye Banking Activity—1985 (EBAA report)*, Eye Bank Association of America, Washington, D. C.

Filatov, V. P., 1935, Transplantation of the cornea, *Arch. Ophtlamol.* **13:**321–347.

Glowacki, J., Kaban, L. B. Murray, J. E., Folkman, J., and Mulliken, J. B., 1981, Application of the biological principle of induced osteogenesis for craniofacial defects, *Lancet* **1:**959–963.

Gorin, N. C., 1986, Collection, manipulation and freezing of haemopoietic stem cells, *Clin. Haematol.* **15:**19–48.

Graham, L. M., Burkel, W. E., Ford, J. W., Vinter, D. W., Kahn, R. H., and Stanley, J. C., 1980, Immediate seeding of enzymatically derived endothelium in Dacron vascular grafts. Early experimental studies with autologous canine cells, *Arch. Surg.* **115:**1289–1294.

Hardy, M. D., Chabot, J., Tannebaum, G., and Lau, H. T., 1986, Immunomodulation by ultraviolet irradiation, in *Transplantation: Approaches to Graft Rejection* (H. T. Meryman, ed.), pp. 119–138, Alan R. Liss, New York.

Jackson, D. W., and Drez, D. (eds.), 1987, *The Anterior Cruciate Deficient Knee*, C. V. Mosby, St. Louis.

Kaizer, H., Tutschika, P., Stuart, R., Korbling, M., Braine, H., Saral, R., Colvin, M., and Santos, G., 1983, Autologous bone marrow transplantation in acute leukemia and non-Hodgkins's lymphoma: A phase 1 study of 4-hydroperoxycyclophosphamide (4HC) incubation of marrow prior to cryopreservation, in: *Haematology and Blood Transfusion*, Vol. 28, *Modern Trends in Human Leukemia*, Vol. V (R. Neth, R. C. Gallo, M. F. Greaves, M. A-S. Moore, and K. Winkler, eds.), pp. 90–91, Springer-Verlag, Berlin.

Kamp, van der, A. W. M., Visser, W. J., Donger, van, J. M., Nanta, J., and Galjaard, H., 1981, Preservation of aortic heart valves with maintenance of cell viability, *J. Surg. Res.* **30**:47–56.

Kaufman, H. E., Varnell, E. D., Kaufman, S., Beuerman, R. W., and Barron, B. A., 1985, K-Sol corneal preservation, *Am. J. Ophthamol.* **100**:199–304.

Lafferty, K. J., Babcock, S. K., and Gill, R. G., 1986, Prevention of rejection by treatment of the graft: an overview, in: *Transplantation: Approaches to Graft Rejection* (H. T. Meryman, ed.), pp. 87–117., New York.

Langer, F., and Gross, A. E., 1974, Immunogenicity of allograft articular cartilage, *J. Bone Joint Surg.* **56A**:297–304.

Lim, F., 1983, Preparation of substances with encapsulated cells, U.S. Patent #4,409,331.

Loskutoff, D. J., and Edgington, T. S., 1977, Synthesis of a fibrinolytic activator and inhibitor by endothelial cells, *Proc. Natl. Acad. Sci. USA* **74**:3903–3907.

Lovelock, J. E., and Bishop, M. W. H., 1959, Prevention of freezing damage to living cells by dimethylsulphoxide, *Nature (Lond.)* **183**:1394–1395.

McCarey, B. E., and Kaufman, H. E., 1974, Improved corneal storage, *Invest. Ophthalmol.* **13**:165–173.

Mermet, B., Buch, W. S., and Angell, W. W., 1970, Viable heart graft: Preservation in the frozen state, *Surg. Forum* **21**:156–157.

Mochtar, B., Kamp, van der, A. W. M. N., Roza-de Jough, E. J. M., and Nauta, J., 1984, Cell survival in canine aortic heart valves stored in nutrient medium, *Cardiovasc. Res.* **18**:497–501.

Murray, G., 1956, Homologous aortic valve segment transplant as surgical treatment for aortic and mitral insufficiency, *Angiology* **7**:466–471.

O'Brien, M. F., Stafford, G., Gardner, M. Brosnan, A., 1987, The viable cryopreserved allograft aortic valve, *J. Cardiac Surg.* **2**(suppl):153–167.

Patton, R. T., 1945, Sight restoration through corneal grafting, *Sight Sav. Rev.* **15**:3–12.

Polge, C., Smith, A. Y., and Parkes, A. S., 1949, Revival of spermatozoa after vitrification and dehydration at low temperatures, *Nature* (Lond.) **164**:666.

Ross, D., 1987, Application of Homografts in clinical surgery, *J. Cardiac Surg.* **2**(suppl):175–182.

Sachs, S. M., Ricotta, J. J., Scott, D. E., and DeWeese, J. A., 1982, Endothelial integrity after venous cryopreservation, *J. Surg. Res.* **32**:218–227.

Sanfilippo, F. R., MacQueen, J. J., Vaugh, W. K., and Foulks, G. N., 1986, Reduced graft rejection with good HLA-A and B matching in high-risk corneal transplantation, *N. Engl. J. Med.* **315**:29–35.

Tomford, W. W., and Mankin, H. J., 1983, Investigational approaches to articular cartilage preservation, *Clin. Orthoped.* **174**:22–27.

Tomford, W. W., and Mankin, H. J., 1986, Studies in preservation of Bone and Cartilage, *Cryobiology* **23**:568 (abst.).

Urist, M. R., Mikulski, A., and Lietze, A., 1979, Solubilized and insolubilized bone morphogenetic protein, *Proc. Natl. Acad. Sci. USA* **76**:1828–1832.

Watkins, M. T., Sharefkin, J. B., Zajtchuk, R., Maciag, T. M., D'Amore, P. A., Ryan, U. S., VanWart, H., and Rich, N. M., 1984, Adult human saphenous vein endothelial cells: Assessment of their reproductive capacity for use in endothelial seeding of vascular prostheses, *J. Surg. Res.* **36**:588–596.

Weinberg, C. B., and Bell, E., 1986, A blood vessel model constructed from collagen and cultured vascular cells, *Science* **231**:397–400.

Weksler, B. B., Marcus, A. J. and Jaffe, E. A., 1977, Synthesis of prostaglandin I-2 (prostacyclin) by cultured human and bovine endothelial cells, *Proc. Natl. Acad. Sci. USA* **74**:3922–3926.

V

OTHER TOPICS IN ORGAN RETRIEVAL AND DONATION

26

ORGAN AND TISSUE RETRIEVAL AND DONATION
The Ethical Imperative

ALBERT R. JONSEN

1. INTRODUCTION

An organ, as defined in *Taber's Medical Dictionary,* is "a part of the body having special function." The entry goes on to note that, since most organs are in pairs, "one may be extirpated and the remaining one will perform all necessary functions." In the accompanying alphabetical list of 32 organs, however, at least 13 are not paired and, of these, the extirpation of several, such as heart and liver, is fatal (barring their immediate replacement). Nevertheless, the dictionary's remark is well taken, since the human body has a remarkable ability to compensate for the loss of its parts or to generate tissue. For centuries, this was important because parts were lost by accident or by deliberate extirpation in a surgical procedure. One ethical question was consistently asked about deliberate extirpation: Is it morally licit to multilate one's body? The answer, from most moralists during those centuries, was "yes, if the loss of the bodily part is necessary for the health of the whole body." Clearly, the physical and physiological capacity to compensate for loss of an organ, and even more, of tissue made that answer an easy one.

In recent years, however, a new question has arisen: Is it morally licit to mutilate one's body for the sake of the health of another person? This question arose because it became technically possible to take a living organ from one person and place it in or upon the living body of another. Transplantation of the cornea and of skin and transfusion of blood became feasible medical procedures during the first half of the twentieth century. Transplantation of major organs has become feasible during the second half. Thus, the ethical question about mutilation takes on a new dimension: Does the motive of charity or beneficence change in any way the traditional answer? The changes might be threefold: (1) Is it morally permissible to give up an organ for the sake of another?; (2) Is it morally obligatory to give up an organ for the sake of another?; and (3) Is it morally permissible or obligatory for others, such as the state, to take organs from the living or the dead, if those organs are needed?

ALBERT R. JONSEN • Department of Medical History and Ethics, University of Washington School of Medicine, Seattle, Washington 98105.

A poignant case illustrates the relevance of these questions. Robert McFall was suffering from aplastic anemia. A bone marrow transplantation was recommended as potential life-saving therapy. Mr. McFall's cousin, Daniel Shimp, was a medically suitable donor of bone marrow but, on being invited to donate, refused. Mr. McFall sought to force his cousin by seeking a court order. Judge Flaherty denied the order, saying that "forceable extraction of bodily tissue causes revulsion to the judicial mind." But he also noted that Shimp's refusal to help his cousin was "morally indefensible" (*Science*, 1978).

The revulsion felt by the judicial mind is fostered by a long tradition in the Anglo-American common law that favors inviolability of the human body. It is also reinforced by an American constitutional protection of the integrity of the human body. The moral indefensibility that Judge Flaherty attributed to Shimp's legally defensible refusal of help is also deeply rooted in the moral tradition of Western culture. It has long been taught in that tradition that one person has a moral obligation to assist another in danger, particularly if some special relationship exists between the two parties and it is possible to help without great inconvenience. However, the incompatability between the judicial repugnance and the moral indefensibility stems from the fact that even the moralists admit that an obligation "in charity"—or benevolence—differs from an obligation "in justice"—sometimes described as a matter of "rights." Shimp, it could be said, has a moral obligation to McFall; McFall has no "right" to Shimp's marrow.

Against this background, the ethical "imperative" mentioned in the sub-title of this chapter is ambiguous. It is possible to make a strong case that there is an "imperative in charity," but not an "imperative in justice" that governs the obtaining of organs for transplantation. However, even then, there is a further ambiguity, and it appears in the other words of the title, "retrieval and donation." We have adopted the phrase "organ donation," not merely because it has a nice public relations ring, but because it reflects the moral and legal tradition of our culture: the legal inviolability of the body and the moral obligation in charity. However, the question can be asked whether "retrieval" might not be less a matter of charitable gift and more a matter of justice. Can organs be taken or "harvested" even when no person has made a gift of them?

2. PERMISSIBILITY OF DONATION

The first ethical question raised by organ transplantation is whether it is morally permissible to give up, for any purpose, an important body part. This is an ancient question, raised long before organ transplantation was possible: Do persons have the authority to multilate their bodies, that is, to separate from themselves a part or organ that would appear to be a natural constituitive part? Roman Catholicism and Judaism have long forbidden mutilation. The person is but steward of his or her body; dominion over the body is God's alone. Any mutilation is morally justified only if it will contribute to the well being of the person whose body is mutilated. Thus, removal of a diseased limb to save one's life was permitted. The advent of successful transplantation of organs and tissues called for refinement of this traditional position. In both faiths, the predominant opinion at present allows that the removal of an organ for immediate and genuine benefit of another person should not be considered a reprehensible self-mutilation; indeed, it is an act of charity. However, this position envisages that the removal of the organ will not cause serious detriment to the donor; certainly, it would not be tolerated if the removal of the organ was attended with certainty of the donor's death. Thus, donation of one's heart while still living would be forbidden and condemned as suicide (Kelly, 1965; Rosner, 1986).

3. OBLIGATION OF DONATION

The second question is more complex: Is it morally obligatory to give up an organ for the sake of another? Again, this question refers to a debate that long antedates transplantation: What is the stringency and the extent of one's moral duty to come to the aid of another person in need? The Roman philosopher Cicero posed the case of the philosopher and the sailor clinging to a slender piece of flotsam after a shipwreck: was one of these obliged to give up his place for the other? Catholic and Jewish traditions have long debated the problem in other contexts. Their answer is a qualified "yes"—such a duty does exist and the weight of its obligation depends on the degree of affinity to the one in need, on the seriousness of the need, of the risk one must take, and, finally, on the likelihood that the helping action will really help.

This sort of duty has generally been identified as an obligation in charity or beneficience rather than a duty in justice. The meaning of this distinction has been much debated. In general, the distinction was not crafted to differentiate more and less important duties: Both justice and charity are significant in understanding the moral life. Yet, they do designate notably diverse occasions in the moral life: Obligations in justice can be written in precise terms regarding the nature, time, and place of their fulfillment. The persons to whom they are due and who can claim a right to them are identifiable as parties to contracts, promises, loans, or holders of certain offices and positions. The circumstances that exempt or excuse from these duties are rare, weighty, and specific. Perhaps, most significant, sentiment or fellow-feeling have little to do with the origin or the extinction or the attenuation of these obligations. The persons to whom such duties are owed may as frequently, or more frequently, be strangers than acquaintances.

Obligations in charity or benevolence may be equally serious, but they seem to belong more to the realm of fellowship than of commerce. Opportunities for their exercise are more occasional, discretional, and convenient. Usually, no specific other party can claim a right to be recipient of their benefit. Gratitude, rather than demand, is the recipient's attitude. At one end of the spectrum of obligations in charity, certain actions are "supererogatory," literally "beyond what can be asked." These are heroic acts in which the cost to the performer is great; one who performs them is worthy of praise, but one who omits them is hardly subject to blame. At the other end of the spectrum lie certain relationships, such as consensual agreements, which can be defined equally well as legal or moral relationships and which are, in fact, often the object of lawmaking. In the most general sense, then, duties of justice bear on the kinds of moral relationships that are requisite for the very existence and functioning of a human society; their disregard corrodes the social structure. Obligations of benevolence make a society a better place for persons to live well; disdain for these obligations leaves society meaner and rougher (Feinberg, 1984).

The boundary between duties of charity and duties of justice is not sharp. The moral obligation to help another in need starts to turn more specific, relative both to the recipient and to the occasion, when persons are bound by some natural or conventional tie, when the performance is possible without great inconvenience, and when the effect will relieve the recipient of great harm. Thus, in the case of cousins McFall and Shimp, the donation of bone marrow, which poses little risk to the donor, would impose a significant obligation on Shimp. Yet Shimp's fear of adverse effects as well as the possibility that the procedure might fail provide him with a weak excuse; he can be called cowardly and selfish, but not unjust. As a matter of justice, Shimp has as much, indeed more, claim to his marrow as does McFall. Unjust Shimp is not; uncharitable he certainly is.

Against the background of this traditinal distinction, the term "donation" seems appropriate. There is an obligation in benevolence to make a gift of one's organs to assist those who can benefit from them: the stringency of that obligation depends on the relationships between persons, the feasibility of the gift to the donor, and the need of the recipient. But an obligation in benevolence never becomes absolute. Thus, we reject totally the notion, proposed in a short story of several years ago, that the organs of some vigorous youths could be confiscated for the benefit of geriatric congressmen, as in a national "organ draft." We repudiate the application of social and psychological pressure upon potential donors. We even hesitate to use minors as donors for their siblings, unless it can be suggested that the donor, as well as the recipient will be the beneficiary of the "donation."

All of this suggests that, in our culture, organs, no matter how badly needed for persons in danger of death, can be obtained only through gift, implemented by the free choice of a donor. The ethical imperative that bears on that free choice is an obligation in benevolence or charity, not an obligation in justice.

4. FAMILY AND SOCIETAL RIGHTS AND OBLIGATIONS

However, most organs for transplantation do come from cadavers, persons judged dead on the basis of brain-related criteria. During the late 1960s, the Uniform Anatomical Gift Act was passed in every state. This law enables competent adults to indicate their intention to donate the organs of their body at the time of their death by signing a legally valid document. In the absence of such a document and in the absence of contrary indications by the decedent, specified family members may authorize the taking of organs (as stated in the Uniform Anatomical Gift Act, 1983).

The Anatomical Gift Act reflects, even in its title, the ethical belief that organs be obtained only by donation and that the moral imperative is one of an obligation in charity. It makes new law, insofar as it projects the right of a person over his or her body into the future, as if bodily parts were like possessions that could be left by testament. However, it infringes somewhat the ethic of benevolence and voluntary donation by allowing next of kin to authorize the retrieval of organs even in the absence of the decedent's wishes. In this respect, the Anatomical Gift Act reflects old law that gives authority to next of kin over the disposition of the cadaver of their relative and applies that old law to the retrieval of organs, just as it had been applied to the permitting of an autopsy. This departure from the ethical basis in benevolence is barely noticeable, since the law hews quite closely to the traditional authority of the family. Still, the departure is significant: does it suggest that the society's need for organs might override the principle of donation? Can sound ethical reasoning refute that principle or demonstrate that others than the deceased and immediate family have authority of the disposition of the body?

These are reasonable questions in the light of the shortage of organs for transplant. In recent years, concern has grown that the supply of organs is in critical shortage. Approximately 20,000 persons are declared dead each year on the basis of brain-related criteria; organs are obtained from approximately 2000. Yet, the need for hearts, lungs, and kidneys is estimated in the range of 50,000 or more potential beneficiaries (Schwartz, 1985).

Western philosophical and religious ethics contains nothing that would argue against the moral propriety of a person's willing body parts after death. At the same time, there is little in this tradition that would support the requirement that removal of organs must always be sanctioned by an explicit voluntary donation. Indeed, one modern ethical theory, utilitarianism, could provide a plausible argument that any use of the body of a decedent that could benefit society would be mandatory, unless society's revulsion or discomfort at certain uses counterbalanced the advantages. However, one of the difficulties often raised by philosophers against utilitarian theory is the absence of any clear distinction between benevolence and justice.

Can the removal of organs for transplantation, without or even against the explicit wishes of the decedent or the family, be ethically justified? Does the cadaver, in some sense, belong to the state or to society? Should organ retrieval be seen as an obligation in justice rather than an obligation in charity? Can it be shown that the obligation rests not on individuals directly but on the state?

Can it be said that the state has an obligation to retrieve and make available organs as part of its general obligation to provide equal access to an adequate level of health care? (President's Commission for the Study of Ethical Problems in Medicine and Biomedical and Behavioral Research, 1982). Such a position is not, I think, implausible. It is analogous to the state's right to impose death duties toward the general goal of redistributive justice. A significant need exists; a significant benefit can accrue to recipients. At the same time, it is difficult to demonstrate that a significant interest of those from whom organs would be taken is violated. Thus, should we relax the ethic of donation?

Yet, most ethicists have argued against routine salvaging of organs without personal or familial permission. Ramsey proposed that "the routine taking of organs would deprive individuals of the exercise of the virtue of generosity" (Ramsey, 1970). Veatch (1976) also states that, in a "society which values personal integrity and freedom, we must be able to control our bodies not only in our lifetime but within reasonable limits after that life is gone."

Muyskens, a philosopher, has argued against both Ramsey and Veatch. Against Ramsey, he maintains that routine salvaging does not deprive persons of the opportunity to exercise the virtue of generosity simply because there are many ways to demonstrate that virtue. Against Veatch, he counters that salvaging does not undermine individual autonomy of the individual and collectivity, since not all powers vested in the state threaten the autonomy of the individual. Thus, "with regard to organs such as kidneys—given the relatively good chances of successful transplantation—we [pragmatically] ought to be [hence, if acting rationally would be] willing to relinquish our right to be buried intact." (Muyskens, 1978).

Caplan (1984) suggested approaches that, while dispensing with explicit consent, are short of routine harvesting. He proposed that consent be presumed: Unless a person or a family explicitly objects to removal of organs, it can be presumed that a person would be willing to donate for the good of others. Kennedy has made the same suggestion in Great Britain. In France, the law actually approves such an approach: Cadaver organs can be taken unless the decedent has objected or the family objects. However, if the right to refuse is taken seriously, it would require record keeping and coordination that would be complex and perhaps impossible. Caplan recently modified this concept to "required request": hospital personnel would be required by law to request permission of the family. Several states have already enacted legislation to this effect.

Can an argument be constructed that would replace or supplement the ethics of benevolence by an ethic of justice? It is doubtful that, given the background of western philosophical and religious ethics, a persuasive case could be made to replace the ethic of benevolence in the matter of organ donation. However, this ethic of benevolence does rest upon the significant value of personal autonomy and personal bodily integrity. It is more likely that the ethic of justice could be seen as a supplement to the ethic of benevolence. Once personal autonomy and integrity are no longer at stake, after the death of an individual, then organs might be seen as a scarce resource to be distributed according to principles of justice. The living would have a right to the organs of the dead.

Even if thoughtful philosophical consideration were to conclude that social use of organs is ethical and, in general, supersedes the ethical value of individual or familial right to prohibit such use, there might be important policy reasons for not adopting this position. Intrusion into the grief of survivors is repugnant. The use of cadavers for organ retrieval might lead to the use of sources less obviously acceptable, such as anencephalics and persons in a persistent vegetative state. Various religious sentiments against mutilation of the dead and in favor of respectful disposition might be offended. Difficulties in fair distribution of organs might be perplexing. In addition, it is somewhat peculiar to imagine a system in which organs for transplant are readily available while there is no guarantee of access to the system for most, other, less dramatic health needs. Those in danger of death from major organ failure would be helped; those in danger from lack of immunization, malnutrition, and so forth, would remain in the perilous *status quo*. A policy that would afford certain legal protections to the refusal of individuals and families, as well as requiring permission of next of kin when available, might be preferable. Law might be devised that will make organs available with ease, while at the same time respecting these limitations. Yet, the problems encountered in framing such a statute can be seen in the history of such an effort in Virginia (Lombardo, 1981; Caplan, 1983, 1984; Kennedy, 1979; Raymond, 1978; Sadler and Sadler, 1984).

The supply of organs may be increased by means short of routine harvesting. Legislation and social arrangements could tip the balance in favor of donation. The law might favor or mandate request to patients or next of kin of the deceased. Arguments against a market in organs do not rule out certain arrangements that might involve monetary considerations. Tax deductions or reduction in hospital bills might increase the incentive to donate. The idea of organized giving to charity based on similar incentives was probably frowned on in the early twentieth century by those accustomed to giving solely for the sake of charity, unmotivated by anything but generosity.

5. CONCLUSION

Organs for transplantation are, at present and for the forseeable future, in short supply; many persons who might benefit by organ transplantation will be unable to receive an organ. The dominance of the concept of gift and the definition of the ethical imperative relative to the obtaining of organs as an obligation in charity rather than justice does impose certain constraints on the "harvesting" of organs. Even if charity is supplemented by justice, it might be wise to refrain from policies that could maximize efficiency of organ retrieval, if those policies cast a shadow on the "gift relationship" which, as Titmus warned with regard to blood, constitutes a crucial element of our humanity (Titmus, 1971).

REFERENCES

Caplan, A., 1983, Organ transplants: The costs of success, *Hastings Ctr. Rep.* **13**(6):23–32.

Caplan, A., 1984, Ethical and policy issues in the procurement of cadaver organs for transplantation, *N. Engl. J. Med.* **311**:981–984.

DHEW Task Force on Organ Transplantation, 1986, Department of Health and Human Services, Washington, D. C.

Feinberg, J., 1984, *Harm To Others. The Moral Limits of the Criminal Law*, Oxford University Press, New York.

Gaylin, W., 1974, Harvesting the dead, *Harpers* **249**:23–30.

Harrison, M., and Meilaender, G., 1986, The anencephalic newborn as organ donor, *Hastings Ctr. Rep.* **16**:(2)21–23.

Kelly, G., 1956, The morality of mutilation: Toward a revision of the treatise, *Theol. Stud.* **17**:332–344.

Kennedy, I., 1979, The donation and transportation of kidneys: Should the law be changed?, *J. Med. Ethics* **5**:13–21.

Lombardo, P., 1981, Consent and donations from the dead, *Hastings Ctr. Rep.* **11**(6):9–11.

Massachusetts Task Force on Organ Transplantation, 1985, *Law Med. Health Care* **13**(1):8–27.

Muyskens, J. J., 1978, An alternative policy for obtaining cadaver organs, *Phil. Public Affairs* **8**:88–99.

Perry, C., 1980, Human organs and the open market, *Ethics* **91**:63–71.

The Pittsburgh Press, 1985. The challenge of a miracle: Selling the gift. Nov 3–8.

President's Commission for the Study of Ethical Problems in Medicine and Biomedical and Behavioral Research, 1982, Securing Access to Health Care. U. S. Government Printing Office, Washington, D. C.

Ramsey, P., 1970, *Patient as Person*, Yale University Press, New Haven.

Raymond, A., 1978, France, the automatic transplant. *Washington Post* August 16, 1978.

Rolston, H., 1982, The irreversibly comatose: Respect for the subhuman in human life. *J. Med. Philos.* **7**:337–354.

Rosner, F., 1986, *Modern Medicine and Jewish Ethics,* Chapter 19, Yeshiva University Press, New York.

Sadler, A. M., and Sadler, B., 1984, Organ donation: Is voluntarism still valid?, *Hastings Ctr. Rep.* **14**(5): 6–9.

Schwartz, H. S., 1985, Bioethical and legal considerations in increasing the supply of transplantable organs: from UAGA to "Baby Fae," *Am. J. Law Med.* **10**:397–438.

Science 1978, **210**:596.

Titmus, R. M., 1971, *The Blood Relationship,* Vintage, New York.

Veatch, R. M., 1976, *Death, Dying and the Biological Revolution,* Yale University Press, New Haven.

Walzer, M., 1983, *Spheres of Justice,* Basic Books, New York.

27

ATTITUDES TOWARD CLINICAL AND SOCIAL ISSUES IN ORGAN PROCUREMENT

JEFFREY M. PROTTAS and HELEN LEVINE BATTEN

1. INTRODUCTION

Organ supply depends on the active cooperation of several groups. The general public is the ultimate source of all human organs, but certain medical professionals have a key role in the process as well. In fact, the cooperation of these medical professionals antedates in time and overshadows in impact the role the giving public plays. The sequence of organ procurement must start with a referral from a hospital. Within this context, a "referral" contains two elements—a call from a clinician informing an organ procurement agency that one of his patients has been, or shortly will be, declared dead by brain-death criteria and an invitation to determine if that patient is a suitable organ donor. This is the first step in the organ procurement process and, while it is not sufficient, it is a necessary condition for a successful procurement. Its central importance flows from its placement in time and from the difficulty Organ Procurement Agencies (OPAs) have in bringing it about.

The general public is very supportive of organ donation. Various surveys have shown that 50–75% of the population are willing to permit the donation of the organs of a deceased relative (Gallup Organization, 1983, 1985; Prottas and Batten, 1986). Surveys of the actual experience of OPAs indicates that, in fact, permission rates more closely approximate the later than the former figure (Prottas, 1985). Such high levels of cooperation from the public make the step of obtaining permission relatively unproblematic, if not less important. However, obtaining referrals is much more difficult, and so the willingness of medical professionals to make these referrals has the greatest single effect on the supply of transplantable organs (Prottas 1985).

The key players in the professional sphere are neurophysicians, especially neurosurgeons, and nurses in intensive care units (ICUs). Organ donors must be heartbeating cadavers, and the vast majority of these die in ICUs while under the care of a neurosurgeon or neurologist. In this chapter we explore the willingness of these clinicians and the ICU nurses to play their role in organ procurement and consider what could be done to increase their willingness.

JEFFREY M. PROTTAS and HELEN LEVINE BATTEN • Bigel Institute for Health Policy, Brandeis University, Waltham, Massachusetts 02254.

For a medical professional, unlike the family of a donor, cooperation in organ procurement is not a unitary act—a single decision to permit or refuse. Rather, cooperation is a series of concrete actions that require effort, take time and may have risks. Therefore we conceptualize the cooperation of medical professionals in terms of the willingness to engage in specific clinical and social actions. This chapter discusses the attitudes of neurosurgeons and ICU nurses toward the clinical components of organ procurement and toward the interactions with the families of donors that accompany an organ donation. We also compare those attitudes, where appropriate, with the attitudes of the public.

2. METHODS

During 1984 and 1985, we conducted a series of national surveys under a grant from the Health Care Financing Administration. These included a survey of neurosurgeons, a survey of ICU nurses and a survey of the public. Approximately 250 neurosurgeons who were members of the American Association of Neurological Surgeons responded to our mailed questionnaire (with a response rate of 65%). The nurses were surveyed via the hospitals in which they worked. Approximately 350 hospitals were selected for inclusion in the survey design. They included only acute care hospitals with more than 100 beds. Transplantation hospitals were excluded. The sample was national in scope and stratified by region, rural/urban, teaching/nonteaching hospitals. In each, the director of nursing was asked to distribute four questionnaires to the nurses of the ICU, one to its head nurse and one to a nurse on each shift. Some 900 questionnaires were returned. The survey of the public was also national in scope and was conducted by telephone. We obtained 750 respondents.

3. RESULTS

3.1. Personal Levels of Support

Although there is a very large reservoir of support for organ donation among the American public (Gallup Organization, 1983, 1985; Prottas and Batten 1986), that reservoir is even larger among key medical professionals. As Table I indicates, ICU nurses are substantially more sup-

TABLE I. Personal Support

Item no.	Item	ICU nurses (%)	Neuro- surgeons (%)	Public (%)
1	Personally, I strongly approve of organ donation.	93	91	90
2	I would consider donating own organs.	94	91	72
3	I have discussed my feelings about organ donation with my family.	71	52[a]	46
4	I would consider giving permission to have a family member's organs donated.	95	94	53

[a]Differences between professional groups statistically significant.

portive of organ donation than is the general public (with the exception of the first question, in which virtually all respondents express approval of organ donation in broad terms). The same is true of neurosurgeons regarding the questions measuring willingness to donate. However, neurosurgeons were more like the general public in that only about one half had actually discussed their positive feelings with their families. By contrast, more than 70% of ICU nurses had done so. This difference is statistically significant and introduces a theme we shall see repeated in other areas—neurosurgeons are quite uncomfortable with personal interactions regarding organ donation.

This difficulty with, or unwillingness to, communicate on this issue also shows up in the different perceptions of clinicians regarding each others' level of support for organ procurement: 71% of neurosurgeons believe that their colleagues strongly support organ donation, but only 29% of ICU nurses believe that physicians have that level of support! As a successful organ procurement requires the cooperation of both ICU nurses and neurosurgeons, this lack of communication has the potential to pose a serious problem. Not only does it make cooperation difficult, but because ICU nurses look to physicians as a reference group, it undoubtedly has a negative impact on their own willingness to cooperate.

3.2. Clinical Issues

No doubt the personal attitudes of neurosurgeons and ICU nurses influence their willingness to cooperate in organ donation, but that is not our primary concern. The real issue is the willingness of these clinicians to play their professional role in the procurement process, specifically to make the brain-death determination and convey that fact to the family of the patient as well as to broach the subject of donation. There are at least two possible constellations of reasons why clinicians might not wish to undertake these duties. Either they might have reservations regarding the clinical aspects of the organ donation process, or they may be unwilling to confront the family with the death declaration or the request for permission, or both.

The first responsibility of a clinician in organ procurement is to identify potential donors in a timely way. Obviously, this requires knowledge of the criteria by which a potential donor may be recognized. As Table II shows, neurosurgeons are absolutely confident that their colleagues can make such identifications. By contrast, ICU nurses are less sure of the ability of their co-workers, but even here almost 70% believe that the knowledge exists. Strikingly, ICU nurses perceive that physicians are less aware of donor criteria than are their own co-workers and are far less knowledgeable than the neurosurgeons believe themselves to be! If any of the views of the ICU nurses are accurate, a program of education is called for. Even if we accept the physicians' own self-evaluation, there remains some 30% of ICU nurses who may be having trouble even identifying potential donors. Failure to identify a donor is certain to mean failure to obtain needed organs.

Brain death itself is not a controversial medical issue for neurosurgeons. Almost 90% consider that the medical guidelines for brain death are clear, and about the same number consider that the criteria are generally accepted in the medical community. ICU nurses are far less comfortable regarding the medical status of brain death. Barely a majority consider the criteria well established, and only about 60% believe that it is generally accepted in the medical community. Given the neurosurgeons' unanimity regarding the clinical status of brain death, it is striking that some 45% of respondents believe that their colleagues remain uncomfortable making the death declaration. As we shall see, this is probably more a function of social than of medical reservations.

Once brain death has been determined and the family has given permission for a donation to take place, a number of steps remain in the procurement process. Generally, the brain dead cadaver must be maintained for a short period in order for the condition to stabilize, for medical

TABLE II.   Clinical Issues

Item no.	Item	ICU nurses (%)	Neuro-surgeons (%)
1	Physicians are aware of criteria that make a terminally ill patient a possible candidate for organ donation.	49	96[a]
2	Nurses are aware of criteria that make a terminally ill patient a possible candidate for organ donation.	69	—
3	Medical and clinical guidelines for deciding whether a patient is brain dead are well established.	53	88[a]
4	Brain-death criteria are generally accepted by the medical community.	62	91[a]
5	Physicians don't like to become involved in making brain-death decisions.	81	44[a]
6	I am comfortable designating a patient on a respirator as being a potential donor. (percent yes)	92	82
7	Involvement of OPA staff in donor maintenance is appropriate.	—	60
8	Donor maintenance is appropriately part of a nurse's job.	92	—
9	Nurses are resistant to caring for brain-dead cadavers.	28	—
10	Medical protocols for treating a patient who may become an organ donor often conflict with procedures for protecting organs that may be transplanted.	58	59

[a]Differences between groups statistically significant.

suitability to be determined more definitively, and for access to operating room facilities and the arrival of organ procurement teams. All this involves maintaining the cadaver on a respirator in the ICU. The tasks that need to be done during this period fall primarily on the ICU nurses and, to a lesser degree, on the OPA staff. ICU nurses are willing to perform these duties (see Table II). Most neurosurgeons find the involvement of the OPA staff in donor maintenance acceptable, and virtually all ICU nurses believe that donor-maintenance tasks are appropriate to their professional role. However, a substantial minority of ICU nurses do express a certain reluctance for caring for brain-dead cadavers.

Finally, we come to the last question in Table II, regarding the possible conflict that exists between the preferred protocol for treating a potential donor and the steps needed to insure the usability of the organs. A significant percentage of clinicians consider that such a conflict can arise. In circumstances in which such a conflict occurs and in which there is no clinical resolution, the ethical responsibilities of the clinicians are clear and patient care takes precedence. Organ procurement must operate within this medical constraint.

Taken all together, it appears that in the minds of the relevant clinicians, there are only modest medical objections to cooperation in organ procurement. The criteria for brain death have wide acceptance, the criteria for potential donors are reasonably well understood, and ICU nurses are willing to deal with the activities needed to maintain brain-dead cadavers in the ICU. If there is a significant problem for clinicians, it must lie in some other realm.

3.3. Interpersonal Issues

Clinical issues are not the only problems facing neurosurgeons and ICU nurses in the organ-procurement world. Our voluntary system of donation requires that medical professionals deal with the families of organ donors in order for the donation process to be complete. Although the Uniform Anatomical Gift Act allows an individual to arrange to become an organ donor by signing a donor card, in practice all organ donations require permission from the deceased patient's family. For many clinicians, we hypothesized, this encounter with a family represents the most difficult test of their commitment to organ procurement.

In this section, we report on the responses we received from neurosurgeons and ICU nurses regarding their attitudes toward various aspects of their encounters with donor families. In order to better understand their responses, we compare them with the responses we received from a survey of the families of organ donors. Before proceeding, a word about this last survey is in order.

Unlike the other surveys done as part of this research project, the survey of donor families is not a representative sample. It is impossible to define the universe of donor families accurately, and no national data exist from which to draw a scientific sample. However, several large OPAs allowed us access to their lists of donor families under carefully controlled conditions. These agencies were spread across the country and represented a fair mix of regional types. We are reasonably confident that the data on family attitudes are trustworthy, but in the nature of things, we cannot claim for these data the kind of scientific accuracy common to the other more traditionally structured surveys. These are, however, the only such data in existence. These data are analyzed at length by Prottas and Batten (1987).

Both ICU nurses and neurosurgeons find organ procurement emotionally demanding; indeed, ICU nurses find it more so than do neurosurgeons. Considering the tragic circumstances of all organ donation, this is hardly a surprising finding; however, it must not be overlooked. Clinicians see themselves as entering a painful emotional experience each time they choose to initiate an organ procurement. But, as Table III shows, neurosurgeons believe that certain aspects of that encounter are their responsibility. Almost 90% of neurosurgeons surveyed accepted that they have the responsibility for explaining brain death to the family of a potential donor—one of the steps necessary to a successful organ procurement. Question 3 shows that a substantial minority also believe that brain death is a difficult concept to explain to a family. In this, the neurosurgeons' perception is remarkably similar to that of donor families—36% of them report that they did, in fact, find it a difficult concept to grasp. Interestingly, ICU nurses significantly overestimate how hard families will find the explanation.

But brain death is only a part, and not the larger part of the questions that arise for professionals and donor families. As question 5 indicates, both neurosurgeons and ICU nurses are reluctant to approach donor families. However, neurosurgeons are substantially more reluctant than are ICU nurses. Almost one half of ICU nurses perceive that reluctance among their coworkers, while more than two thirds of neurosurgeons surveyed believed that their colleagues were reluctant. And as in other areas we have reported, ICU nurses believe that physicians seriously overestimate the support of their colleagues. (Almost 90% of nurses believe that physicians are reluctant to approach donor families.) In any case, their own reported reluctance is not easily attributable to brain-death issues—a far larger percentage of neurosurgeons accept the need to explain it to families, and a far smaller percentage anticipate that the explanation will be difficult.

Part of the reason for their reluctance might lie in the way they believe the family will respond to their raising the donation question. Almost one half of surveyed neurosurgeons believe

TABLE III. Concerns of and about the Families of Donors

Item no.	Item	Families (%)	ICU nurses (%)	Neuro-surgeons (%)
1	My professional colleagues find organ procurement emotionally demanding.	—	84	74[a]
2	It is the neurosurgeon's responsibility to explain brain death.	—	—	88
3	Brain death is hard to explain (or was hard to understand).	36	66	40[a]
4	My professional colleagues are some-what reluctant to approach families about organ donation.	—	49	68[a]
5	Donor families would see somewhat of a conflict for involved physicians to request organ donation.	20	—	48
6	Organ donation helps families grieve.	79	79	66

[a]Differences between the professional groups statistically significant.

that families might see that they had a conflict of interest if they were directly involved in asking for a donation. Presumably they are concerned that the family might call into question their commitment to saving the patient's life if they raised the possibility of organ donation. Indeed one of the most common reasons the public gives for not being willing to donate (the 30% or so who are not willing) is a mistrust of the medical profession and a concern over the quality of care a potential donor might receive (Prottas and Batten 1986). In that sense, the neurosurgeons' worries are well founded. However, as the families' responses to question 5 shows, the neurosurgeons' concern is also exaggerated. Neurosurgeons are almost two and a half times as likely to believe families will see a conflict of interest as families are to report such a belief.

Not only do neurosurgeons overestimate the likelihood of conflict with donor families, but they also underestimate the benefit families obtain from organ donation. Only 66% of neurosurgeons believe that an organ donation helps the family deal with its grief. By contrast, 80% of donor families report that they were, in fact, helped. An almost identical percentage of the general public (81%) (Prottas and Batten, 1986) answer that they believe that organ donation would help mitigate grief, and about 80% of ICU nurses answer in the same way.

3.4. Intragroup Difference among Professionals

All neurosurgeons and ICU nurses are not the same. In each group we found important differences in 50–60% of responses we obtained. We wished to understand how to account for these different levels of expressed support and concern. We wanted to know, for example, why some neurosurgeons are more concerned about approaching donor families than are others. We found that, for neurosurgeons, one factor predominated—the acceptance of organ procurement as a professional responsibility. All neurosurgeons were asked the degree to which they believed that they had a professional responsibility to cooperate in organ procurement. We found that the answer to this question had a great influence on all other attitudes expressed. The neurosurgeons who strongly believed they had such a professional responsibility were more personally supportive of organ donation, saw clinical conflict to be of less importance, were less reluctant to approach families, and saw families as supportive of their involvement in organ procurement. In short, once organ procurement became a professional duty, all other aspects of the process became less threatening and more endurable.

We also examined the relationship between the workplace of our respondents and their attitudes. We expected the neurosurgeons who worked in teaching hospitals and those who saw more potential donors might have more positive attitudes. We did find this to be somewhat true, but the effects were small compared with those of professional responsibility. Finally, we hypothesized that older neurosurgeons would be more conservative and, in general, less supportive of organ procurement. This was not true. Indeed, older neurosurgeons were less intimidated by donor families and less unwilling to approach them. As a result they were, in fact, somewhat more supportive of organ procurement than were their younger colleagues.

ICU nurses followed a pattern similar to that of neurosurgeons, but with some interesting differences. Like neurosurgeons, ICU nurses were very strongly influenced by their perception of their professional responsibility. Like neurosurgeons, ICU nurses comprise a highly "scientific" specialty within their profession. Both routinely deal with life and death situations, and both depend on and must master highly technical equipment and skills. Therefore, the congruence on this matter is comprehensible. However, "professional responsibility" was not the most important factor influencing ICU nurses' attitudes; actual donation experience was. ICU nurses who had actually assisted in an organ donation were, on most measures, more willing to cooperate in the future than those who had not had that experience. Clearly the donation experience, for all its difficulties, is so satisfying to ICU nurses that it strongly motivates future behavior. Interestingly, donation experience had no meaningful effect on neurosurgeons' attitudes. Finally, we found that ICU nurses were strongly influenced by their perception of physician attitudes. Although ICU nurses were, as a group, more supportive than were neurosurgeons, those ICU nurses who saw physicians as more supportive were, themselves, more supportive than their colleagues. As in almost all medical contexts, the physician is a primary reference for what is and what is not proper behavior.

4. CONCLUSIONS

Medical professionals are the most critical link in the organ procurement process. It is they who control access to potential donors, they who first identify suitable candidates, and they who must take responsibility for declaring death and informing the family. In many instances, it is their expertise that maintains a donor during the critical period between death and organ removal.

They perform these tasks without compensation and at some emotional costs to themselves. Moreover, organ procurement tasks differ in kind from those medical professionals are trained for and dedicated to. An ICU (where virtually all donors die) is dedicated to saving lives in desperate danger—organ donors are their failures. Despite all this, we have found a heartening willingness to cooperate among all the professionals surveyed.

It is clear from our findings that increasing cooperation from medical professionals does not require extensive re-education or the application of new and complex incentives. Rather, it requires a sensitive appreciation of their needs and concerns. Medical issues do not predominate. The medical profession has incorporated into its technological repertoire those steps needed for organ donation. Social and interpersonal issues are central. It is, by and large, hesitation about dealing with donor families that looms largest for medical professionals. This is particularly true of physicians. Our data also shows that other professionals are influenced by the stance of doctors.

This is not to say that other groups are unimportant. Efforts toward education regarding organ procurement have traditionally been aimed at nurses, and the extraordinarily high levels of support found among them implies considerable success. Indeed, organ procurement efforts to maintain and increase their support are justified. Nor have we found that nurses are solely dependent on doctors for the definition of their responsibility for organ donation. They take their clues from their own professional peers and from their experiences in their own workplace.

Nevertheless, doctors remain critical. Their own involvement is necessary for the success of organ procurement, and their attitudes influence all those around them. Moreover, they are the weakest link in the chain, and so the one most in need of strengthening. Our data on neurosurgeons show that they take their clues regarding organ procurement from their professional peers. As a profession, they perceive that they have resolved the major medical issues. But the profession has not, at least for many neurosurgeons, provided clear guidance on other matters. In particular, it has not communicated that active assistance in organ procurement is a positive professional duty.

Virtually all neurosurgeons have reservations about dealing with the families of organ donors. In fact, who would not hesitate to encounter a family of strangers in the midst of profound tragedy? But neurosurgeons, more than other clinicians involved, underestimate the benefits to families of organ donation (compared to the perceptions of families themselves). They resist involvement in brain-death decisions for social rather than medical reasons. Yet these fears loom less large once a physician acknowledges professional responsibility. This body of men and women take their professional duties very seriously. Persuading those with doubts on where their professional responsibilities lie is likely to have a substantial effect on the entire organ-procurement process. All indications from our research are that they are open to such persuasion.

REFERENCES

Gallup Organization, 1963, *Attitudes and Opinions of the American Public Toward Kidney Donation*, Princeton, New Jersey.

Gallup Organizaton, 1985. *Attitudes and Opinions of the American Public Toward Kidney Donation*, Princeton, New Jersey.

Prottas, J., and Batten, H., 1986, The Attitudes of the American Public Toward Organ Donation, Report to the Health Care Financing Administration.

Prottas, J., Batten, H., 1987, Kind strangers: The families of organ donors, *Health Affairs* **16(2):** 35–48.

Prottas, J., 1985, Structure and effectiveness of the American organ procurement system, *Inquiry* Winter **22:**365–376.

Prottas, J., 1986, ''Asking and answering: The role of law in organ donation, *Univ. Detroit J. Urban Law*, **63(1):**183–193.

28

Effect of Organ Donation on Families of Brain-Dead Patients

Roberta G. Simmons, Robert Fulton, and Julie Fulton

1. INTRODUCTION

The shortage of cadaver organs for transplantation is serious (Levey *et al.*, 1986). Yet, few studies have been made of the psychological reactions of families after they donate the organs of a relative (see Chapter 27, this volume). Most of the literature in this area deals with the ethical and medical aspects of brain death (Simmons and Abress, 1988), the attitude of the general public (Manninen and Evans, 1985), and the logistics of approaching physicians and families. The study reported here is a small exploratory investigation of one of the first cohorts of families who donated organs of their brain-dead relatives. Relatives were interviewed in depth 1 year after the donation.

Here, we report both the positive and negative aspects of the experience at the time of the decision-making and over the long term. We explore the nature of the family decision-making process and the long-run impact of donation on grief.

2. METHOD

2.1. The Sample

We defined as our basic population all families whose relatives had served as cadaver donors at the University of Minnesota Hospitals during the period January 1971 to May 1972 and who, at the time of the interview (1½ years later) still lived within a 20-mile radius of the Twin Cities

See a similar version of this report by J. Fulton, R. Fulton, and R. Simmons, 1977, The cadaver donor and the gift of life in: *Gift of Life: The Social and Psychological Impact of Organ Transplantation* (R. G. Simmons, S. D. Klein, and R. L. Simmons, eds.), Wiley (Interscience), New York. New edition, Transaction, New Brunswick, New Jersey, 1987.

ROBERTA G. SIMMONS, ROBERT FULTON, and JULIE FULTON • Department of Sociology, University of Minnesota, Minneapolis, Minnesota 55455.

of Minneapolis and St. Paul. Seventeen families met these criteria, 12 of whom agreed to be interviewed. The interviews were unstructured and open-ended. Among the families interviewed was one extended family unit in which there had been two separate accidents resulting in two separate donations. We have also included, for purposes of this analysis, earlier interviews conducted with two families whose relatives had served as cadaver donors prior to January 1971.

We attempted to interview all members of the donor's immediate family who were in the Twin Cities area as well as other relatives who played a significant role in the decision to donate. A total of 35 relatives from 14 families were interviewed: Spouses, parents, siblings, grandparents, and in-laws were among those who participated. The respondents ranged in age from 8 to over 65 years of age.

2.2. The Cadaver-Patients

Table I shows the age, sex, and cause of death of the cadaver-donors. They are predominately male, young, and single. The sudden unexpected character of their deaths is evident.

3. FINDINGS

3.1. The Period Prior to the Decision

3.1.1. The Suggestion of Donation

Most of the family members interviewed were unprepared to accept the death of such young persons. The suddenness of the events as well as a refusal to relinquish hope were significant factors in the initial response of family members to the idea of donation. In 12 cases, the initial

TABLE I.   Cause of Death of 15 Cadaver-Patients[a]

Sex	Age	Cause of death
Self-inflicted injury		
Male	21	Suicide (gunshot wound to head)
Male	26	Suicide (gunshot wound to head)
Congenital weaknesses		
Male	24	Aneurysm
Male	30	Aneurysm
Male	8	Aneurysm
Female	3½	Pneumonia following open heart surgery
Accidental injury		
Male	19	Two-car collision
Male	16	Car–truck accident
Male	15	Car–train accident
Male	20	Motorcycle accident
Male	20	Motorcycle–car accident
Male	6	On bicycle, hit by motorcycle
Male	17	Fell off car trunk when car started to move in parking lot
Female	15	Pedestrian, hit by car
Female	10	Suffocated in snowdrift while playing

[a]Only three patients (all male) were married, and each was the father of young children.

suggestion to donate organs was made by the physician in the local hospital to which the patient had been taken. In the other three cases the donation was brought about (1) by the suggestion of a hospital staff member who was a friend, (2) by the parents themselves, and (3) by the cadaver-patient himself who had written a suicide note directing that his entire body be given to the university. In most cases, the idea of donation was not originally activated because of the patient's prior desires but because of the physician's suggestion. Given the family's state of shock and disbelief following the accident, it is not surprising that they were not the ones to suggest the donation. An additional reason for the physician suggesting organ donation may be that it helps him to inform the family that the patient will never recover. The suggestion, in other words, becomes tantamount to a declaration of death.

3.1.2. Initial Response to the Suggestion of Donation

Therefore, the reactions of the relatives to the physician's suggestion of donation may reflect more than just their feeling about the donation *per se;* their initial response may also reflect their readiness or willingness to accept the inevitability of the death. In at least one half of families interviewed, one or more of the relevant family members experienced initial reservations about the donation but then changed their minds in the time they had to think about it. Of the 35 respondents considered individually, four indicated they were definitely against the idea of donation initially, five needed time to think about it because they had some serious reservations, three said they were ambivalent, and 23 felt basically positive toward the idea.

Thus although most were immediately disposed to donation, approximately one third needed more time before they were prepared to permit the donation. Eventually each of these persons— or at least each of the relevant decision-makers—came to accept the idea of donation. The determination of who among the possible decision-makers *were* relevant decision-makers is of interest.

3.1.3. Which Families Members Were Included in the Decision

The living donor's decision to give his own organ to a relative can be made without the concurrence of anyone else. But interpersonal strictures mitigate against a person unilaterally deciding to donate the organs of a dead relative, if there are other survivors who may be affected by this decision. The exception to this rule seems to be the case in which the cadaver-patient is married, for then the surviving spouse may be viewed as legitimately making the decision alone. In only one of the 12 cases in which the patient was not married did a surviving relative make a unilateral decision to donate organs. This was a case in which the parents of the dying child had been divorced and the custodial parent made the decision without consulting the other parent, who, she implied, had ignored the family and therefore had not earned the right to be consulted. The decision to donate someone else's organs is therefore usually a group decision. What becomes critical in the decision process is the determination of whose wishes prevail. Who among all possible survivors are thought to be the legitimate decision-makers with regard to the question of donation?

In fact, there are strong feelings about the right to decide such an issue. Usually marital ties are the strongest factors, and blood and age also play significant roles. If the patient is married, the spouse, in both a normative and a legal sense, is seen to be the major decision-maker. This holds true despite the fact that the marriage may be of short duration and despite the fact that the parents may also be present.

In each of the three cases in which the cadaver-patient was married, the wife became the primary decision-maker, although this fact presented difficulties to the parents in two of the three instances. In one of these two cases, the wife made the decision to donate the organs and swore the physicians to secrecy because she was afraid of the response of her husband's father. In the other case, the family members felt distressed that the decision seemed to be left up to the wife, because she had been estranged from the patient. Although the wife was willing to make the donation and the physicians believed that legally her permission was sufficient, both she and the physicians were responsive to the feelings of discontent among the husband's family members. Together the physicians and the wife decided that unless all the family members agreed, the donation would not take place. With some difficulty, the husband's parents and siblings decided to "allow" the donation.

In the third case of a married cadaver-patient, the legitimacy of the wife's authority to make the donation decision was accepted by her husband's mother who was with her at the time. In fact, the patient's mother desired this choice, but she indicated that if the wife had not approved of the donation, she would have remained silent. In fact, when the wife agreed to donate the kidneys and the pancreas but refused to donate her husband's eyes, the mother was somewhat surprised but said nothing because of her belief that this was properly the wife's decision.

If the patient was not married, the strength of the blood ties seemed to determine which relatives could be "legitimate" decision-makers. Parents figured prominently in the decision-making processes of the remaining 12 cases. In four cases, the parents alone made the decision for the donation. In two other cases the parents included the siblings in the discussion but indicated that they would be willing to donate even if the children were not willing. Their inclusion was an apparent attempt by the parents to be considerate of them as family members rather than to respond to any of their contradictory feelings. In one family, for instance, the mother reported:

> We [parents] *knew* right away, but didn't *decide* right away so as not to hurt my older daughter and my father. We let it sink into them. . . . Now the older girl thinks it was her decision. If she had said no or something, I think her father and I would have gone on anyway. My father didn't express any opinion, he said, "It's your son."

In these cases, the disapproval of other family members would probably not have made a difference to the parents in the final decision.

In four other cases, the parents specifically wanted to include siblings of the cadaver-patient in the decision-making process. These interviews suggest that the parents were truly concerned about the responses of their children and would not have decided to donate if family consensus on the donation could not be reached. Age of siblings was a factor in these and other cases, however. The parents were careful to include the older children in the decision but never considered the opinions or feelings of the younger children. The age cutoff seemed to be around 14 or 15 years; anyone younger was not seriously included in the donation decision.

Although there is uncertainty about the role of older children in the decision-making process, the role of grandparents seems clearly defined as irrelevant. The opinions offered by grandparents frequently reflected traditional beliefs and strong objections to the proposed transplantation. Larger surveys have also indicated that older persons are less positive toward organ transplantation and toward nontraditional methods of handling death (see Simmons *et al.*, 1974, 1987). In seven cases, one or more of the grandparents expressed a profound resistance to the idea of the donation. One respondent said, "My mother had absolute fits. She is extremely religious and she feels you are given one set of organs and if something goes wrong with them, that's it. Horrible to go putting somebody else's organs in another body. She'll never come around." Obviously, since each of these interviews was conducted because the family did agree to donate organs, the resistance of the grandparents was overcome or, more likely, ignored. In one case in which the grandparents expressed strong objections, an 18-year-old son stood up in the hospital waiting room and announced, "The decision is on the basis of what we [that is, father, mother, and older sister] want, and whether you [grandparents] want it or not doesn't matter." In several other cases, the irrelevance of the feelings of grandparents was also clear. One father reported, "Well, my wife's mother did say something but we shut her off real quick on that. It was our decision and she would have had nothing to do with it." Sometimes family members were significantly upset by the disapproval of grandparents, but their nonsupport did not dissuade them from their final decision. In none of our cases was the opinion of the grandparents specifically sought. Whether grandparents played a larger role in cases in which parents did not allow donation remains to be investigated.

Usually, then, among the family, only the closest blood relatives or the patient's spouse are included in the decision-making process. In two out of the three cases in which the dying child had a stepparent, the stepparent was left out of the decision-making. But the data indicate that in an intact family both parents of the unmarried cadaver-patient must ultimately agree if the donation is to take place. As one mother said, "If he says 'no' and I say 'yes', I'm not going to push my 'yes'. After all, if there's any disagreement, it has to be the 'no' one, then."

Of the 14 situations that were clear enough to categorize, four induced significant family stress during the decision period above and beyond the grief all were experiencing. These situations included (1) a family that felt locked into donation, (2) the family in which the parents were angry at the estranged wife, (3) one family in which the grandparents' opposition was strongly expressed and was upsetting to the parents, and (4) the family in which the wife concealed the donation from her husband's family. In the latter case the cadaver-donor's brother who suspected the truth expressed great anger to the wife.

3.1.4. Role of Friends, Medical Staff, and Clergy

The question of outsiders' influence in the decision-making process is relevant. Did those who deliberated about the decision turn to any type of expert for advice?

Although in some cases friends were present throughout the ordeal and their tacit approval was clear, in only three cases were we aware of a larger role on their part. In all three cases, the friends were either medical personnel themselves or were closely affiliated with medical staff and thus felt free to argue in favor of donation. The major nonfamily member involved in each process, however, was the local physician himself, and his primary role seemed to be to initiate and explain the idea of donation. In two cases, the physician also assumed the role of temporizer: he refused to accept immediate consent from the potential donor's family and directed them to think the issue over more carefully.

In three cases, local physicians assumed a more active role in urging the donation in order to help families bring themselves to turn off the machines. One father reported that the physician said to him:

> When do you want the machines turned off? Your whole family is here now and you have been going through this for three days. We're just conducting a charade. We could do this for the next two weeks. The hospital bills are very high. If it's comforting for you to sit here and hold her hand when she's in a coma, OK. She's breathing, but she's essentially dead. You might as well agree to the fact that she's dead. It's costing like $700 to $800 a day to go through this.

The clergy played a supportive but not influential role for these families. Their role in the decision process seemed to be more a matter of supporting a decision once made than of providing information or guidance in making the decision. In almost all cases, either a hospital chaplain or their own clergy was in contact with the family during the decision-making process, but in only three families of 15 were the clergy said to have had some role in the decision-making process.

Thus the decision to donate cadaver organs is a group decision made by key family members in a crisis situation. At the time of the decision, these key members, both at home and in the hospital, are likely to be surrounded sporadically or continuously by other individuals who are defined as having less right to make the choice but who provide emotional support—the hospital medical staff, clergy, friends, younger children in the family, grandparents, in-laws, stepparents, and so on. Of these persons, only the grandparents are likely to express an opposing view. The factors that make the decision easy for these key family members, as well as the factors that make it difficult for others, must be explicated.

3.1.5. What Factors Made the Decision Easy?

3.1.5a. **Prior Knowledge of Transplantation.** Only one family indicated that they knew nothing of transplantation prior to this incident. In fact, transplantation had been a subject of family discussion previously in seven families and, in these discussion, five of the cadaver-patients (all male and all over 17) had indicated their desire to donate organs in the event of their death. In view of the fact that four of the sample of cadaver-patients were 10 years of age or younger, it is interesting that five of the remaining 11 had expressed some prior interest in donation.

In these cases, the decision of the family was made easier because once the issue of donation was raised, they remembered the cadaver-patient's own desires concerning the subject. A father reported:

> It's a funny thing. We had talked about organ transplants no more than two weeks before. He said he would like to do something great with his life. Our thought went back to that conversation. I guess I was feeling that that was about as great as you can do when you are going to die. . . . I think that made it easier to feel as we did. That he had a desire to make a contribution of some kind and that he had expressed it.

Even though the patient's expressed interest in donation did not lead the family to suggest the gift themselves, the recollection of such wishes did facilitate their decision to allow the donation.

3.1.5b. **Altruistic and Empathic Motivation.** Altruism and humanitarianism play a major role in the family members' decision to donate. A few of the respondents said that in the decision process they empathized with the recipient's family and thought about what it would be like if their own child were "lying there, waiting for an organ."

One wife was convinced by hearing of the need of some patients for the kidneys. "I figured if he had two good kidneys there are two people who need them to stay alive with their family. I said OK . . . I don't know what he would have said [the dead husband], but I figured if he could save two lives, I'm going to do it."

3.1.5c. **Feelings about Immortality.** Certain feelings about immortality also sometimes made the decision to donate an easier one. At least five of the survivors took comfort in the idea that part of the cadaver-patient would still be alive. In the words of one mother:

> I think we generally got approval from most people but kind of like "Isn't that nice of her to do this?" I didn't do it because I thought it was nice to do. I did it because I thought [crying], I guess, something to help him [son]. Perhaps he was alive as far as I was concerned. So his death wasn't totally a death.

A sense of extended life was echoed in the worlds of another father, "Well, it's a funny feeling. In a sense you think they're still around and yet they're not. [As long as his kidneys still function] he isn't dead down there."

Another family of a young girl viewed the transplant as a continuation of "life" in another way. The mother explained:

> We had the privilege of having all the children in on the decision. There was very little discussion. The decision was "yes"; we really didn't have to go into it much at all. Then my

nineteen-year-old son had this beautiful thought that it was two transplants. As her family who knew her joy and knew what her life was, it was up to us to do a psychological and a spiritual transplant. The doctors would do a physical transplant and we would live her joy and implant it in others.

3.1.5d. Relief from Deciding to "Turn off" Machines.

Once the death was accepted as a reality, the prospect of donating organs was felt by some family members to be a solution to their dilemma of when to turn off the "life-maintaining" respiratory and circulatory machines. In a way, the decision *to* turn them off was made by them, and yet they were relieved at not having to decide *when*.

One father said:

> [The physician] put the termination in a very clear light, and the fact that he hated to be the person that would turn off these machines. I don't think he would hesitate to take the responsibility, but, I mean, he's a human being too, just like the rest of us. We didn't want to put him in that position. So [with the decision to donate] everything just pretty much fell into place.

The mother in this case describes the situation more emotionally. When they had to put her son back on the machine to sustain his breathing, the doctors told her that it was "sort of a waiting game." "You mean," she replied, "waiting to decide who's going to turn the switch off?," and the doctors admitted, "Well, sort of like that." Then, said the mother, the doctors began "tossing it [the decision of when to turn off the machines] back and forth like a football." Finally she asked, "Well is the ball game really over?" and one doctor replied, "Well, yes, unless you want to sustain him on the machines, which isn't really much of a choice, for his sake." For some period of time, while this realization set in, the family paced the halls asking questions such as "Who's going to play God here?" When one of the doctors suddenly seemed to realize that organ donation would be an alternative and suggested this, the mother said, "We [she and her husband] both just jumped for joy. The pressure was off of us, you know. It was just like a shot in the arm. We both even smiled."

3.1.6. What Factors Make the Decision Difficult?

3.1.6a. Problem of Brain Death.

In each case, as in all cases of transplants using cadaver organs, the patient experienced sudden and irreversible brain damage at the time of the accident. Sometimes later the family was told that, despite appearances of life, the patient was dead because his brain had ceased functioning. Without the artificial respirator, he would not be able to maintain a heartbeat or respiration. The concept of brain death, however, was sometimes very difficult for family members to comprehend in the presence of other signs of viability such as breathing and a pulse rate. One woman said, "[My husband's] mother couldn't get it through her head—she felt that as long as his heart was beating and he was breathing, he was alive."

A definition of death relying upon the absence of certain neurological signs not only is a departure from the traditional definition of death (i.e., no heartbeat or breathing) but also is a departure from the concept of a "moment" of death. Brain death suggests a death process, something extending both forward and backward from the moment of a verbal declaration. To decide at what point in this process they wish to discontinue the efforts to keep the other systems functioning has been the task of the family or physician. But many family members, tied as they are to an "instant" notion of death, are reluctant to make any decisions until they are told that this "instant" has taken place and that their relative is "dead."

One mother reported that the physician said to her, " 'We wanted to approach you about a transplant. Would you consider it if her organs were still intact?' He did a beautiful job of presenting it but she hadn't been declared dead [as far as we knew]. It was kind of a shock."

Paradoxically, therefore, the suggestion of donation becomes this "announcement," and the family is then led to realize that the decision to discontinue "life-saving" measures will soon be made. The family members seem to have had to deal with both "kinds" of death in their response to the initial suggestion of donation. They have to accept the emotional shock that the instant when life ceases and death begins has already passed; and they have to confront the fact that part of the process of death is still to occur.

Several respondents commented that it was difficult to talk about taking organs (or making funeral arrangements) when the patient still seemed alive. The 14-year-old sister of a cadaver-patient said:

> That night we discussed what we were going to do and someone said that they were going to donate some of his organs. And I was just shocked. You know he's dead but he's still alive. I was just shocked, I couldn't believe it.

Not being present at the "instant" of death is difficult for some family members. In our culture, this moment has assumed a sacred and fundamental quality and its absence is disturbing. As one mother said:

> For the most part, people said, "Well, great." They thought it was a tremendous thing to do. But I think the majority of them say this not knowing that you give up their organs before their heart has stopped beating. My mother died seven months before he [son] did and I stood at her bedside and felt her pulse until it was completely gone. It's a different kind of thing when you walk into a room and see the kid is breathing. You know the difference.

An 18-year-old sister stated that she never had any regrets about the decision to donate. Rather, she said:

> I think it was harder trying to decide at what point we would say that he was dead when he wasn't. But I never felt that they should just have kept on the machines for an indeterminate period, just to prolong his life so that he could exist. I knew that this wasn't the kind of life that he would want to live. And I felt that rather than being a vegetable all his life, or being in a coma, or whatever, I think that would have been harder on us if that would have been the way he would have lived.

The word *vegetable* is mentioned in several of the interviews. Although the family member may not have been able to comprehend the notion of *death* from the definition of brain death, the extent of the brain injury slowly penetrated their thinking to the point that they were able to talk about the continued existence of their relative (were the machines to be kept on) in terms that seems to them to mean a subhuman condition.

Sometimes, however, the definition of the patient as a potential "vegetable" ("subhuman" but "alive") brings with it other religious and ethical problems for the survivors.

A father confided:

> The one reluctance I had [to the donation] I think may have been kind of a religious question— wrestling with the concept of death, either as I am used to thinking of it or as one might legally define it, as a plain death. I guess basically in my mind I wondered, "OK, if we, by our decision, are going to terminate his life, where is he in terms of salvation?" I don't have any guilt feelings, but I wonder if we were short on patience.

Several relatives could only partially accept the certainty of brain death and felt some guilt at making the decision that would absolutely ensure death. A mother elaborated:

> I guess I have no regrets other than the fact that I would have liked to have a better knowledge of what could have happened to him had he been left the way he was. Of course, they did tell us it would have been 24 hours and this type of thing, but I guess you always have the question that man isn't always right. You always hear about the miracles and this type of thing, where

a doctor thinks that someone is just about dead and he lives. I guess you kind of have some of these things in the back of your mind.

Two other mothers put their feelings even more bluntly. One lamented ''I think the hardest part is the fact that she didn't die. I had to tell them to 'pull the plugs,' I willed her to die.'' And another said, ''There he was, right around the corner, still breathing on a machine and we were signing his life away in here.''

Their decision to allow donation and the cessation of the machines is an irreversible one, while the condition of the heartbeating cadaver appears capable of being reversed despite physicians' assurances to the contrary.

3.1.6b. Timing. The timing of the decision process seems to be crucial. Not only must the decision to give the organs be made within a reasonable period of time (so as not to jeopardize the organs unduly), but also the family must be given sufficient time to overcome their initial feelings of shock and disbelief. Because the request for donation is frequently tantamount either to a declaration of death or an announcement that the case is hopeless, family members sometimes respond only to the announcement rather than the request. The grief at the realization that the patient's condition is, in fact, hopeless is so overwhelming that the donation issue cannot be handled at that moment. In fact, to be making future plans of any type appears in some cases to be inappropriate before the shock of the death or impending death has been assimilated.

Thus in some cases the initial negative reaction to donation was not necessarily a negative judgment of donation but rather a feeling that this was not the time to consider such issues. One father remembered telling the doctor:

> There's such a shock to think that there's no hope for her living, that I can't bear to make such a decision right now. . . . After about a day, I'd say, when the whole idea kind of developed in my thinking, then I was a little more apt to consider it on a rational basis, that it might be a worthwhile thing to do.

There seems to be in the brain-death donation experience certain stages of acceptance and awareness that family members go through that somewhat parallel the grieving process (but in the donation process the timing is, of necessity, accelerated). Dealing with the family members as if they are in one stage of grief when they may in fact be in another, can lead to strained communication. The 18-year-old brother of a cadaver-patient summarized:

> [The doctor] was just saying ''If she's going to die, then I think you should think about this.'' . . . But as far as my mother and father, it was way too early to say something like that. . . . There were certain stages you go through the whole time, and each thing needs a little bit of time. It seems kind of ridiculous, but maybe just an hour, maybe after each thing, an hour or half-hour. . . . When my sister came [from out of the country] . . . well, she was at a different stage than us [the rest of the family who had been together in the hospital since the accident]. You know, it was strange to try and talk to her, well and try to explain things.

Even when family members experience the accident and the hospital events at the same time, their stages of personal acceptance may differ greatly from one another. In one case when the parents were approached with the idea of organ donation, the father agreed to the transplant and the mother refused. The father told the physician no, and the physician went away but said, ''I'll be around anyway in case you change your mind.'' The father commented, ''The only thing I can say is if he [the physician] had talked much longer after the first refusal, he never would have gotten it. It was the wrong time and the wrong place.''

3.1.6c. Limited Information. One of the reasons that some families believed they needed more time to decide is that despite knowledge that transplantation existed, they really knew very little about details involved. Although local physicians were able to satisfy the queries of many individuals, five respondents who were very anxious to have their questions answered found that the medical staff did not seem to have time to give them the answers they sought. One father said, "I think the initial reaction was that we wished we knew more about it so that we could have a better basis for making a decision. The doctor didn't stay long or provide much information."

One mother suggested an educational approach for other donors. "I would think that a pamphlet or a brochure [for the family to read in the waiting room] would allow them not only to be clear in their own minds as to what certain procedures are but also help answer the thousands of questions they are asked by friends and relatives." Donors' families need information not only for their own decision but also to help them explain the process to interested others.

3.1.6d. Attitude toward Special Body Parts: Body Image. A decision to allow the donation of any organs at all for transplantation is the first decision that must be considered by the family, but in addition, they can decide which organs they will allow to be donated. A willingness to donate certain organs was arrived at without too much feeling of body disturbance or body mutilation, but the idea of removing certain other organs sometimes aroused great emotion. Most respondents did not have any feelings one way or another about the spleen, pancreas, liver, or kidneys. But hearts and eyes, particularly, were organs of the body that sometimes provoked very strong images and association; these organs possess special significance even after death for many people.

3.2. After the Transplant

3.2.1. Body Image

Almost all families interviewed (12 of the 15) put the body on view either at the funeral home or at the funeral ceremony, or both. In five families, there were specific complaints about the appearance of the cadaver. In one family, this was blamed on the mortician, but in four families it was blamed on the experience in the hospital and on the procedures necessary for the transplant operation. One mother said, "Even if that look were normal, we would naturally associate it with the transplant." Some of the others believed that the head or face did not look right partly because the lips were swollen from having had tubes in them and the face was puffed. Many of these patients, however, had had direct injuries to the head that in and of themselves might have been disfiguring.

3.2.2. The Funeral

In some other ways, the donation made the funeral a more positive experience than it might otherwise have been. In two cases, the fact of the organ donation was mentioned by the clergy as part of the sermon at the funeral service. The official praise was comforting to the concerned family members, as was the praise of friends at that time. In the words of one of these mothers, who had discussed the sermon with the minister the night before the funeral:

> The minister read this into the sermon. . . . I wanted him to get across in there loud and strong . . . that there has to be some meaning . . . that it [the death] wasn't just a wasted thing, and so [the minister] weaved this through his sermon. . . . [My son] was . . . an outstanding leader . . . and so there had to be some meaning for why He would take a boy who's never been in trouble . . . and so I think this transplant was a good substitute . . . just to hold everybody together.

3.3. Long-Term Reaction to Cadaver Donation

Throughout the period in which the decision to donate is made and the transplant operation is performed, the concerns of the family have been largely focused on the cadaver-patient. During the weeks and months that follow, their focus begins to shift. The long-range issues associated with the donation center more clearly on the welfare of the survivors, particularly with their own grieving processes. Our question was whether the donation eased or intensified the grieving process. Were the long-term attitudes toward the donation primarily positive or negative?

3.3.1. Overall Evaluation

Although the donation was not equally salient to all family members a year or more after the death, most respondents appeared to hold a primarily positive attitude toward it at the time of the interview. Table II indicates that 23 out of the 28 adults were still favorable toward the donation. Whether this proportion would have been reduced had we been able to interview all the families in the targeted population is a question that cannot be answered here.

For all five of the ambivalent or negative respondents, the negative reactions were very much attributed to the transfer of the body to or administrative problems at the university hospital. Two of the respondents were from families that had been erroneously billed by the University, and one of these persons had also been upset by the lack of communication from the hospital during the time they were waiting for the transplant to be completed. Two others were parents who reported that they had felt "locked into" donation before completely making up their minds, and at this point they were concerned they had not been patient enough. The fifth respondent was one of the parents who believed the estranged wife of the cadaver-doner had assumed too much authority in allowing the donation. Many of the factors responsible for these complaints have already been corrected, either by changes in the university protocols for communication with cadaver-donor families or by the introduction of the preservation machines, which allow the body to remain at the original hospital.

All but four of the respondents whose attitudes were other than "clearly positive" are thus identified above. The four remaining persons were classified as "primarily positive," although they held some reservations. For example, a patient's sibling and his wife were very positive toward the actual donation of their sibling's organs but were not certain of whether they would be willing to donate their own child's organs if an accident were to happen to him.

TABLE II. Ratings of Attitudes of Cadaver-Donor Family Members 1 Year or More after the Donation[a]

	Adults		Children under age 14 (N)	Total	
	N	%		N	%
Clearly positive attitude	17	60	7	24	68
Primarily positive, with a few slight reservations	6[b]	22		6	17
Ambivalent	1	4		1	3
Negative	4[c]	14	—	4	11
	28	100	7	35	100

[a]Two of the authors made these ratings independently.
[b]Four of six of these persons are from the same family
[c]Two of these persons are from the same family.

All in all, the 11 respondents who reported other than "clearly positive" attitudes were from six out of the 14 families. Several of the respondents who maintained very favorable attitudes over the long run commented on the donation as the one positive aspect of the death. The following remarks were typical:

> The transplant was one of the few bright spots in the whole experience.
>
> The death was not a total loss. There was something good that came out of the whole thing.
>
> If we can't save him, we can save someone else.
>
> Maybe that's why he was here, or something. Maybe the other children [recipients] will do something, make a contribution or something.

For many respondents, then, the donation seemed to give meaning to an otherwise meaningless death.

3.3.2. Long-Term Salience of the Donation

At the time of the interview, families varied in the degree to which the donation was still salient in their thoughts or talk. While most family members still thought about the death often, even daily, the donation occupied their thoughts only occasionally; some respondents reported that they no longer think about it at all. In one family, however, the donation was still a relevant part of their thinking. More than 200 people had sent in donor cards because of the death of the child in this family, and the mother often talked about the donation in her contacts with friends— so often, in fact, that the other sons in the family were upset with their mother's preoccupation.

3.3.3. Easing Grief

Did the respondents believe that the donation had played any role in easing their grief? Of the 17 respondents who were asked explicitly whether they felt that the donation had helped them in their own grieving, nine indicated that it had, and two others were not sure whether it had made any difference. Of the six respondents who reported that the donation had not played such a role, two claimed that if they could have had knowledge that the transplant was a long-term success, their grief might have been eased. Without such knowledge, the donation affected their grief very little.

In sum, for various reasons, most respondents remained quite positive in their feelings about the donation. For a significant number of individuals, the donation appears as the one good thing in the death, and for several others, it served to ease their grief. In fact, one father believed the donation had actually had a positive impact on the interaction of the family. He explained,

> [Donation] has probably made us more appreciative of his [the son's] memories, and I think that probably all our kids look up to us with a little bit more respect. I think they probably accept us and evaluate us more than the older generation. I think it served to bring us closer together.

For other respondents, however, the donation, while viewed positively, is seen to have little current salience in their lives and little impact on their grief. In the words of one mother who had made an instantaneous decision to donate:

> Donating hasn't made any difference . . . neither easier to accept the death nor more difficult. Nothing one way or the other. If I had not donated . . . I don't know how to say it . . . as long as she was dead I'm glad that medical science has advanced to the point where some use can be made of the organs, but that's all.

3.3.4. Thoughts about the Transplant Recipients

At some time or another, the thoughts of virtually all the survivors turned to questions about the recipients of the donated organs. Fifteen family members specifically indicated that currently or previously they wanted more information about the recipients than they had received. In fact, for many relatives, this desire for more information was quite strong. The current policy of the University Transplant Services is to send a letter to the family of the cadaver-patient shortly after the surgery thanking them for their donation and telling them something about the operation(s). Although the recipients are not named, the letter generally mentions which organs were used, the sex and age and some other basic information about the persons who received them, and some statement about the success of the transplants.

The University does not give the name of the recipient so as to protect the recipient from the well-meaning but possible guilt-provoking concern of the cadaver-patient's family. While many recipients have stated that they would like to thank the donating family, the University staff feels that the stress of being a transplant patient is significant enough without exposing the patient to the grief of the donor's family.

The first families interviewed, however, received no information about the recipients, and because of the concerns expressed in our interviews basic information was added to the letter. As one mother said, "If you want people to do it, they have to be told more . . . they've given so much and they want something back." Without some information, the gift appears unreciprocated.

The letter from the transplant services was usually the only information that the family received following their donation, and however inadequate the information may seem in light of their questions, the letter was eagerly received. One wife said:

> When I received the letter, it was about a month and a half after. In my case I was just feeling so terribly down and I've never been a down person in my whole life. But I would say that was one of the most rewarding things, to hear that something good came out of his death. Just the way it was written and everything. It really pleased me. You don't get very many rewards out of something like this.

Many family members took pleasure in sharing this letter with friends, especially if the letter implied that the transplants were successful. One mother reported, "I got a letter from the University stating that two people in their thirties had received them, and I took it to a wedding and I let 'em all read it and they thought it was just great that you could do something like that in the circumstances where he was, to help two people." Obviously, the praise and support of other people may be a significant ancillary gain of having made the decision to donate organs.

Many respondents at 1 year or more after the death still wanted to know how well the recipients were dong. One woman, for example, felt that following the transplant, in fairness to the cadaver-patient's family, as well as to encourage others to donate, the transplant service should send the family periodic reports on the recipient's progress.

One reason that families are not always informed about the success of the operations is that not all of the organs are tolerated by the body of the recipient. Seven family members were asked whether they would like to know about the recipient's health if the transplant had not been successful. Upon reflection, six of the seven realized that they only wanted information if the operations had been a success.

One woman remarked:

> I have mixed emotions about knowing who the recipients have been. I would like to know only if it was successful. If there were some complications or if it was rejected or didn't work, then I wouldn't feel as satisfied as I do right now just from having that first letter that gave me just a little bit of information.

And another mother concurred:

> If the patients weren't doing well, we [the parents] wouldn't want to know. It still gives you a
> little bit of hope that he didn't die for nothing, and maybe somebody is getting some help from
> this. Maybe somebody else has a child that is alive on account of my son and they can live a
> normal life.

Even at a year after the transplant, many cadaver-donor families feel a need to know whether
the donation was successful or, in other words, whether the death had any meaning. Such positive
information would serve as reciprocation to the families that gave this major gift. Yet, the hospital
staff has not instituted any such long-term feedback, because they are uncertain how to handle
the cases in which the transplant has failed.

3.3.5. Reaction of Others

There is information about others' reaction to the donation for 12 families. In all of these
cases the family received some positive reaction to the donation, and this praise may have functioned as an additional reward for them. One mother said:

> It made me feel good that other people knew. I didn't know how other people would react.
> Everybody thought it was marvelous. They thought it was big of me. . . . Some of them
> didn't know if *they* could do it but they thought it was wonderful.

Yet not all comments of outsiders were completely favorable. Many families reported some
less than positive feedback as well. After one mother noted a lot of positive support from friends
we asked:

> INTERVIEWER: Did anyone say anything the other way?
> MOTHER: Only one . . . a friend of ours . . . he doesn't be-
> lieve in playing God, and if someone is sick, "let
> 'em die" . . . he feels very strongly that we
> shouldn't be messing around with lives . . .
> INTERVIEWER: How did you feel when he said [this]?
> MOTHER: Hurt. I felt real bad.

In one case, a family received unpleasant crank phone calls when some persons read the
news about the transplant in the paper and checked the obituary to find a child the age of the
reported cadaver donor. These calls generated much unnecessary stress.

4. CONCLUSION

This small, exploratory in-depth study of cadaver-donor families 1 year after the donation
showed that most family members maintained positive attitudes toward this gift. Their prime
motivations were altruistic and empathetic—a desire to help the ill recipients. Some felt that the
donation gave a type of immortality to their dead relative. Several indicated that the donation had
served as the one bright moment in an otherwise tragic event.

Yet, negative aspects of the experience were noted. Brain death was a difficult concept for
several family members, despite careful explanations. Therefore, a few relatives felt guilty because they had given consent to disconnect the respirator.

Some conclusions relevant to policy can be made. The physician's role in initiating the idea
of donation appeared important at the time of the study, and seems to still be so (Simmons *et al.*,

1987). It is not surprising, therefore, that required request laws are apparently increasing the volume of donation. Families who do not think of donation during the initial period of grief are willing to make the gift when it is suggested by the physician.

The role of donor card campaigns in securing donors may be of more indirect than direct importance. That is, the medical staff does not appear to search for donor cards in the patient's wallet very frequently. However donor-card campaigns increase discussion of donation in the family and later, at the time of brain death, it is easier for the family members to make the decision to donate when they recall the positive attitude the patient expressed during such discussions (whether or not a card was actually signed).

This study also points to the need to be careful about the timing of the request for a donor—to allow the family to separate the announcement of death from the request for organs. Also, the double-edged sword of publicity is clear. On the one hand, publicity increases positive and gratifying responses from others; on the other hand, it allows for unpleasant crank calls and correspondence.

Finally, the desire of the cadaver-donor family for continued information about the well-being of the recipients should be noted. As the successes of organ transplantation increase, it should be easier and easier to send anniversary announcements indicating that their donation continues to benefit the lives of others. It is our impression that few, if any, centers send letters to cadaver-donor families a year or more after the donation.

From our point of view, actual face to face contact between organ recipients and donor is not advised, since such contact may place too great a burden of guilt on the recipient. We recommend anonymity of recipient and donor insofar as possible, but increased correspondence between the center and the donor family. Anonymous letters of thanks from the recipient to the donor should also be beneficial (Bartucci and Seller, 1986).

REFERENCES

Bartucci, M. R., and Seller, M. C., 1986, Donor family response to kidney recipient letters of thanks, *Transplant. Proc.* **18**:401–405.

Levey, A. S., Hou, S., and Bush, H. L., Jr., 1986, Kidney transplantation from unrelated living donors: Time to reclaim a discarded opportunity, *N. Engl. J. Med.* **314**:914–916.

Manninen, D. L., and Evans, R. W., 1985, Public attitudes and behavior regarding organ donation, *JAMA* **253**:3111–3115.

Simmons, R. G., and Abress, L., 1988, Ethics in organ transplantation, in: *Organ Transplantation and Replacement* (J. Cerilli, ed.), pp. 691–702, J.B. Lippincott, Philadelphia.

Simmons, R. G., Bruce, J., Bienvenue, R., and Fulton, J., 1974, Who signs an organ donor-card: Traditionalism versus transplantation, *J. Chronic Dis.* **27**:491–502.

Simmons, R. G., Marine, S. K., and Simmons, R. L., 1987, *Gift of Life: The Effect of Organ Transplantation on Individual, Family and Societal Dynamics*, Transaction, New Brunswick, New Jersey.

29

LEGAL ASPECTS OF ORGAN TRANSFER

H. RICHARD BERESFORD

1. INTRODUCTION

Once it is assumed that society generally favors organ transplantation as a treatment for impaired, sick, or dying persons, it is appropriate to ask whether applicable laws help or hinder the process. The following discussion considers several questions: What are the existing legal constraints on organ transfers? What changes in law can or should be made to augment organ transfers? What role should law play in achieving just allocation of organs? No attempt will be made to catalogue laws of various states or to replay debates about "brain death." Suffice it to say here, all participants in organ transplantation should be knowledgeable about local legal standards concerning consent to organ transfer and "brain death." For more detailed information, the reviews of Schwartz (1984) and Stuart *et al* (1981) are recommended.

2. LEGAL CONSTRAINTS ON ORGAN TRANSFER

2.1. Direct

2.1.1. Requirement for Consent

Under the widely adopted Uniform Anatomical Gift Act (1985), competent persons 18 years of age or older may donate an organ by will, donor card or other document. The donation becomes effective on the death of the donor, and the act does not require that surviving family members also agree to the donation. The act also empowers specified surviving family members to authorize organ donation on behalf of the deceased donor, provided the donor has not expressed a contrary intention and provided that certain specified family members do not object. Thus, under existing law, consent of the donor or certain family members ordinarily must be proven or obtained before an organ can be taken for transplantation. A few states, however, permit medical

H. RICHARD BERESFORD • Department of Neurology, North Shore University Hospital, Manhasset, New York 11030; Cornell University Medical College, New York, New York 10021.

examiners to remove corneas, pituitaries, and some other organs from decedents during autopsy if there is no evidence that the donor would have opposed this (Areen *et al.*, 1987*a*).

The practical effect of requiring consent of donor or family to organ transfer is to reduce availability of otherwise transplantable organs. Despite extensive educational efforts, many persons do not sign organ donor cards or other authorizations. Even if a donor has executed an appropriate consent, family members may nevertheless refuse permission for organ donation. In this circumstance, health care providers are usually unwilling to proceed further (Overcast *et al.*, 1984). Health-care providers may also simply not try to persuade grieving family members to agree to organ donation. For these reasons, and perhaps others, the principle of consent operates as a constraint on organ transfers. This has evoked a variety of proposals of alternative approaches to the problem of how to obtain transplantable organs after death.

If a living person is to serve as an organ donor (e.g., a kidney donor), the issue of competency to make such a decision assumes paramount importance. Under existing informed consent standards, the potential donor is entitled to disclosure of the risks of serving as an organ donor and must make a voluntary choice to proceed. If the potential donor has cognitive or psychiatric difficulties or is a minor, serious concerns arise about the validity of any consent to serve as a living donor. Concerns of this nature have led transplant centers to reject offered donations of kidneys from persons who are not related to potential donees (Overcast *et al.*, 1984), apparently because of a perception that psychiatrically normal persons would not volunteer important body parts. Moreover, transplant centers have been unwilling to rely on consent by parents to organ transfer from one of their minor children to another, and have sought judicial authorization. For example, in *Hart v. Brown* (1972), transplant physicians refused to operate without a court order, even though the parents had consented to a kidney transplant from their healthy 7-year-old daughter to her identical twin with end-stage kidney disease. After hearing medical testimony that the transplant had a high probability of success, posed only "minor" risks to the donor, and would result in psychological benefit to the donor, the court agreed to allow the parents to substitute their consent for that of the donor twin. In a sharply criticized portion of its opinion (Goldstein, 1977), the court indicated that approval of parental consent should rest on favorable judicial appraisal of parental "motivation and reasoning." The decision in *Hart v. Brown* is but one of several in which courts have approved intrafamily organ donations among minor children (Schwartz, 1984).

When incompetent adults are potential live donors, the question arises as to whether anyone has the right to consent to transfers of their organs. Assuming that they did not express themselves about organ donation before becoming incompetent, there is little basis for invoking the substituted judgment rationale for achieving "consent" to organ transfer. Also, it would be difficult to sustain the argument invoked in cases involving donations between twin siblings that the donor will derive psychological benefit from a transplant. Thus, in *Lausier v. Pecinski* (1975), the court refused to permit the guardian-sister of an adult schizophrenic to consent to his donation of a kidney to another sister with end-stage renal disease. The majority opinion emphasized his inability to consent and the lack of benefit to him from an organ donation, while the dissenting opinion suggested that a substitute consent would be proper because organ donation did not pose a major risk to the potential donor. Some authority for allowing substitute consent to organ donation may be derived from judicial decisions authorizing removal of life support from persons with severe and permanent neurological impairment (Beresford, 1984). It might be argued, for example, that if it is justifiable to end someone's life because there is no hope of recovery, it is even more justifiable to allow their organs to be used for altruistic purposes if family or legal representatives agree. In a sense, this argument introduces a utilitarian concern into a calculation about how best to respect a person's autonomy. But it is a reminder that the substitute judgment approach has been applied in cases involving adults whose preferences are unknown and cannot be determined.

2.1.2. Authority of Family Members

Our legal system confers on surviving family members the authority to decide how a decedent's body should be treated. They can either agree to or refuse autopsy, organ donation, or use of the body in research, unless there is evidence that the decedent had expressed a contrary intent or that there is an overriding state interest at stake (e.g., autopsy as part of a criminal investigation). The survivors' authority rests in part on the notion that the body is property that "passes" to them when a person dies and in part on the view that a family's religious and other strongly held sentiments must be respected (May, 1985). The effect of conferring this type of authority on family members is to empower them either to override a decedent's wishes about how his or her body should be handled or to assert their own views in the situation where the decedent's wishes are unknown. Although the Uniform Anatomical Gift Act (1985) permits competent persons to consent to organ donations after their deaths and provides immunity from civil and criminal liability to donees who act in "good faith" under the provisions of the act, the practice of transferees has been to secure the consent of appropriate family members before taking organs for transplantation.

2.1.3. Prohibition against Sale of Organs

Perhaps the number of organs available for transplantation could be augmented by allowing a market to develop for purchase and sale of organs. But legislatures that have addressed this matter have concluded that allowing sales is an unacceptable approach to the shortage of transplantable organs. For example, California makes it a criminal offense to remove any organ "with intent to sell it," and recent federal legislation bans interstate sale of human organs (Schwartz, 1984; Areen et al., 1987b; National Organ Transplant Act, 1984). Opponents of organ selling assert that a free market in organs would discriminate against those whose ability to pay for a needed organ is limited and would undermine the altruism that is responsible for past successes in obtaining organs (Areen et al., 1987b).

2.1.4. Residual Uncertainty about Brain Death

Most states now have legislation or judicial decisions that adopt the principle that irreversible cessation of functions of the brain constitutes death (Beresford, 1984; Stuart et al., 1981). While this has undoubtedly been helpful for obtaining organs from those who are "brain dead", problems in implementation of the "brain death" concept continue to arise. For example, death is not defined in the Uniform Anatomical Gift Act, and potential transferees in the few states without laws regarding brain death may be reluctant to remove organs until the heart has stopped beating. Moreover, existing criteria for brain death are rigorous—as they must be—and physicians who are inexperienced in applying them may err on the side of delaying determination of death beyond the point at which certain organs can be salvaged. There are also lingering uncertainties about whether generally accepted criteria for brain death are valid for infants and very young children. An additional disincentive to declaring brain death occurs when the potential donor's death has major legal implications, as might be the case if the brain injury resulted from criminal assault or medical malpractice. Thus, even though law now generally reflects the medical consensus about brain death, situations may still arise in which physicians are reluctant to make the determination.

2.2. Indirect

2.2.1. Autonomy Principle

A prominent feature of American jurisprudence is its emphasis on protecting individual persons against harm by the state or by others more powerful than they. This is reflected in doctrines relating to informed consent, criteria for involuntary hospitalization or treatment of the mentally ill, and the evolving constitutional right of privacy. Within this context, there is little reason to expect much support for a suggestion that individuals, or those best situated to speak for them, should subordinate to interests of the larger society their autonomous right to say what is done with their bodies after their death. One can argue that organ transfer is a special case because it confers a positive benefit on another, and that the autonomy of an involuntary source is not much offended by what is done with his body once he can no longer perceive any intrusion. But here symbolism may be more important than logic.

2.2.2. Defensive Medicine

Debate about the malpractice crisis has generated assertions that health care providers are so fearful of its litigation they forego actions that are medically appropriate. Whether or not this is generally true, it seems reasonably clear that physicians are wary about making determinations of brain death and recognize that families may vacillate considerably in attitudes about brain death or about whether to agree to organ transfer. This can only reinforce their sense of vulnerability to later legal actions, even though the Uniform Anatomical Gift Act (1985) affords immunity for "good faith" conduct.

3. CHANGING LAW TO AUGMENT ORGAN TRANSFERS

3.1. Consent Rules

3.1.1. Mandated Choice

In a system that emphasizes voluntarism as the proper basis for securing transplantable organs, any rule or procedure that contains coercive elements will be suspect. But if one of the shortcomings of the existing system is that persons who are willing to serve as organ donors do not bother to express this willingness (Overcast et al., 1984), a minimally coercive tack is to require them to opt in or out of organ donation in a formalized way. This approach does not force them to become organ donors; it simply asks them to declare themselves on the matter (Starzl, 1984). One state, Colorado (1981), has pursued this approach by requiring applicants for drivers' license to declare, as a condition of issuing a license, whether they agree to serve as organ donors after their deaths. Other states ask applicants to indicate a choice but do not deny licenses to those who fail to do so. Given evidence that a majority of adult Americans are willing to serve as organ donors on their deaths (Areen et al., 1987a), a law that asks them to opt in or out of organ donation does not seem particularly offensive. Nevertheless, it represents a compromise with the principle of voluntarism.

3.1.2. Presumed Consent

If organ transfer is perceived as a social good and most persons are willing to be donors, a reasonable legislative response might be to enact laws that permit organs to be removed on death unless there is evidence that the potential donor (or perhaps his or her next of kin) would oppose this. Such laws would preserve a person's right to opt out of organ donation but would presume consent to organ donation unless a contrary intent is expressed. A rationale for presuming consent in this circumstance is that, since most persons favor organ donation, it is likely that the particular person would have consented to organ donation had he or she been asked. Moreover, by concentrating on the donor's assumed preferences, less emphasis is placed on trying to obtain consent from next of kin under circumstances where making an informed, voluntary choice is difficult

(Caplan, 1983). Several states have adopted a presumed consent approach in permitting medical examiners to remove certain organs (e.g., corneas, pituitary) in situations where no evidence of donor or family opposition exists (Areen *et al.*, 1987*a*; Schwartz, 1984), but other state legislatures have rejected presumed consent laws. Arguments against them include their reliance on a fictional consent, their undermining of the principle of voluntarism, and their blatant utilitarianism (Areen *et al.*, 1987*a*; Feinberg, 1985; May, 1985). However, as Feinberg (1985) indicated, presumed consent laws need not have "coarsening effects" if existing legal and ethical norms are heeded.

3.1.3. Abolish Consent Requirement

To some extent, the same arguments that support presumed consent laws justify complete abolition of the requirement for consent to organ transfer. If there is, indeed, a critical shortage of urgently needed organs and if there is general agreement that organ transfer if desirable, the most straightforward solution is to allow the taking of any transplantable organs once a person has died. While some nations other than the United States have adopted this strategy (Schwartz, 1984; Stuart *et al.*, 1981), the arguments that have defeated presumed consent laws would carry even greater weight when the right of a person to determine what happens to his or her body is directly threatened.

3.2. Required Request Laws

Given a widespread perception that physicians have been less than diligent in seeking to obtain transplantable organs, several states have followed the lead of Oregon (1985) in imposing on physicians and hospitals a legal duty to seek consent to organ donation from the next of kin of medically suitable organ donors (Areen *et al.*, 1987*a*). No request need be made, however, if there is evidence that the decedent or the next of kin would have been or are opposed to organ transfer. These laws directly address an important weakness in the existing system for obtaining organs and their principal coercive effect is on those health care providers who, for whatever reasons, have been lax in seeking organ donations. While some families may resent being asked to consent to organ donation or may experience guilt over any choice they make, once they indicate a choice the required request laws contemplate no further efforts to persuade them.

3.3. Strengthened Immunity for Transplanters

If one reason for the reluctance of physicians to seek organ donations is the fear that the Uniform Anatomical Gift Act does not provide sufficient protection against later legal actions, consideration might be given to strengthening the immunity already afforded. The problem here is to demonstrate that such a step is either necessary or desirable. Laws relating to brain death clearly authorize determinations of death where specified criteria are met, and the Uniform Anatomical Gift Act clearly indicates what constitutes an adequate consent to organ donation. Short of granting immunity for negligent application of brain-death criteria or negligent failure to obtain consent, it is difficult to see how more formal immunity than already exists could be provided. A preferable approach would be to educate wary physicians about the protections already available to them.

3.4. Relaxation of Brain-Death Criteria

Scrupulous observance of the generally accepted criteria of brain death may necessitate a variety of clinical and other examinations over a period of days. This may result in some organs becoming unsuitable for transplantation or may discourage evaluators from even attempting a determination of brain death. But even if the criteria are conservative, it is not clear that they are so conservative as to require explicit relaxation. Within this context, it is important to distinguish efforts to update criteria in light of new scientific data from efforts to expand the range of persons who might be considered as organ donors. For example, if the goal is to use living anencephalic infants or adults in a vegetative state as organ donors, the issue ought to be addressed directly rather than through efforts to alter criteria for defining death. Although hopelessly ill and as good as dead in the minds of some, they retain detectable neurological functions and are variably capable of prolonged survival. It would distort the meaning of the word to categorize them as dead. Moreover, using flexible formulations of death for the frankly utilitarian purpose of harvesting human organs carries with it some rather offensive and ominous implications (Capron 1987).

3.5. Greater Allocation of Resources to Transplant Programs

A variety of legislative programs can be devised to maximize the effectiveness of organ transplantation as medical treatment. These might include financial assistance to procurement programs, direct subsidies of transplant centers, expanded reimbursement of the medical and other expenses of transplant recipients under federal and state programs, and support of research aimed at controlling rejection reactions. To some extent, programs of this nature are already in effect, and the recently enacted National Organ Transplant Act (1984) contemplates support of organ procurement and research relating to immunosuppression.

4. ROLE OF LAW IN JUST ALLOCATION OF ORGANS

4.1. Rights of Recipients

Under the existing rather pluralistic system of organ transplantation, allocations of organs are usually based on a mixture of "objective" criteria (e.g., histocompatibility, prognosis without a transplant) and less precise standards (e.g., age, support systems, ability to cooperate in complex treatment). A recipient has no legally protected entitlement to due process in the selection procedure or any defined remedy if another recipient who is less well suited by "objective" criteria receives an organ that might otherwise have been given to him. However, if federal and state governments increase their support of transplant programs, it seems inevitable that standards will emerge that provide potential recipients with something akin to procedural due process in the selection mechanism. For example, as suggested by the Report of the Massachusetts Task Force on Organ Transplantation (1985), the state should require uniform medical screening criteria to be reviewed by a committee representative of the public and available for public inspection in the files of a state agency. Once formal standards are promulgated, individuals may then be able to bring private actions against those who violate them.

4.2. Interest of the State in Distribution of Resources

As is apparent from the report of the Massachusetts task force (1985), governmental decisions to support organ transplantation programs will occur against the backdrop of a broad consideration of how many social resources are properly allocable to a specific form of medical treatment. One implication is that those who control funding may make a more or less deliberate choice to support only certain types of transplants (e.g., hearts but not livers), to emphasize less "halfway" approaches to treatment of disease (e.g., low-cost prevention over high-cost transplants), or even generously to fund transplant programs in preference to less dramatic forms of health care. Any resulting legislation will reflect lawmakers' perspectives about how strong a claim transplant programs should have on the public purse. These perspectives can obviously be shaped by the quality and depth of information provided by those who seek particular allocations of resources.

5. SUMMARY

Whereas existing public policy favors organ transfers, our legal system protects the power of individuals to determine whether or not to serve as organ sources. Despite laws designed to encourage voluntary organ donation, neither potential donors nor health-care providers have taken full advantage of them. Various modifications of these laws have been proposed, including attempts to make potential donors exercise a choice or to implement the notion of presumed consent. But the principle of voluntarism remains the dominant force. Little support has surfaced for approaches that would limit the authority of potential donors or their families to control organ transfer or to expand the power of health care providers to obtain more transplantable organs.

REFERENCES

Areen, J., King, P. A., Goldberg, S., and Capron, A. M., 1987a, Law Sci. Med.: 157–159.
Areen, J., King, P. A., Goldberg, S., and Capron, A. M., 1987b, Law Sci Med.: 163–166.
Beresford, H. R., 1984, Severe neurological impairment: Legal aspects of decisions to reduce care, Ann. Neurol. 5:409–414.
Caplan, A. L., 1983, Organ transplants: The costs of success, Hastings Ctr. Rep. 13:23–32.
Capron, A. M., 1987, Anencephalic donors: Separate the dead from the dying, Hastings Ctr. Rep. 17:5–9.
Colo. Rev. Stat., 1981, sec. 42–2–106(5).
Feinberg, J., 1985, The mistreatment of dead bodies, Hastings Ctr. Rep. 15:31–37.
Goldstein, J., 1977, Medical care for the child at risk: On state suprvention of parental autonomy, Yale Law J. 86:645–675.
Hart v. Brown, 29 Conn. Sup. 368, 289 A. 2d 386 (1972).
Lausier v. Pescinski, 67 Wis. 2d 4, 226 N.W. 2d 180 (1975).
May, W. F., 1985, Religious justifications for donating body parts, Hastings Ctr. Rep. 15:38–42.
National Organ Transplant Act, 1984, Pub. Law 98–507, 98 Stat. 2339.
Ore. Rev. Stat., 1985, 97.268.
Overcast, T. D., Evans, R. W., Bowen, L. W., Hoe, M. M., and Livak, C. L., 1984, Problems in the identification of potential organ donors, JAMA 251:1559–1562.
Report of the Massachusetts Task Force on Organ Transplantation, 1985, Law Med. Health Care 13:8–26.
Schwartz, H. S., 1984, Bioethical and legal considerations in increasing the supply of transplantable organs: From UAGA to "Baby Fae," Am. J. Law Med. 10:397–437.
Starzl, T., 1984, Implied consent for cadaveric organ donation, JAMA 251:1592.
Stuart, F. P., Veith, F. J., and Cranford, R. E., 1981, Brain death laws and patterns of consent to remove organs for transplantation from cadavers in the United States and 28 other countries, Transplantation 31:238–244.
Uniform Anatomical Gift Act, 1985, Unif. Law Ann. 8A:15.

30

ANATOMICAL GIFTS EFFECTIVE AT DEATH

CARL H. LISMAN

1. INTRODUCTION

Recognizing the humanitarian, educational, and scientific needs to encourage the donation of human organs and tissue at death, the National Conference of Commissioners on Uniform State Laws (the National Conference) promulgated, in 1968, the Uniform Anatomical Gift Act.

It is the purpose of the National Conference to promote uniformity in state law on all subjects where uniformity is desirable and practicable. Organized in 1892, it is one of the oldest state organizations designed to encourage interstate cooperation. (See the *1983 Handbook of the National Conference of Commissioners on Uniform State Laws and Proceedings*, pp. 220–221.)

Public acceptance of the 1968 Act was overwhelming; the Act, or a substantially similar version of it, was adopted in every state and in the District of Columbia. (8A *Uniform Laws Annotated*, Master ed.)

The Act applies only to anatomical gifts that become effective upon death. The common law—brought with the first colonists—was quite firm as the validity of gifts; subject to exceptions not applicable generally, the rules of the common law provide that a valid gift requires both donative intent and delivery, and gifts to be effective at or after death can be made only by will and only with the formalities of a will.

As a consequence, anatomical gifts to be effective at or after death would fail under the strict examination of the common law: Although there may be donative intent, delivery does not occur until after death and, unless the document evidencing the gift is a Last Will and Testament that satisfies all the statutory requirements for wills, the gift would be ineffective. As noted by the National Conference in its prefatory note to the 1968 Act,

---

CARL H. LISMAN • Private Law Practice, Burlington, Vermont 05402.   The Chairman of the Drafting Committee of the National Conference of Commissioners on Uniform State Laws on Amendments to the Uniform Anatomical Gift Act is Glee S. Smith, of the Kansas bar; other members of the Committee are Mr. Lisman, Mary Joan Dickson, of the New Jersey bar; Ronald W. Del Sesto, of the Rhode Island bar; Robert G. Frey, of the Kansas bar; David T. Prosser, Jr., of the Wisconsin bar; Robert E. Sullivan, of the Montana bar; and William H. Wood, of the Pennsylvania bar. Nothing in this chapter is intended to express the position or opinion of the National Conference of Commissioners on Uniform State Laws or the Drafting Committee.

> If utilization of bodies and parts of bodies is to be effectuated, a number of competing interests
> in a dead body must be harmonized, and several troublesome legal questions must be answered.

The application of these common law rules was a primary motivation behind the Act's original
adoption. If nothing else, the Act authorized and legitimized anatomical gifts made during life to
become effective at death.

However, following adoption of the Uniform Anatomical Gift Act by state legislatures during
the late 1960s and early 1970s, the Act became less "uniform" due to local amendments. In
short, the Act, intended to provide an identical law throughout the country, became less and less
identical. This lack of uniformity, as well as a perception that the Act should be measured against
medical and technological advances, were primary motivations for the decision by the National
Conference to revisit the Act and to consider whether amendments to it should now be proposed.
At its annual meeting in 1987, the National Conference approved a revised Act, to be known as
the Uniform Anatomical Gift Act (1987).

2. EXPLANATION OF THE ACT

The text of the Act is short; it contains merely 17 sections. Six of the sections are common
to most legislative enactments: title, repealler, time of taking effect, uniformity of interpretation,
severability. Section 1 contains definitions. The following is a brief summary of the substantive
provisions of the revised Act.

2.1. Who May Make an Anatomical Gift?

An anatomical gift to take effect upon death of all or part of an individual's body may be
made by (1) an individual [Section 2(a)], or (2) others according to priorities specified in Section
3(a).

The Act no longer contemplates a single standard of competency and age but assumes that
most states will opt for 18 years of age. This approach is intended to enlarge the class of potential
donors. The common age of majority is now 18 years.

Even though Section 2(a) in the 1968 Act clearly stated that a competent adult could make
a gift to become effective upon death, it had become increasingly common for doctors and hospitals to defer to the desires of surviving family members to prevent implementation of the gift.
This willingness to defer—spurred in part by threat of litigation—ignored the desires of the deceased individual. Consequently, the Act now provides that a gift made during life by a donor,
and not otherwise revoked by the donor during life, is not revocable by another after death and
does not require the consent or confirmation of any person.

Section 2(h): If a person has not made an anatomical gift of all or part of his body, at death
any of the following persons, in the order of priority stated, may make the gift:

1. The spouse
2. An adult son or daughter
3. Either parent
4. An adult brother or sister
5. A grandparent
6. A guardian of the person of the decedent at the time of his death

Section 3(a): This legislative surrogacy places family members in the position to make gifting
decisions. No such rights existed at common law, there being no property right in a dead body in
a commercial sense. Nonetheless, the law does recognize that family has a duty to bury the dead,

including the rights to possession and custody of the body for that purpose (American Jurisprudence, second edition). Section 3(a) is a natural extension of that analysis; if family is responsible for burial, organ and tissue gifting by family is an incidental right.

Nonetheless, Section 3(b) imposes limits on the right to make such a gift. If a person in a prior class is available at the time of death to make the gift, or if the person has knowledge of contrary indications by the decedent, or if a member of the person's class or a prior class objects to the gift, the gift will not be effective.

There has been little controversy regarding the various family classes; the categories are self-defining. The 1968 Act also contained a sixth clause of surrogate donor: "any other person authorized or under obligation to dispose of the body" [Subsection 2(b) (6)]. This provision has been troublesome. In the common instance, the executor or administrator of the decedent's estate will see to proper disposition of the body; in the absence of a will or probate administration, family or friends frequently undertake this task. As a general rule, a member of a higher class is likely to be available to make a gift; subsection (6) addressed the exception. It applied to local public health officials and medical examiners who come upon a deceased person in their official capacities, either because the decedent had no family and assets or because death occurred outside a hospital and no person claimed the body. The commonality of interests of the first five categories was absent from this category.

Frequently, the decedent has been a "street person" whose death passed unnoticed by society; family may have been long estranged and, in any event, could not be located because the decedent carried no identification or erroneous information. The decision to donate by the medical examiner or public health official cannot be viewed as a surrogate family decision.

Section 4 has been added as a substitute for the sixth class. It delegates decision-making to the public official likely to be responsible for disposal: the coroner or local public health official. Pursuant to Section 4(a), these officials may make the anatomical gift in the absence of contrary indications by the decedent (a lesser standard than affirmative refusal) or by family members in the step process. If a request for an anatomical gift has been received, removal will be accomplished by a qualified person, removal will be in accordance with accepted medical practices, and appropriate cosmetic restoration will be done.

2.2. In What Manner Does the Act Encourage Anatomical Gifts and Increase the Likelihood of Anatomical Gifting?

"Tissues and organs from the dead can be used to bring health and years of life to the living" (Prefatory Note to the 1968 Act). The demand for anatomical parts for transplantation far outpaces the supply. The 1968 Act brought order from the chaos of disparate state enablement and regulation; it set forth simple rules for making anatomical gifts.

However, by creating a framework within which anatomical gifts become effective at death throughout the nation, the 1968 law failed to comprehend the extent of the demand for anatomical parts spurred on by medical and scientific advances. In short, it is no longer sufficient to rely on the passive encouragement of gifts enabled by the 1968 Act.

Various states have addressed the need for more active encouragement with a variety of techniques. Following this lead, the National Conference has revised the Act to incorporate *routine inquiry* on hospital admission, *required request* at or near the time of death, and *search* for documents of gift by emergency rescuers.

Routine inquiry will add one more subject matter during the typical hospital admission procedure. Each incoming hospital patient must be asked whether he or she is an anatomical donor. If the answer is positive, a copy of the document of gift is to be requested for insertion in the patient's file; if the answer is negative (and only if the attending physician thereafter consents), discussion of the possibility of making an anatomical gift will follow. Various alternatives to routine inquiry exist at this time. Perhaps the most common are provisions requiring operators of motor vehicles to identify themselves as donors on an operator or chauffeur's license, as is the law in Colorado. Other suggestions include mandating health insurers to include donation as an item on policy applications and renewal forms or state tax officials to include donation as an item on statewide tax forms. Each of these approaches has its failings. Not all persons operate motor vehicles, a sizable portion of society is without the benefits of health insurance, and not all states employ a broadly based statewide taxing mechanism. Inquiry at hospital admission is, however, an appropriate technique; it has been applied in New Jersey, apparently without problem. Routine inquiry is not synonomous with required request. Its purpose is to identify existing donors, not to preach the merits of donation.

Required request will occur at or near the time of death, but only if there is nothing in the patient's file identifying the patient as a donor or as a person who has refused to make an anatomical gift. Unlike routine inquiry, required request is addressed to family, not the patient. This process "is to be made with reasonable discretion and sensitivity to family circumstances" [Section 5(b)]. No request is required if the gift would be unsuitable, as judged by accepted medical standards.

Search is consistent with the goal of identifying persons who have evidenced their desire to donate by carrying a card or other form of document or gift. The duty to search will apply to police officers, fire department personnel, and emergency rescuers, if they believe a person to be dead or near dead. Search also will apply to hospitals for admissions at or near death.

Finally, hospitals must notify specified recipients or procurement ogranizations if a patient or person in transit is identified as a donor. Notice must be given to the specific recipient or, if none, to a procurement organization.

2.3.   What Is a Proper Subject of an Anatomical Gift?

The Act comtemplates that all or any part of a human body may be the subject of an anatomical gift to take effect on death [Section 1 (1)]. Part is defined to mean an "organ, tissue, eye, bone, artery, blood, fluid, or other portion of a human body."

Section 1(7): When death occurs is not defined by the Act. A "decedent" is described as "a deceased individual and includes a stillborn infant or fetus" [Section 1(2)]. This definition remains unchanged from the 1968 Act. Greater reliance on life-prolonging machinery raises serious ethical and religious concerns; the Act is neutral with regard to those concerns. In recent years, a substantial number of states have added, by statute or judicial decision, the concept of brain death to the traditional death definition of cessation of circulatory and respiratory functions. [See, e.g., Uniform Determination of Death Act, *Uniform Laws Annotated* (master ed.).] As a general rule, the occurrence of death is not controversial. The exception may be anencephaly—children born without brains or, more accurately, without most of the brain. These children do have a heartbeat and respiratory function, which can be sustained for a matter of days after birth, if properly nourished. Here the legal definition of death, which presupposes life, is not helpful because death is a medical and scientific phenomenon, not a legal conclusion.

2.4.   For What Purposes May an Anatomical Gift Be Made?

The Act describes in broad terms the purposes for which anatomical gifts may be made. Section 6 specifies that gifts may be made for transplantation, medical or dental education, research, advancement of medical or dental science, or therapy. It is clear that gifts for other purposes are prohibited.

2.5.   To Whom May an Anatomical Gift Be Made?

The Act identifies, as appropriate recipients, hospitals, surgeons and physicians, accredited medical and dental schools, colleges and universities; banks and storage facilities; and specified individuals [Section 6(a)]. The Act also permits donations to facilities licensed, accredited or approved under state laws for procurement, distribution, or storage of human bodies or parts. Inasmuch as transplantation is a primary use of parts, the clear mandate is reassuring.

An anatomical gift may be made to a specified recipient. Contrary to common law principles, a gift will be effective even if a donee is not specified [Section 6(b)]. If so, the gift may be accepted by any hospital. Inasmuch as the intention is to make a gratuitous transfer for positive social reasons, implementation of the gift, by delivery to a recipient, can be achieved by others after death.

2.6.   What Steps Must Be Followed to Make, Amend, or Terminate an Anatomical Gift?

2.6.1.   Making a Gift

2.6.1a.   By the Individual. An individual may make an anatomical gift of all or any part of his body by a Last Will and Testament or by a document (Section 2). If the gift is made by will, the Act recognizes that the probate process cannot interfere with implementation of the gift. Consequently, the gift is effective upon death, without waiting for probate. If the will is not probated or is invalid as a will (e.g., because statutory formalities for execution were not followed), the anatomical gift is nonetheless valid and effective [Section 2(e)].

An individual may make, or may refuse to make, an anatomical gift [Section 2(a)]. The Act now employs the phrase "document of gift" to describe "a card, a statement attached to or imprinted upon a motor vehicle operator's or chauffeur's license, a will, or any other instrument used to make an anatomical gift" [Section 1 (3)]. A gift must be made by "a document of gift" [Section 2(b)]. This document must be signed by the donor (or, if the donor cannot sign, by another person, in the presence of two witnesses and the donor); otherwise, there is no witness requirement. The original witnessing requirements for signed documents of gift were not consistent with social policy. The Uniform Probate Code, for instance, calls for only two witnesses for wills. Nonprobate transfer devices at death (e.g., joint bank accounts) are increasingly common and require no witnesses. The Uniform Simplification of Land Transfers Act abolishes the requirement of witnesses for real estate deeds. Some states have already deleted the witness requirements from the 1968 Act.

2.6.1b.   By the Surrogate. A gift by a person specified in Section 3(a) is made by a document signed by him or made by his "telegraphic, recorded telephonic or other recorded message" [Section 3(d)]. There is no requirement of witnesses.

2.6.2.   Amendment and Termination

Section 6 of the 1968 Act distinguished the method by which amendment or revocation could be made. If a nonwill document of gift had been delivered to a specified recipient, an individual could have amended or revoked his gift before death by communicating the amendment or revocation to the specified donee. If the nonwill document of gift had not been delivered to a specified donee, the individual could have revoked it by notice to the specified donee or by destruction, cancellation, or notification. A gift by will could have been amended only by employing the means to amend or revoke a will. The Act did not specify how an anatomical gift made by others at or after death could be revoked.

The 1968 Act's dependence on delivery of the document of gift was incorrect in light of gifting patterns. The widespread solicitation and collection of donor cards has served primarily to educate potential donors. Most persons who complete and return a donor card solicited while at a supermarket or in a shopping mall quickly forget the gift and, more significantly, there is no procedure by which the donor can be identified immediately before death.

The better approach, now embodied in the Act, is to permit amendment or revocation by an individual in the same manner as a gift made by him. A signed statement in the donor's possession, an oral statement in the presence of two witnesses, or any form of communication to a physician or surgeon during a terminal illness should be sufficient to amend or revoke in addition to notice to a specified recipient.

The method by which a surrogate family member may revoke a gift made by him or by another surrogate in an equal or lower priority has also been clarified. The means permitted should be identical to that required to make a surrogate gift. More significant, however, is the time within which the revocation must be made. In order to ensure that surrogate gifts cannot be revoked after delivery, the Act now makes clear that revocation is ineffective if the physician, surgeon, technician, or enucleator performing the removal has commenced the procedures for the removal.

2.7. Does the Act Recognize the Rights of Persons Who Do Not Wish to Make an Anatomical Gift?

The universe in anatomical gifting contemplated by the 1968 Act was too narrowly drawn:

Persons who are donors
Persons who have made no decision about donating
Persons who have "proxy" or "surrogacy" rights as to others

The law simply failed to recognize that there are persons who do not wish to be anatomical donors. As the Act empowers others to make anatomical gifts of or from a decedent, it must incorporate the concept of "refusal to make a gift" and recognize the rights of persons who do not wish to donate.

Furthermore, the Act now provides a procedure by which a person can refuse to be a donor. The manner of refusal is sufficient if done in the same manner as a gift. Under some circumstances, such as during a terminal illness or injury, the refusal can be oral [Section 1(i)].

Affirmative refusal during life will preclude gifts by family. If a decedent fails to make a gift but did not refuse to make a gift during life, the family may still make a gift [Section 3(a)].

2.8. Does the Act Provide for Coordination among Hospitals and Procurement Organizations?

There is clearly a need to coordinate procurement and utilization procedures among hospitals and procurement organizations. Just as important as this need may be, it is equally difficult to legislate a solution. Recent federal legislation requires hospitals receiving Medicaid or Medicare to establish protocols to encourage donation, including a form of routine notification to procurement agencies of persons identified as donors and membership in the national organ transplant network, if performing transplants. Regional cooperation is now required, although definition of that cooperation has been left to the hospitals and procurement organizations (Section 9).

2.9.   Does the Act Prohibit the Sale of Anatomical Parts after Death and Define the Limitations on the Determiner of Death to Participate in Transplantation?

Both matters have generated substantial adverse publicity. Sale is contrary to the voluntariness of gifting. It is reasonably clear that voluntary gifts will be substantially diminished if an active economic marketplace were to be tolerated. Similarly, sale at the highest price or on the best terms, although appropriate for some products and services, in this area smacks of impropriety and lack of principled allocation of resources.

Neither the attending physician nor the person determining the time of death may participate in the procedures for removing or transplanting a part. Here, the appearance of impropriety, whether or not it exists, demands that the standard demanded of Caesar's wife be followed.

2.10.   Will Nondoctors Be Permitted to Remove Anatomical Parts?

In addition to doctors and surgeons, persons licensed for that purpose are now permitted to perform removal and processing of a limited class of parts [Section 9(c)]. The eye enucleator is a good example of a person who is neither a physician nor a surgeon but who, if properly trained and licensed, can perform a useful and vital function.

3.   CONCLUSION

More than ever before, the explosion in the number of transplantations and the expanding category of parts for use in transplantation demand encouragement and simplification of the gifting process. The Uniform Anatomical Gift Act (1987) should serve both of these goals.

REFERENCES

Dead Bodies, 1988, *American Jurisprudence* 2:22.
Uniform Anatomical Gift Act (prefatory note), (1968), *8A Uniform Laws Annotated* (1987 Master Ed.).
Uniform Anatomical Gift Act, 1968, *8A Uniform Laws Annotated* (1987 Master Ed.).
Uniform Anatomical Gift Act, 1987, *National Conference of Commissioners on Uniform State Laws.*
Uniform Determination of Death Act, *12 Uniform Laws Annotated* (1987 Master Ed.).

31

Fragile Trust

The Success and Failure of Required Request Laws, and the Procurement of Organs and Tissues from Children and Adults

Arthur L. Caplan

1. INTRODUCTION

This chapter addresses two topics that may appear, at first, to have very little in common: (1) the question of whether required request laws have been successful with respect to organ procurement, and (2) the morality of using infants born with anencephaly as a source of organs and tissues. Despite the apparent incommensurability of the two subjects, I believe that the topics are intimately related.

Required request refers to laws that have been enacted in a number of states mandating that hospital adminstrators must ask or designate someone to ask family members or legal guardians about the possibility of organ donation when death has been pronounced. More than 40 states have enacted such legislation since July 1985. These laws typically require that those persons designated by administrators to make requests receive appropriate training as to the manner and content of such requests. Most state laws do not carry explicit penalties for noncompliance, but they do require that a "certificate of request" be filed with the death certificate to indicate whether consent to donate was given or refused.

A somewhat related policy—routine inquiry—has been enacted into law at the federal level as part of the National Organ Transplant Act and as part of recently created standards of the Joint Commission on Hospital Accreditation. Routine inquiry requires hospitals to create protocols aimed at encouraging organ donation but leaves the specific details of such protocols up to individual hospitals.

Required request and routine inquiry may appear to have little to do with matters pertaining to organ donation from infants born with anencephaly. These children suffer from a fatal congen-

Arthur L. Caplan • Center for Biomedical Ethics, University of Minnesota, Minneapolis, Minnesota 55455.

ital neural tube defect in which all portions of the brainstem fail to develop. Since such children cannot live long with such a massive defect and, since they are incapable of feeling any stimuli or having any awareness of the world around them, some medical professionals have wondered whether they are bound by required request or routine inquiry laws to mandate that parents of children born with anencephaly be approached about the possibility of organ donation.

The answer to this question is a simple No. It is only after death has been pronounced that requests are to be made. And in most cases when the use of an anencephalic child is being considered, death has not been pronounced. But even if required request laws were not intended to include requests to the parents of infants born with anencephaly, the link between required request and the possible use of anencephalics as sources of organs and tissues would still be present. For it is only if the transplant community insists that required request laws be strictly enforced that there is even the remotest of possibility of directing public policy in the direction of utilizing anencephalic infants as the sources of organs or tissues.

The use of anencephalic infants as the source of organs or tissues for transplantation, research or education is a prospect that fills many inside and outside the transplant community with dread (Capron, 1987). The use of such sources would violate a longstanding moral prohibition against the removal of life-supporting organs from anyone other than those who are dead.

To endorse such a proposal, society would have to be persuaded that the benefits of such utilization would far outweigh the risks and dangers inherent in expanding the concept of donorship to include those who are neither dead nor cannot consent to such a use. Society will also have to be persuaded that all other avenues for obtaining organs and tissues have been exhausted before allowing such a practice. This is why the use of anencephalic infants as sources of organs and tissues is so intimately related to the assessment that is made of required request policies.

2. THE SHORTAGE OF ORGANS AND TISSUES AND PROPOSALS TO REMEDY THE SITUATION

It is well known that there is a severe shortage of organs and tissues available for transplantation to those with end-stage organ failure (Caplan, 1984). This shortage is even more acute where infants and children are concerned.

In recent years, a number of proposals have been made for increasing the supply of organs and tissues for very young children who might benefit from a transplant. Some have urged following the experimental path pioneered by Dr. Leonard Bailey and his team at Loma Linda University Medical Center by using primates as a source of organs or tissues (Caplan, 1985). Others have suggested that abortuses, which occur as a result of both spontaneous and elective abortions, might be used as either tissue or organ donors (Caplan, 1987; Mahowald et al., 1987). And it has also been suggested that anencephalic infants might be used as a source of organs and tissues, a source of organs that has already been used in the United States in the past and that continues to be used in both Europe and Japan today (Harrison, 1986a,b).

In thinking about these proposals for increasing the supply of organs and tissues from very young children or fetuses, it is important to remember that a number of proposals have been advanced for alleviating the shortage of organs and tissues for adults. For example, some have suggested that the definition of brain death be modified so as to equate death with neocortical death (Veatch, 1975). Those in a permanent vegetative state would be eligible to donate organs as long as their capacity for conscious thought, sentience, and feeling had been irreversibly destroyed.

Others have called for the creation of specialized wards where so-called *neomorts*—those who have been declared either brain dead or in a permanent vegetative state—could be kept on artificial life support for as long as anyone desired to withdraw organs or tissues from them.

People could simply carry a card indicating their interest in being used in such a fashion for transplantation, research, or teaching purposes.

Other proposals have called for the examination of the use of those declared dead on arrival (DOA) at hospital emergency rooms as organ or tissue donors. Still others are actively engaged in attempts to broaden the donor pool for certain organs and tissues to include donors who are spouses or those who are strangers but have the requisite biological characteristics to serve as a donor for another (Rapaport, 1986).

These efforts cannot be separated from those directed at pediatric and fetal organ and tissue procurement. The success of newer forms of organ and tissue transplantation will lead to increasing pressures from both potential recipients and those in the field of transplantation to modify public policy in ways that will permit increases in the supply of organs and tissues available for transplantation or research. The public, if it has not already come to the opinion, will soon begin to view those in the transplant field as eager, perhaps distastefully so, to find ways to expand the donor pool.

The fact is that the public will not be as astute as many patients and transplant professionals in drawing distinctions between proposals aimed at increasing donations from infants and those aimed at increasing donations from adults. The prospect of utilizing anencephalic children will make many wonder whether adults who are not dead might be used as organ donors as well. Similarly, calls for the creation of neomort wards will convince a public already nervous from movies such as *Coma* that matters are not always what they are claimed to be in the realm of organ procurement.

The point is that any effort to expand the donor pool, be it the use of anencephalics or those who are DOA at the hospital door, will depend on the degree to which the public feels it understands transplantation and can trust those who are involved in procurement, research, or therapy in this area. The more transplantation seems exotic, strange, or bizarre, the less contact the general public has with the need for and realities of organ and tissue donation, the more suspicion, doubt, fear, and fantasy will come to dominate law and regulation regarding organ and tissue procurement.

3. USING ANENCEPHALICS AS ORGAN DONORS

Arguments about the use of anencephalic infants have centered on the desirability of declaring them dead as soon as the diagnosis is confirmed (Harrison, 1985a,b). Others have worried about the morality of procuring organs or tissues knowing that the death of the child, at least on existing views of brain death, will be hastened if not directly caused by the procurement team (Capron, 1987). Still others have asked how donations can be refused when the need for them is great and there are many parents who would like to see their child serve as a donor.

All these arguments fail to address the central issue in using infants born with fatal and massive congenital defects as sources. The central issue is whether the public trusts transplant professionals enough to believe that, if granted the right to use anencephalics, they will not abuse their authority to procure organs from other children or adults who have neither fatal diseases nor massive intellectual deficiencies.

My own view is that the public does not have the degree of trust requisite for seeing public policy move in the direction of using anencephalics as sources. A credible argument can be made that would permit the use of such children on ethical grounds. But as long as organ donation is a subject that affects the lives of a relatively small percentage of the public, the understanding, compassion, and trust necessary to translate a moral argument into law or policy reality will not exist.

In part, but only in part, this is a result of the perception that transplant surgeons and their teams are interested in more than saving lives—they want to make money from these operations. More importantly, the lack of trust stems from a lack of familiarity on the part of the general public with existing procedures and practices regarding organ and tissue procurement.

If one asks friends or relatives who are not in the transplant field what their views are about what happens to a body when an organ or tissue is procured or what state a person must be in in order for tissue or organ procurement to proceed, it quickly becomes evident that there is much work still to be done in the field of public education. The public is not well informed about organ and tissue donation.

4. SUCCESS OF REQUIRED REQUEST LAWS

The only way to fully and adequately inform the public about organ and tissue procurement in a way that will create a kind of understanding and, as a result, the trust that is a prerequisite to any modification of existing laws governing the definition of who may donate, is to make sure that the public is involved to as great an extent as is possible with organ procurement and transplantation. The easiest and most efficacious way to do this is to make sure that the public is fully informed of their right, as created by required request laws at the state and federal levels, to be given the option of donation when a family member dies (Caplan, 1984; Caplan and Bayer, 1984).

The point of required request laws is not simply to obtain more organs and tissues for transplantation. While it is often claimed by critics of these laws that such policies place utilitarian objectives ahead of individual autonomy, such a charge is simply nonsense.

The goal of required request legislation is to both insure people have the option to donate, knowing that the chances are good that if they are asked they will give and thereby increase the supply of organs and tissues, and to stimulate discussion of organ donation prior to the occurence of a tragedy, so that more informed, more thoughtful choices can be made about donation, whether it be to donate or not.

The first goal is motivated as much by a respect for autonomy as it is the utilitarian goal of having more organs and tissues available for transplant. The second goal is motivated solely by a desire to promote autonomous choice by allowing those who must make hard choices about donation to do so in an informed, deliberate and rational manner. Simply increasing the supply of organs and tissues available has never been the underlying value behind required request laws (Caplan and Bayer, 1984).

The first goal, that of increasing the opportunity to donate, has met with moderate success. In many states, organs and tissues are being obtained from hospitals that have not previously had an organ or tissue donor.

There have been obvious increases in the donation rates for both skin and corneas which are directly attributable to the passage of required request legislation. New York has experienced a 67% increase in corneal donations since the enactment of the law (O'Neil, 1986). Oregon has enjoyed a 135% increase (Burris *et al.*, 1986). Alabama and Arizona have had similar increases.

Donations of skin have increased by similar percentages or in some cases significantly more. Oregon has had a 300% increase in donors since required request went into effect in February 1986. These increases are the result of more people being asked about tissue donation.

Figures on solid organ donation are much more difficult to come by. But there is some evidence that required request laws have had a positive impact in this area. Stanford University's heart and heart–lung programs and the heart transplant program at Columbia Presbyterian Medical Center, both in "required request" states, report increases in the number of donors and donor referrals nearing fifty per cent over previous years. In Arizona, the rates of donation for the last part of 1985 and the latter part of 1986, when a required request law was enacted, show significant increases in organ donation.

TABLE I.   Total Referrals and Donors in 1985 and 1986

Period	Arizona		Las Vegas, Nevada	
	Total calls	Donors[a]	Total calls	Donors
1985 (before required request) 1/1/85–12/2/85	262	45	14	6
1986 (after required request) 1/1/86–12/2/86	734	97	23	16
Percentage change	280%	216%	164%	267%

[a] Includes kidney, bone, heart, multiorgan.

The total number of calls received by the Arizona Organ Bank increased by a factor of seven or eight times between the last 4 months of 1985 and the same period in 1986. The total number of donors of organs and tissues increased by about 20% over the previous year (Arizona Organ Bank, 1986). The number of kidneys obtained more than doubled during this period, whereas earlier in the year kidney procurement had actually been slightly lower than the previous year's experience (Tables I–IV).

These figures are encouraging. However, some critics of required request have suggested that perhaps the increases observed in tissue or organ donation to date are not the result of the laws themselves but rather of other factors. The most popular alternative cause for an increase appears to be increased public education.

I am not in a position to know whether there have been improvements in the quality or quantity of public education efforts between 1985 and 1986 that might be reflected in the numbers cited above. But there are three other facts that would indicate that required request has had much more to do with the increases that have been seen in both tissue and organ donation in 1987.

First, those hospitals that have adopted protocols in response to required request are obtaining more organs at rates that are higher than hospitals which have not complied with these new laws. Eye bank officials in both New York and Oregon note significant patterns in the hospitals serving as sources for new donors that correlate with the creation of required request protocols in particular hospitals within both states. When hospital personnel at facilities that have never before supplied a donor are asked why they have now done so, they frequently mention the influence of required request laws.

Second, the nations involved in the Eurotransplant program have actually seen a drop in the number of donors of kidneys from 1984 rates. In 1984 there were 1415 kidney donors. In 1985 the number dropped to 1300. In 1986 it had risen to only 1373. There was only one more kidney

TABLE II.   The Impact of Required Request for Organ and Bone Donors: The Last Quarter of 1985 and 1986[a]

Period	Arizona		Las Vegas, Nevada	
	Total calls	Donors	Total calls	Donors
1985 9/3/85–12/2/85	86	15	5	2
1986 9/3/86–12/2/86	310	37	2	2
Percentage change	360%	247%	−250%	0%

[a] For the last quarter, after required request enacted.

TABLE III.   Overall Referrals in Arizona and
Las Vegas for Cornea Donors

Period	N
Total: 1985	56
1/1/85–12/2/85	
Total: 1986	234
1/1/85–12/2/86	

TABLE IV.   The Impact of Required Request
for Eye Bank Referrals: Arizona and
Las Vegas, Nevada Combined in 1986

Period	N
1985	26
8/13/85–12/2/85	
1986	76
(before required re-quest)	
8/13/86	
1986	158
(after required request)	
8/13/86–12/2/86	

actually transplanted in 1986 then was transplanted in 1984 (Cohen, 1986). The general trend in donation in this system, which has emphasized public education but has not had a required request policy, has been one of stability in both the number of donors and the number of kidneys transplanted.

The last and most interesting data supporting the impact of required request laws as causally responsible for the increases in tissues and organs seen last year are the comparison of donor rates in Arizona with donor rates in the city of Las Vegas, Nevada—a state with no required request law (Tables I–IV). As is clear from the data presented, there have been more referral calls from hospitals, more overall donors, and more referrals to the eyebank as a direct result of required request legislation. Since the law only went into effect in August 1986, one should see even more impressive differences between 1985 and 1987 donor rates as the law is better understood by the public and health care professionals.

5.   FAILURE OF REQUIRED REQUEST LAWS

The statistics available on tissue and organ donation provide convincing evidence that if people are asked to donate, many will do so. Donation rates can be increased by the creation of a systematic practice wherein people are afforded the opportunity to make a donation either by discussing the subject with their families before their death or by giving families the opportunity to donate when no guidance has been forthcoming from the deceased.

However, another way to look at these statistics is that they represent a dismal failure of the laws to achieve their intended goals of increasing the supply of organs and tissues while also maximizing the opportunity for informed choice concerning donation. The statistics are not as impressive as they should be if public opinion polls can be trusted concerning the willingness of families to give permission for donation. (Tissue donation rates have done far better than organ donation, yet there is no real reason that this should be so.)

There are many grounds for complaint concerning the implementation of required request laws by both public officials and hospital personnel. The sound of feet dragging can be heard throughout the land where these laws are concerned. The public is not being given the opportunities it has requested through the implementation of required request laws to consider the option of donation.

The harsh fact of the matter is that many organizations, including medical examiners' offices, health departments, and hospitals, have not complied with state legislation requiring that requests be made. In those states that enacted laws first, Oregon, New York and California, there are obvious regional differences in the degrees of compliance and enthusiasm brought to the subject of requesting donations by various hospitals. In Oregon and New York, urban hospitals are clearly trailing behind rural and suburban hospitals in implementing protocols or carrying out requests.

Many state health departments have been slow to issue regulations implementing state laws governing required request. Organizations of hospital-based clergy and social workers have not pressed for educational programs on this topic. Nor have hospital associations and boards of trustees assigned high priority to required request.

Much of the brunt of required request implementation has fallen onto the shoulders of nurses. In many states, this need not be the case. In New York, the required request law explicitly allows clergy or social workers to become involved in making requests. There is no evidence that they have done so.

Professional education efforts aimed at those who will most likely be making requests—in medical schools, nursing schools, and continuing education forums—are simply lagging behind where public rhetoric about donation would indicate they should be. In many hospitals, emergency room personnel still do not understand the procedures they are to follow under a required request law.

Neither government officials nor health-care professionals have complained about the lack of compliance with required request laws shown by many institutions and providers. Despite all the rhetoric devoted to the need for donations, even those within the transplant community have not tried to do what needs to be done to jog hospitals and medical personnel into compliance with existing laws. It is still easier to point the finger of blame at the general public for lacking altruism or public-spiritedness when it comes to donation than it is to put the blame squarely where it belongs—on the medical community for its failure to ask about donation.

The failure of the transplant community to seek zealous compliance with required request laws is evident in many ways. Public education campaigns, or at least those I have heard or seen on radio and television, never mention required request. The fact is that families must be taught they have a right to be given the opporunity to donate. This message is not being communicated. It would be sad if the only way it could be emphasized would be by withdrawing federal funds from a hospital that fails to have a required request policy in place or by a lawsuit from an outraged family who wanted to donate but whom no one thought to ask.

The transplant community has not sought cooperation in its efforts to push for compliance with the law from public officials or the media. After an initial spate of stories, very little coverage has been given to the impact of required request laws. And few if any curriculum reforms or educational programs appear to have been initiated in our churches or schools to let people know about required request and the rights and obligations it creates. As far as I know, only one public hearing has been held by government officials to urge hospital associations, health departments, and other responsible agencies to make sure that all hospitals are making a good faith effort to assure families their right, and to assure those who have died their opportunity, to make a donation.

Most peculiarly, there is a desire on the part of some in the transplant community to deny the impact of required request laws on donor rates or to impute increases to other factors besides an increase in the number of families being asked. I have heard distinguished transplant surgeons on more than one occasion on both radio and television in the New York area deny that increases in skin and corneal donation have anything to do with required request laws. Their evidence for such beliefs was simply personal authority.

6. CONCLUSION

The resistance to requiring requests within the transplant community is both surprising and morally outrageous. The data available to date indicate that the laws will work if hospitals and transplant personnel enthusiastically support their implementation.

The only possible explanation for balking at required request is that old habits die hard. There are many within the transplant community who are still committed to the notion that organ donation should be voluntary both for those doing the giving and for those doing the asking (King, 1986). There are others who still believe that donation is an act of heroism or supererogation and that families ought not be forced or coerced into being heroes.

These beliefs are simply out of place in a world in which progress in transplantation is accelerating, research needs are increasing daily, and public expectations are on the rise. The beliefs reflect the fact that it is professionals as well as the public who have doubts or reservations about the harvesting of organs and tissues. Paternalism based on professional doubts and reservations (Younger et al., 1985), rather than on a concern for the sensitivities of the families of donors, is hard to acknowledge and harder to avoid in implementing public policies aimed at giving potential donors and their families the best possible opportunity to discuss and consider donation.

Moreover, returning to the issue of whether anencephalics ought be used as sources, the only conceivable way the transplant community can hope to effect any public policy at broadening existing definitions of who may provide organs and tissues is to maximize public trust in organ and tissue procurement. Required request holds the best hope of cementing that trust, since it is a policy that will enable the transplant community to communicate its needs, hopes, and procedures to the broadest possible audience. The failure to implement such a policy enthusiastically means that organ and tissue procurement is a subject that affects relatively few people at a time of tremendous emotional crisis—not a fertile political climate for effecting controversial changes in public policy.

Yet, the communities of more than 40 states have said that people ought be given the option of donation when a death in a hospital occurs. The federal government has agreed and asked that eligibility for funding be tied to the creation of donor protocols. The public has been persuaded by the transplant community that transplants are important and that every effort should be made to maximize the chance of obtaining a donation.

Sadly, the transplant community and the health care professions have not responded with a similar level of concern and enthusiasm for required request. The lackadaisical attitude shown by many hospitals and health care providers toward making requests for donation is morally wrong. For if such attitudes are not changed, many organs and tissues will be lost from those who would have wanted the opportunity to give with a consequent alleviation of disability and death for others. Nor will it be clear why the public should trust the transplant community to apply new standards carefully in the realm of donation when it is not making every effort to see that existing laws and policies are zealously complied with and responsibly enforced.

REFERENCES

Arizona Organ Bank, 1986, Cadaver Donor Activity Report, December 9.

Burris, T. E., Marquette, M., Gordon, M., and Tanne, E., 1986, Impact of Required Request Legislation in Oregon, unpublished manuscript, Oregon Lions Eyebank, October 8.

Caplan, A. L., 1984, Organ procurement: It's not in the cards, *Hastings Ctr. Rep.* **14**(5):6–9.

Caplan, A. L., 1985, Ethical issues raised by research involving xenografts, *JAMA,* **254**:3339–3343.

Caplan, A. L., 1987, Should foetuses or infants be utilized as organ donors?, *Bioethics* **1**(2):119–140.

Caplan, A. L., and Bayer, R., 1984, Ethical, legal and policy issues pertaining to organ procurement, pp. 1–25. *Hastings Ctr.*

Capron, A. M., 1987, Anencephalic donors: Separate the dead from the dying, *Hastings Ctr. Rep.* **17**(1): 5–9.

Cohen, B., 1986, Statistics, Eurotransplant Newsl. **40**:1–2.

Harrison, M. P., 1986*a,* The anencephalic newborn as organ donor, *Hastings Ctr. Rep.* **16**(2):21–22.

Harrison, M. P., 1986*b,* Organ procurement for children: The anencephalic fetus as donor, *Lancet* **1**:1383–1385.

King, A. B., 1986, Preliminary analysis of the size and characteristics of the donor pool in Northeastern Ohio and the influence of neurosurgeons' attitudes on the death process, *Transplant. Proc.* **13**(3):57–60.

Mahowald, M. B., Silver, J., and Ratcheson, R. A., 1987, The ethical options in transplanting fetal tissue, *Hastings Ctr. Rep.* **17**(1):9–15.

Rapaport, F. T., 1986, The case for a living emotionally related international kidney donor exchange registry, *Transplant. Proc.* **13**(3):1–5.

O'Neil, M. J., 1986, Testimony before assembly committee on health, Hearings on Required Request Legislation, New York State Assembly, Committee on Health, New York, New York, October 21, 1986.

Veatch, R. M., 1975, The whole-brain oriented concept of death: An outmoded philosophical formulation, *J. Thanatol.* **3**:13–23.

Younger, S., Allen, M., Bartlett, E., Cascorbi, H., Hau, T., Jackson, D. L., Mahowald, M. B., and Martin, B. J. 1985, Psychosocial and ethical implications of organ retrieval, *N. Engl. J. Med.* **313**:322–323.

32

RECONSIDERING THE BAN ON FINANCIAL INCENTIVES

NORMAN FOST

1. A PRELIMINARY QUESTION: IS THE ENTERPRISE AS A WHOLE JUSTIFIED?

Few policies attract wider support than the prohibition of financial incentives to prospective organ donors. In order to challenge this taboo, a preliminary observation on transplantation as a whole is required. This book has been predicated on an implicit assumption that organ transplantation, on the whole, is a good and just activity. That is a necessary condition for proposals to improve the supply of organs in ethically acceptable ways. In this chapter, I argue that financial incentives can be justified and that arguments banning such incentives are faulty. This argument depends on support for the enterprise as a whole: Why else would we want to improve supply? For the purpose of this discussion, I concede this approval but would like to register a few concerns before proceeding.

The enterprise of organ transplantation is surely a beneficent one. It expresses many values, most importantly respect for life. It strives to respect the rights and interests of donors and their families, through increasingly strict attention to consent requirements. Established programs, such as kidney transplantation, do well on cost–benefit analysis. Transplantation is generally less expensive than dialysis and less expensive than allowing such patients to die, if one considers the medical costs as well as potential loss of earnings. How, then, could one object on ethical grounds to such a well-meaning and successful effort?

The answer depends, in part, on considering the health system as a whole. Most important is the reality that 20% of Americans—40–50 million people—are without health insurance, i.e., cannot afford private insurance and are ineligible for either Medicaid or Medicare. This means that a woman with a lump in her breast must anguish over whether to see a doctor, with a possible expense of hundreds or thousands of dollars, and thereby forgo food, clothing, or some simple pleasure, or take the possibly fatal risk of avoiding medical care. It means that a parent whose child has a fever and headache must weigh the risk of meningitis against other sacrifices. For tens

---

NORMAN FOST • Department of Pediatrics, University of Wisconsin, Madison, Wisconsin 53792.

of thousands of pregnant teenagers, it means forgoing prenatal care, with the attendant risks of prematurity and neonatal death and disability.

How can one test the fairness of a system in which everyone has access to a kidney, but in which one in five lacks access to routine health care? One way is to ask what we would agree to before we knew what hand fate would deal us. How would we choose to allocate health-care resources if we were about to enter society without knowing whether we would end up rich or poor, with insurance or without? An analogy can be made with a poker game, in which you discover the deck holds five aces. It is difficult to divine a fair solution to this problem if the cards are already dealt, but it is useful to ask what a fair solution would be if one didn't know who stood to gain or lose.

I suggest that a rational consumer would not opt for a system in which rescue was guaranteed for a highly improbable event but that left him with a 1 in 5 chance of having no coverage for common events, many of them life-threatening. We have at least one test of this question. A consumer panel of a large health maintenance organization (HMO) was told they would have to choose between coverage for all solid organ transplantation or more basic services; they rejected full transplantation coverage.

It does not follow from these observations that discontinuing public funding for established transplantation programs would be desirable or even justified. We cannot, for example, assume that the savings would go toward universal health insurance or providing a decent minimum of routine health care for those presently without it. We could not even assume that the savings would go toward health care. We could not even predict whether the dividend would accrue to the benefit of those least well off, or would instead further improve the status of those presently well off. Because of these uncertainties, and the clear benefits of transplantation, it may be prudent to continue the present program while simultaneously trying to close the more disturbing gaps in access to routine health care. In a closed financial system, however, such as an HMO or a state Medicaid budget, providing coverage for liver transplantation might require forgoing mental health services beyond a bare minimum. A rational consumer, or an administrator claiming to serve the interests of the majority, might reasonably be against coverage for transplantation, even though a predictable number of lives could be saved with transplanted organs.

Finally, it should be noted that this example of publicly financing expensive high-technology services, while basic health-care needs are unmet, is not unique to transplantation. It is typical of the American system, which prefers health care to health, crisis intervention to prevention, and technology to more effective and efficient means to health (Knowles, 1977). Transplantation at least has the virtue of being medically and economically effective. Since its abolition would almost certainly result in worse health and more economic hardship for the poor and the affluent, it is reasonable to support it. With that as background, we can turn to the question assigned: Is the prohibition against payment for organs justified?

2. FINANCIAL INCENTIVES FOR DONATING ORGANS

It has become a shibboleth that financial incentives for donating organs are immoral. They are clearly illegal, since the passage of the Organ Procurement and Transplantation Act (1984), which prohibits the "sale for valuable consideration of human organs for use in human transplantation." Since financial gain is not generally prohibited in health care in general, or transplantation in particular, some justification is needed for this exception. Kidney transplantation alone is a multibillion-dollar business, with considerable economic incentives for all involved except the donor. Surgeons, procurement officers, hospitals, and recipients are all allowed economic benefits; only the supplier—the donor—is excluded from profit.

The arguments that have been used to support this special exclusion are as follows:

1. *Financial incentives would be coercive for poor people.* Many opponents of financial incentives refer to concerns about adverse effects on the poor. Some are explicit about coercion as their concern (Carpenter *et al.,* 1984). Others state more vaguely, that such a system "would likely be prejudiced against the poor." (Dougherty, 1986). Another concern for the poor emphasizes the injustice of a system in which "the good health of one privileged group is achieved at the expense of the certain discomfort and possible ill-health and death of a less privileged group" (*Lancet* editorial, 1986). It is unclear whether this latter concern assumes inequities in distribution of organs that would result from a free market. Offering incentives to improve supply would not imply any particular method of distribution once the organs were obtained. Theoretically, it would be possible to achieve an equitable distribution system independent of the mode of procurement.

The concern about coercion is misplaced at least in the sense that it involves a misuse of the word, which conventionally implies the use or threat of physical force, as defined by the *Oxford Universal Dictionary.* I know of no proposal that intends or even alludes to the use of force. Implicit in the definition of coercion is a threat that the subject will be worse off than he is if he does not comply. Financial incentives for organ donation seem more like an offer, which presents the subject with an opportunity to be better off than he is, or at least gives him the option to decide whether, according to his own value system, he would rather have more money and fewer kidneys, with the attendant risks of the operation and its sequelae.

All this implies that it would be improper to truly coerce someone into organ donation, with or without a financial compensation. Taking organs from minors or other nonconsenting subjects, with payments to parents or guardians, would therefore be prohibited. It does not follow that coercion for organ donation would always be morally indefensible. Consider, for example, a child with a fatal hematological condition, for whom bone marrow transplantation offered the only reasonable chance of survival, and the father were the best or only available donor. As the Supreme Court of Pennsylvania stated in refusing to force a man to donate bone marrow to his dying cousin, it would be morally reprehensible to refuse to come to aid of a dying person in this setting *(McFall v. Shimp),* particularly one's own son. There is a trend for requiring women to undergo unconsented surgery, such as cesarean section, for the benefit of a full-term fetus and child-to-be (Robertson, 1987). The analysis that finds it a duty for a mother to undergo physical intrusion for the benefit of her own child-to-be would seem applicable to organ donation for a postnatal child (Fost, 1983). But these complex issues take us afield from our original question.

Perhaps critics have in mind a different ethical concern, i.e., exploitation, i.e., taking unfair advantage of another's needs for personal or selfish gain. But why is this particular form of offering money for a risky act morally different from other compensable dangerous activities. All blue collar work involves risks, often more serious and more common than those associated with organ donation. Coal miners, construction workers, and football players are all induced to undergo risks of disability and death in exchange for money, often to the economic benefit of others who gain far more than the exploited worker. It should go without saying that such risky ways of earning money are typically associated with poverty or a lack of alternatives. Most people would prefer a job with less risk, given the choice. To the degree that our society does not offer equal opportunities, it may be considered unfair, and we should support and promote social change to reduce such inequality. It does not follow that eliminating risky work while waiting for the utopia of equal opportunity is in the interests of those exploited or is a policy that they would appreciate. Those who advocate a prohibition of selling organs owe us at least an explanation as to whether they would also prohibit construction work and football on the grounds that it exploits the same people who would be likely to sell their organs.

The sale of organs, as compared with other risky work, is, if anything, less troublesome, in that it is less risky and offers more immediate social benefits than do many jobs. Death or disability are remarkably uncommon among organ donors, in contrast with, say, football, in which permanent disability is common and death not rare.

The objection to prohibiting an individual from selling his organs can be criticized in another way: It is an unjustified act of paternalism, interfering with a person's liberty on the grounds that we know better than he what is good for him. We start with the presumption of autonomy: A person of sound mind is entitled to be left alone in deciding what risks to take in exchange for the benefits available. Those who would interfere with this choice have the burden of justifying their intrusion on this most basic liberty.

2. *Even if voluntary, organ donation involves unreasonable risks and people should not be induced to take such risks.* The opposition to paid organ donation sometimes assumes that organs would necessarily be removed antemortem, presenting risks to living persons. This concern could be largely eliminated by restricting retrieval to post mortem donors. This would add payment to the present system of asking adults to make such a commitment by a signature on their driver's license. Payment could be made to the donor, as an incentive for signing a donor card, or to his family or estate at the time of organ removal. The only medical risk of such commitments is that it could theoretically affect decisions regarding the vigor with which life support was maintained during possibly terminal illness. Whether this in fact would occur is uncertain, but such a concern would seem to apply equally to voluntary as well as paid donations.

Even antemortem donations, however, involve very low risks. Physicians have been asking and encouraging live related donors to take such risks for decades. It would be hypocritical to now argue that the risks are so great as to make it unethical to ask someone to undertake them. Whatever the risks, they are clearly less than many other activities that we allow people to pursue in exchange for financial inducements, including mining, construction, football and the like. These arguments were reviewed in the previous section on coercion. To put this risk in perspective, the mortality of kidney donation is less than driving 8 miles to work for 1 year. Unless one wishes to defend the claim that it is immoral to offer someone money in exchange for work which entails greater risk than kidney donation, some other justification will be needed to prohibit such offers.

Whatever the risk of live donation, it is greater than postmortem donation. It would therefore be preferable, other things being equal, if the need could be met from postmortem donors, with or without financial inducements. The success of cadaver grafts is now closer to that of live-related donors, due to advances in prevention and management of rejection. This, along with the recent expansion of required request laws (see Chapter 31), may make it unnecessary to consider live related organ donation.

3. *There would be adverse effects on recipients, due to a decline in the quality of organs.* There is concern that paid donors would include a higher proportion from lower socioeconomic classes than would live related donors and that this would entail a higher incidence of infectious and other diseases, including acquired immune deficiency syndrome (AIDS) and hepatitis.

The empirical basis of this claim is disputed. Caplan, who opposes payment, concedes that "hepatitis rates are high in the blood system of Japan which utilizes a voluntary, altruistic approach . . . [and] low in Sweden where a market system prevails" (Caplan, 1985). He points out that the crucial variable may be race, not payment (Drake *et al.*, 1982). It is certainly plausible that payment would skew the distribution of donors toward racial groups that are poorer and that have higher rates of transmissible infectious disease. These risks can be reduced by laboratory tests, which have virtually eliminated the HIV virus from the blood supply, and by screening potential donors for risk factors, with criminal penalties as a deterrent to misrepresentation, at least for antemortem donors.

Whatever the risks, for some recipients, who face imminent death or unacceptable suffering without an organ, the risk–benefit ratio of receiving an organ with the possibility of hepatitis is preferable to the alternative of no organ. Paid donors would not preclude the use of unpaid donors. Many family members would presumably not insist on payment, although it is possible that their willingness to donate may be lessened if they thought a paid donor were available.

4. *A free market would result in a misallocation of organs to the rich.* It should be noted again that misallocation of organs is one of the least important on the long list of health-related services which are distributed unevenly in this country. It is puzzling why this aspect of organ distribution is raised in a country which already relegates so much of the health care system to the marketplace. Indulging in debate about inequities in access to organs while one on five Americans has financial and other barriers to routine health care is akin to rearranging the deck chairs on the Titanic. Transplantation happens to be one area, however, where justice may be easier to achieve.

There is no reason why the method of procurement should or must be linked to the method of allocation. Some believe that the present system already has structural biases favoring those in the upper classes. In some cases, particularly those involving liver and heart transplantation, this has been explicit, when centers have allowed wealthy patients, including some from foreign countries, to jump the queue awaiting liver transplantation. Similarly, American families who are adept at gaining access to the mass media seem to have an advantage in raising necessary funds for the considerable costs of transplantation in facilitating directed donations—procurement of an organ intended for a specific patient. If the poor are not going to participate equitably in the distribution of organs, there is an argument that they should at least be paid, to reduce the inequity. If there were a system of access to organs which did not favor the rich, there would be a stronger argument for not paying poor donors: they would be contributing their organs to a system in which they had a fair chance to benefit.

Whether the present or proposed allocation systems are fair is not the subject of this discussion. Procurement methods and policies need not be linked to allocated policies. Financial incentives might even reduce the inequities of allocation if they increased the supply and thereby increased the probability that all would have access to necessary organs. If it were already the case that a poor person would be more likely to be a donor than a recipient, payment would at least reduce the imbalance of benefits between classes of poor and rich.

Opponents of payment commonly assume a system in which an identifiable and affluent recipient would pay a poor and vulnerable donor. A preferable arrangement would be a government sponsored system in which potential donors would received payments, either premortem to themselves, or postmortem to their estates, and the organs so recovered would be distributed according to established criteria, without regard to social class or ability to pay. There are variations on this theme (Schwindt and Vining, 1986).

5. *It would be immoral for brokers to profiteer on the health needs of dying patients and the economic needs of the poor.* This concern is either disingenuous or naive. Medicine has always been in the business of making money (Fost, 1987). It is a bit late to protest profiteering in an industry that is increasingly profit oriented and employs marketing practices that make it increasingly difficult to distinguish it from industries that have no connection with health care. Treatment of end-stage renal disease is a multibillion-dollar industry, stimulated by the availability of money made possible when the Congress decided to subsidize the treatment of end-stage renal disease through Medicare. Everyone makes money from transplantation except the supplier: the donor. With all respect to the altruism of the many doctors, procurement officers, nurses, researchers, and others who devote their lives to the betterment of those with organ failure, I cannot imagine that the system would have developed to its present extent unless the participants were making money, i.e., profits.

6. *The availability of payments will have an adverse effect on altruism (i.e., there will be a decline in voluntary donations).* The corollary is that life-saving gifts should not be commercialized; life should not become a commodity. Here again, there are empirical and conceptual assumptions that require support. The assumption that allowing the market of a commodity would have a serious deterrent effect upon gift giving may be true in some situations and not in others.

Whether it would in fact occur with organs is untested. The availability to make money from blood products, in commercial plasma centers, for example, has not "dried up" the blood supply in the United States. The opportunity to sell food, shelter, and clothing has not put an end to charitable donations. It is possible that markets in these commodities and services reduce the incidence of gift giving, without ending it, but it is not self-evident that those most likely to donate organs gratis antemortem—the relatives of patients in need—would be less likely to do so in favor of selling their organs to a stranger.

It is not clear whether those concerned with the possible reduction of altruism are primarily concerned with that for its own sake, or because of the consequence it would have on supply of organs. The latter concern would seem avoidable by setting the price at the level required to meet the need. If the worry is rather a more formal concern for a decline in altruism per se, several explanations are needed: (1) Why should the incidence of altruism be more important than saving lives?, and (2) Why should this particular opportunity for altruism be more important or more regulated than other life-saving commodities? It is ironic that the medical community opposes payment in the name of altruism but also opposes altruism in its purest form, i.e., the individual who seeks to donate a kidney—while still living—to a stranger (Fellner, 1973; Fellner and Schwartz, 1971).

3. CONCLUSIONS

Health care is big business. Many individuals and organizations earn large profits, although that is not always the primary goal. For most health professionals, varying mixtures of altruism and self-interest determine behavior. It would be admirable if organ transplantation were selected as a special case, a demonstration project, in which profit were not allowed. But that is not what we have. Only the suppliers—the donors—have been systematically excluded from making money in the enterprise. The United States is not against a commercial market in organ transplantation; it is only against paying the suppliers.

There are two arguments in favor of eliminating this restriction and allowing payments to potential donors. The weak argument is that it may increase the supply of organs, and thereby improve the quantity and quality of life for tens of thousands of patients in need. Such a system would almost certainly have a favorable cost–benefit ratio in economic terms, as well as provide humanitarian benefits for the recipients and their families. A stronger argument is that payments would be consistent with our tradition of respecting autonomy—allowing competent people to decide for themselves what risks they wish to take in exchange for available benefits. It would avoid the problems of paternalism and inconsistency that encumber the present system.

The present system is riddled with double standards. Donation is said to involve low and acceptable risk when it is voluntary, but payment is opposed on the grounds that the procedure is too risky to justify permitting sale. Consent is considered crucial for live-related donation, but studies suggest that donors do not in fact freely consent and do feel coerced (Fellner and Marshall, 1970). There is an insistence that donors be motivated by altruism, but unrelated altruists are labeled as mentally ill and systematically rejected. Proclamations and laws prohibit commercialization, but billions of dollars change hands to the financial benefit of all concerned.

These criticisms do not lead to a conclusion that transplantation should stop. While there are strong arguments that it is unfair and unreasonable to allow so many citizens to go without a decent minimum of routine health care, ending transplantation is not likely to change that. The dollars saved will not predictably go to the basic health-care needs of the underserved. My purpose has been to challenge the assumptions of the present system, particularly the prohibition of payments to donors, and to argue that such a change would be consistent with our traditions and widely shared moral values.

ACKNOWLEDGMENTS. Dan Wikler made many helpful comments, and introduced me to some central concepts and issues.

REFERENCES

Caplan, A., 1985, Blood, sweat, tears and profits: The ethics of the sale and use of patient derived materials in biomedicine, *Clin. Res.* **33**:448–451. (4)

Carpenter, C. B., Ettenger, R. B., and Strom, T. B., 1984, "Free-market" approach to organ donation. (Letter.) *N. Engl. J. Med.* **310**:395–396.

Dougherty, C. J., 1986, A proposal for ethical organ donation, *Health Affairs* **5**:105–110.

Drake, A. W., Finkelstein, S. N., and Sapolsky, H. M., 1982, *The American Blood Supply*, MIT Press, Cambridge, Massachusetts.

Editorial, 1984, Kidney brokerage: A glimpse of the future?, *Lancet* **2**:1081.

Fellner, C. H., 1973, Organ donation: For whose sake?, *Ann. Intern. Med.* **79**:589–592.

Fellner, C. H., and Marshall, J. R., 1970, Kidney donors—The myth of informed consent, *Amer. J. Psychiatry* **126**:1245–1251.

Fellner, C. H., and Schwartz, S. H., 1971, Altruism in disrepute: Medical versus public attitudes toward the living organ donor, *N. Engl. J. Med.* **284**:582–585.

Fost, N. 1983, The new body snatchers: On Scott's *The Body as Property*, *Am. Bar Fdn. Research J.* **3**:718–732.

Fost, N., 1987, Ethical considerations of hospital–physician joint ventures, in: *Joint Ventures Between Hospitals and Physicians* (L. A. Burns and D. M. Mancino, eds.), Dow Jones–Irwin, Homewood, Illinois.

Knowles, J., 1977, *Doing Better and Feeling Worse*, Norton, New York.

McFall v. Shimp, July 26, 1978, No Gd 78-17711 (Eq. Ct. C. P. Allegheny County, Civ. Div., Pennsylvania).

Organ Procurement and Transplantation Act, 1984, No. 98-1127, Oct 2, 1984, 42 USC 274.

Robertson, J. A., and Schulman, J. D., 1987, Pregnancy and prenatal harm to offspring: The case of mothers with PKU, *Hastings Ctr Rep.* **17**(4):23–33.

Schwindt, R., and Vining, A. R., 1986, Proposal for a future delivery market for transplant organs, *J. Health Politics, Policy Law* **11**:483–500.

VI

FUNDING OF TRANSPLANTATION

33

FUNDING OF TRANSPLANTATION
The Health Care Financing Administration

BERNADETTE SCHUMAKER

1. INTRODUCTION

The focus of this chapter is an overview of federal funding of transplantation, specifically of the operations of the Health Care Financing Administration (HCFA)—its structure vis-à-vis decision-making on transplantation issues, the status of funding for various types of transplants, and current and future activities involving transplantation services.

2. HCFA STRUCTURE

2.1. Medicare

HCFA consists of two health-care programs, Medicare and Medicaid. Medicare is available to three basic groups of insured individuals: the aged, the disabled, and those with end-stage renal disease (ESRD). To be eligible for hospital insurance (HI), an individual must be insured based on his or her earnings or on those of a spouse, parent, or child. The worker must have a specified number of quarters of coverage earned through payment of payroll taxes under the Federal Insurance Contributions Act (FICA). The precise number required is dependent on whether the person is filing for HI on the basis of age, disability, or ESRD:

1. To be eligible for HI
    a. A person must be age 65 or older and eligible for social security or railroad retirement cash benefits
        OR
    b. Have been entitled to social security or railroad benefits on the basis of disability for 29 months,
        OR
    c. Receive dialysis or a kidney transplant (after a 3-month waiting period).

BERNADETTE SCHUMAKER • Division of Dialysis and Transplant Payment Policy, Health Care Financing Administration, U.S. Department of Health and Human Services, Baltimore, Maryland 21207.

2. Individuals entitled to premium-free HI are automatically enrolled in supplementary medical insurance (SMI). Those who do not want SMI coverage may refuse enrollment. Individuals who are 65 or older and who are not entitled to premium-free HI may enroll for SMI during prescribed periods.

For fiscal year 1986, Medicare payments totaled 78.1 billion:

Part A	Dollars (in billions)
Inpatient hospital	$45.7
SNF	0.6
Home health care	2.5
Hospice	Negligible (<$50 million)
Administrative expenses	0.7
	$49.5
Part B	
Physician	$18.8
Outpatient hospital	5.0
Group practice	0.7
Independent laboratory	0.6
Administrative expenses	1.0
ESRD	2.5
	$28.6
Total	$78.1

A prominent characteristic of Medicare is its national scope, providing health care to approximately 25 million beneficiaries, approximately 100,000 of whom are renal patients. These benefits do not vary by geographical region. For example, by statute, a kidney transplant patient entitled to Medicare remains a Medicare beneficiary eligible for all program benefits for 3 years following a successful transplant. This is true regardless of where the Medicare beneficiary resides. Medicare benefits are administered by local contractors, i.e., insurance plans familiar with Medicare national policies as well as local medical practices.

By law (Section 1862(a)(1)(A) of the Social Security Act), Medicare may only pay for reasonable and necessary medical procedures. This is generally interpreted to bar coverage of experimental medical procedures. As new procedures are developed, such as transplantation, HCFA requests an examination of the medical practice by the health arm of the Department of Health and Human services, namely the Public Health Service. Following this analysis, a decision on Medicare coverage is made.

Currently, Medicare covers kidney, cornea, and bone marrow transplants. There is limited coverage of liver transplants. Final regulations extending Medicare coverage to heart transplants were published on April 6, 1987, in the *Federal Register*.

2.2. Medicaid

By contrast, Medicaid is a state-directed health-care program. In all states, Medicaid is available to individuals receiving aid to families with dependent children (AFDC). In most states, individuals also receive supplemental security income (SSI), which is a federal benefit program for the aged, blind, and disabled. Federal funds for Medicaid totaled $23.5 billion in fiscal year 1986.

While the federal government contributes a certain percentage of funds to run each state Medicaid program, a number of decisions, such as which transplants to pay for and the method of payment, are basically under state control.

2.3. Administration of Medicare and Medicaid

Medicare and Medicaid are administered in the Department of Health and Human Services, which has a total staff of 131,000 and includes the Social Security Administration, the Public Health Service and HCFA. HCFA is the federal government agency that specifically administers the Medicare and Medicaid programs. It has a total staff of 4000 located in its central office and 10 regional offices.

Within HCFA, health policy is directed by one of four associate administrators, i.e., the associate administrator for program development. Payment policy for HCFA is developed in the Office of Reimbursement Policy, which consists of five divisions, one of which is concerned with dialysis and transplant issues (Division of Dialysis and Transplant Payment Policy).

3. PAYMENT FOR TRANSPLANTS

Funding for Medicare kidney transplants totaled $292 million in 1985. This amount consisted of approximately $150 million for the transplant procedure, $97 million for organ procurement services, and $45 million for related services. The number of independent organ procurement agencies participating in the Medicare program increased from 36 in 1983 to 62 in 1986. In 1985, there were 7695 kidney transplants, a 10% increase from 1984. Living related transplants accounted for 24% of the total; cadaveric transplants represented 76% (HCFA, 1985).

In more recent years, the number of kidney transplants has increased at a higher rate (12% for 1981–1985) compared with earlier years (6.3% for 1974–1981), based on internal HCFA data. While the Medicare ESRD program continues to be dominated by dialysis patients, the distribution of patients into dialysis and functioning graft categories has changed significantly. For example, in 1978, only 11% of the total ESRD population had a functioning graft, while in 1985, this figure has risen to 19%. Similarly, the patient group with a functioning graft grew by 20% in 1985, compared with a 5.8% increase for the dialysis group.

Detailed statistics are not maintained for Medicaid transplants. However, the results of a recent survey (HCFA, 1986) indicate the following:

1. Forty states and the District of Columbia pay for liver transplants (an increase of eight states from the previous year).
2. Thirty-two states and the District of Columbia pay for heart transplants (an increase of eight states from the previous year).
3. Eight states pay for pancreas transplant (an increase of four states from the previous year).
4. Forty-seven states pay for immunosuppressant drugs (an increase of three states from the previous year).

In general, then, Medicaid benefits for transplant services have increased significantly in recent years.

4. CURRENT AND FUTURE ACTIVITIES

In the Medicare program, three significant issues are currently being discussed and will likely impact on the future direction of HCFA transplant policy. These issues include:

1. Proposed Medicare coverage and payment for heart transplants
2. Reconsideration of adult liver transplantation by Medicare
3. Statutory coverage and payment for outpatient immunosuppressant drugs

In October 1986, proposed regulations were published in the *Federal Register* to extend heart transplant coverage to Medicare beneficiaries. Features of the proposed regulation included:

1. Use of designated centers to provide this service
2. A formal application process for centers requiring minimum survival rates and number of transplants performed (i.e., experience criteria)
3. General patient selection criteria
4. Use of a diagnostic related group (DRG) for the heart transplant procedure to determine a prospective payment (organ procurement would be paid on a cost basis, paralleling payment under the kidnehy transplant program).

Final regulations were published in the *Federal Register* on April 6, 1987.

The second major activity with future implications is the recently enacted provision (Section 9335 of the Omnibus Budget Reconciliation Act of 1986, Public Law 99–509) authorizing payment for patients for immunosuppressant drugs following their discharge from a hospital for an approved transplant. Although coverage is limited to one year, it is historic Medicare policy to authorize payment for such drugs. Instructions on billing and payment methods have been issued to our contractors (HCFA, 1987). The approved immunosuppressants may be furnished by a hospital outpatient department, a pharmacy (including mail order), or a physician's office. Payment is on a reasonable cost basis if provided on an outpatient hospital basis, and on a reasonable charge basis in all other cases. Because of the significance of this benefit, we are instructing our contractors to report to HCFA monthly on the number of beneficiaries, number of claims, and amount paid for this new Medicaire service.

As of December 1986, the FDA had identified and approved for marketing only four specifically labeled immunosuppressive drugs. They are cyclosporine (Sandimmune), Sandoz Pharmaceutical; azathioprine (Imuran), Burroughs Wellcome; antithymocyte globulin (Atgam), Upjohn; and Muromonab-CD3 (Orthoclone OKT3), Ortho Pharmaceutical.

In administering this benefit, Medicare contractors have been instructed to furnish the patient with a nonrefillable 30-day prescription for the immunosuppressive drugs. This is because the dosage of these drugs frequently diminishes over a period of time; furthermore, it is not uncommon for the physician to change the prescription from one drug to another because of the patient's needs. Also, these drugs are expensive, and the coinsurance liability on unused drugs could be a financial burden to the Medicare beneficiary.

Regarding liver transplants, Medicare coverage is currently limited to children under 18 years of age with biliary atresia and other congenital diseases. HCFA has asked the Public Health Service to re-examine the issue of adult liver transplants. A notice was published in the *Federal Register* in February 1987 (Public Health Service, 1987) announcing this assessment and requesting information on the types of patients and diagnoses suited to this therapy as well as the types of diseases for which this is the treatment of choice. Following a report from the Public Health Service, HCFA will determine whether coverage of and payments for adult liver transplants will be provided by the Medicare program.

Medicare is about to begin a new era in transplants in paying for heart transplants, implementing a new program for payment of outpatient immunosuppressant drugs and re-examining adult liver transplants. These changes, along with the continued increase in kidney transplants, is resulting in a very dynamic transplant program. We hope to benefit from our knowledge and experience with the kidney program and to continue to provide efficient, economical, and high-quality patient care to transplant patients.

REFERENCES

HCFA, 1985, End State Renal Disease Program Highlights, Bureau of Data Management and Strategy.

HCFA, 1986, Medicaid Coverage and Payment Policies for Organ Transplants, Bureau of Eligibility, Reimbursement and Coverage, Division of Dialysis and Transplant Payment Policy.

HCFA, 1987, Medicare Carriers Manual Transmittal No. 1177.

Public Health Service, 1987, Reassessment of adult liver transplantation, *Federal Register* **52:**5191–5192.

34

MEDICAL TECHNOLOGY EVALUATION AND COVERAGE

SUSAN GLEESON

1. INTRODUCTION

The Blue Cross Association was established in 1948 as a national organization representing non-profit state and local insurance plans that offered Blue Cross coverage for hospital services. Two years earlier, the National Association of Blue Shield Plans (NABSP) had been established to represent nonprofit state and local plans that offered Blue Shield coverage for physician services. In 1982, the Blue Cross Association merged with NAPSP to form the Blue Cross and Blue Shield Association. The merger reflected a systemwide trend of state and local Blue Cross Plans merging with Blue Shield Plans to enhance their responsiveness to account expectations. Today, the Blue Cross and Blue Shield Association provides advice and services to 78 state and local Blue Cross and Blue Shield plans. With each plan serving an average of one million subscribers, the collective sum of 78 million Blue Cross and Blue Shield subscribers makes Blue Cross and Blue Shield the largest private health insurer in the United States. In 1986, Blue Cross and Blue Shield plans paid a total of $40.6 billion in claims.

Most contracts between Blue Cross and Blue Shield plans and provider and subscriber include two provisions that affect a medical technology's coverage status. One coverage provision requires all new and emerging medical technologies to be generally accepted medical practice. Technologies in the experimental or investigative stage are excluded as covered benefits. The other coverage provision requires an established medical technology's use to be medically necessary. Technology uses without an appropriate medical basis are excluded as benefits.

Although individual Blue Cross and Blue Shield plans are responsible for implementing these contract provisions, valuable advice and guidance is provided by the Blue Cross and Blue Shield Associations Technology Management Department. Two programs are relevant: the Technology Evaluation and Coverage (TEC) Program and the Medical Necessity Program. The TEC Program determines the clinical status of new and emerging medical technologies. This focus addresses whether a new and emerging medical technology has progressed to the generally accepted medical

---

SUSAN GLEESON • Technology Management, Blue Cross and Blue Shield Association, Chicago, Illinois 60611.

practice stage or whether it remains in the experimental or investigative stage. The Medical Necessity Program determines the clinical indications for the appropriate use of medical technologies
that are established and considered generally accepted medical practice.

The Association's TEC Program has a long history. Its predecessor programs have been
providing advice to plans on the clinical status of new and emerging technologies for nearly 30
years. The process employed in today's Program, however, differs significantly from the informal
processes of previous programs. Today, the TEC Program and its formal decision process places
a premium on scientific objectivity. Such a basis is especially important in today's litigious health
care environment.

Providing guidance to the TEC Program process is a Medical Advisory Panel (MAP) composed of medical directors from selected Blue Cross and Blue Shield plans. Recently, the MAP
adopted explicit decision criteria for determining whether a new and emerging medical technology
has progressed to the generally acceptable medical practice stage. To our knowledge, this is the
first national technology assessment body to adopt explicit decision criteria.

The Medical Necessity Program was originally established in 1977. On April 2, 1987, at a
joint news conference with the American College of Physicians in New Orleans, the President of
the Blue Cross and Blue Shield Association, Bernard Tresnowski, commemorated the Program's
10th anniversary by introducing its newest product, the Diagnostic Testing Guidelines. The guidelines address the clinical indications for the appropriate use of chest roentgenograms, electrocar-
diograms (ECGs), and selected laboratory tests. Previously introduced guidelines from this series
include the Respiratory Care Guidelines, the Diagnostic Imaging Guidelines, and the Cardiac Care
Guidelines.

2. TECHNOLOGY EVALUATION AND COVERAGE CRITERIA*

At the core of TEC criteria is whether a technology improves health outcomes such as length
of life, ability to function or quality of life. Technologies that specifically meet each of the
following criteria are recommended for coverage consideration. These criteria are as follows:

1. The technology must have final approval from the appropriate regulatory bodies.
   a. A device, drug, or biological product must have Food and Drug Administration (FDA)
      approval to market for those specific indications and methods of use that Blue Cross
      and Blue Shield Association is evaluating.
   b. Approval to market refers to permission for commercial distribution. Any other ap-
      proval that is granted as an interim step in the FDA regulatory process, e.g., an
      Investigational Device Exemption, is not sufficient.
2. The scientific evidence must permit conclusions concerning the effect of the technology
   on health outcomes.
   a. The evidence should consist of well-designed and well-conducted investigations pub-
      lished in peer-review journals. The quality of the body of studies and the consistency
      of the results are considered in evaluating the evidence.
   b. The evidence should demonstrate that the technology can measure or alter the phys-
      iological changes related to a disease, injury, illness, or condition. In addition, there
      should be evidence or a convincing argument, based on established medical facts, that
      such measurement or alteration affects the health outcomes.
   c. Opinions and evaluations by national medical associations, consensus panels, or other
      technology evaluation bodies are evaluated according to the scientific quality of the
      supporting evidence and rationale.

3. The technology must improve the net health outcome.
   a. The technology's beneficial effects on health outcomes should outweigh any harmful effects on health outcomes.
4. The technology must be as beneficial as any established alternatives.
   a. The technology should improve the net health outcome as much or more than established alternatives.
5. The improvement must be attainable outside the investigational settings.
   a. When used under the usual conditions of medical practice, the technology should be reasonably expected to satisfy criteria 3 and 4.

3. HUMAN ORGAN TRANSPLANTATION

Blue Cross and Blue Shield Association's present position on human heart, liver, and kidney transplantations is that each procedure has progressed beyond the investigational stage and should be considered covered benefits. While this position predates use of the TEC criteria, application of the criteria would result in a similar conclusion.

Of particular interest, however, is the final TEC criterion, which addresses the diffusion of a technology. The explosive growth in the number of institutions performing human heart and human liver transplantation procedures has been a concern to the Blue Cross and Blue Shield organization. For example, in 1983 only 12 institutions performed heart transplants. By 1986 a fivefold increase had occurred resulting in 65 institutions carrying out these procedures. During this same three year period, the number of institutions performing liver transplantations increased from 12 to 29. There is no question that heart transplants and liver transplants are generally accepted medical practice at many of these institutions. To maintain, however, that these organizationally complex and resource intensive services, when performed by these new institutional programs, will result in outcomes comparable to those of experienced institutions in an open question. An important consideration underlying the final TEC criterion is the provider's ability to achieve an improved outcome. Indeed, when a medical technology is classified as generally accepted medical practice, an implicit assumption is that improvement in patient outcome will occur across providers. For most technologies, this will likely be the case. For some technologies, however, such as organ transplants, this assumption may not be reasonable. As such, providers may be expected to demonstrate their abilities.

This emphasis on provider demonstration, in addition to being consistent with the last TEC criterion, represents the substance our position on human heart and human liver transplantations. Nearly 2 years ago, we advised Blue Cross and Blue Shield plans that coverage for human heart and human liver transplants as benefits should be limited to those institutions with demonstrated capabilities. To assist Plans in evaluating institutional capability, specific structure, process, and performance criteria were developed for plan use. One of our documents, entitled "Criteria for Evaluating Institutions for Liver and Heart Transplants," has received wide distribution both inside and outside the Blue Cross and Blue Shield Organization. For example, it was used as an important reference document in the deliberations of the Organ Transplant Task Force established under the National Organ Transplant Act (P.L. 98–507) of 1985.

Another relevant publication series, whose distribution has been limited to Plans because of the obvious sensitivity of the information it contains, is our organ transplant registry. Our first registry document, Organ Transplant Registry 1983–1985 contained the number of transplantation procedures and associated survival rates for all U.S. institutions performing human heart, liver, heart–lung or pancreas transplant procedures in 1983 and 1984. The registry was recently updated to include information from 1985 and part of 1986. Sample data from an unidentified institution appear in Fig. 1. The updated document Organ Transplant Registry 1983–1986 is the only one of its kind to our knowledge.

INSTITUTION ORGAN TRANSPLANT EXPERIENCE

STATE: _____

CITY: _____

INSTITUTION: _____

ORGAN: Heart

	1983 01/01—06/30	1983 07/01—12/31	1983 TOTAL	1984 01/01—06/30	1984 07/01—12/31	1984 TOTAL	1985 01/01—06/30	1985 07/01—12/31	1985 TOTAL	1986 01/0—06/30
Number of transplants performed	3	4	7	2	7	9	6	10	16	6
Percentage survival at least										
1 month	100% (3)	100% (4)	100% (7)	100% (2)	86% (6)	89% (8)	83% (5)	90% (9)	88% (14)	100% (6)
6 months	67% (2)	100% (4)	86% (6)	100% (2)	86% (6)	89% (8)	83% (5)	90% (9)	88% (14)	
12 months	33% (1)	75% (3)	57% (4)	100% (2)	86% (6)	89% (8)	83% (5)			
18 months	33% (1)	25% (1)	29% (2)	50% (1)	71% (5)	67% (6)				
24 months	33% (1)	25% (1)	29% (2)	50% (1)						
30 months	33% (1)	25% (1)	29% (2)							
36 months	0% (0)									
Survival status as of 06/30/86	0% (0)	25% (1)	14% (1)	50% (1)	71% (5)	67% (6)	83% (5)	90% (9)	88% (14)	100% (6)

FIGURE 1. Sample data for Blue Cross and Blue Shield Association's Organ Transplant Registry, 1983–1986.

4. CURRENT COVERAGE STATUS

Funding for renal transplants is mainly covered by the Federal End-Stage Renal Disease Program, and is therefore not an important issue. Coverage for other transplants is variable. In a recent survey of Blue Cross and Blue Shield plans, it was found that only 6% of the plans consider liver transplants to be investigative and only 9% of the plans consider heart transplants to be investigative. Heart–lung and pancreas transplant procedures were considered to be investigative by 15% and 42% of the plans, respectively. While such medical policy positions are usually indicative of benefit coverage, exceptions do occur. For example, a plan could consider a technology investigative but still offer coverage to accounts through special riders. A number of plans have done this for heart–lung and pancreas. Thus, 92% of the plans offer coverage for heart–lung transplants and 60% of the plans offer coverage for pancreas transplants, even though many of these plans consider both procedures investigative.

Regarding institutional capability, 58% of the plans have limited coverage of heart and liver transplants to specific institutions. Similarly, 57% of the plans have limited heart–lung transplants to specific institutions, and 46% of the plans offering pancreas coverage have limited coverage to specific institutions.

Plan payment for inpatient institutional services has averaged $69,999 for heart transplants and $96,055 for liver transplants. Average professional payments were $9,931 for heart transplants and $15,312 for liver transplants. Most tissue transplants, such as those for corneas and bone, are covered.

5. ISSUES AND CONCERNS

An increasing concern among consumers in our rapidly developing competitive health care environment is access to new and costly medical technologies. This concern is not misplaced. The linkage between medical technology access and expenditures is direct. Expenditures can be controlled by controlling access.

Two strategies are being employed in today's environment to control expenditures through medical technology access. The first strategy has stressed the elimination of unnecessary medical technology use. Both government as the major public payer and employers as the major private payer have strongly supported elimination of unnecessary medical technology access as an appropriate cost control mechanism. Most of the newer insurer products, including health maintenance organizations (HMOs), preferred payment organizations (PPOs), and Managed Care, address unnecessary medical technology access as a specific objective.

The second strategy, having either an implicit or explicit basis, is controversial. It is, nevertheless, becoming more prevalent because of the unrelenting pressures to achieve health care savings. In this strategy, specific and usually costly medical technologies are eliminated as subscriber benefits. This may be done implicitly through physician decisions indicative of "silent rationing," or it may be done explicitly through employer decisions to purchase health insurance products with special medical technology exclusions. This latter strategy is an integral aspect of a larger societal issue receiving increased national attention: the growth of the underinsured.

Improving protection for the underinsured raises a fundamental questions which will not be easily resolved. Who should pay? Is appropriate health-care coverage a responsibility of the employer, government, or the individual? How this question is answered will determine access to both current and future medical technologies.

6. CONCLUSIONS

The Blue Cross and Blue Shield Association has two programs that address medical technology coverage. The Medical Necessity Program is concerned with the indications for appropriate medical technology use and the Technology Assessment and Coverage or TEC Program is concerned with the clinical status of new and emerging medical technologies.

Recently, the TEC Program introduced specific Technology Evaluation Criteria for determining if a new technology has progressed beyond its investigative stage and should be considered for coverage as a subscriber benefit. The criteria are expected to enhance the TEC Program's ability to communicate its medical technology coverage recommendations effectively to providers, manufacturers, and subscribers.

Blue Cross and Blue Shield plans have been advised that human heart and human liver transplantation procedures have progressed beyond the investigative stage and should be considered for coverage. Currently, 97% of the plans offer coverage for human heart and 99% of the plans offer coverage for human liver transplants.

Plans have also been advised that the administrative and resource requirements to establish a successful transplant program are sufficiently demanding that payment for heart and liver transplants should be limited to proven sites. Fifty-eight percent of Blue Cross and Blue Shield plans have implemented such policies to date.

Access to medical technology services is beginning to emerge as one of our society's leading health-care issues. Its prominence will likely become more pronounced as we approach the 1990s. Central to the issue is controlled or limited access. Both public and private payers are increasingly placing constraints on medical technology access to control their health care costs. Containing cost by eliminating access to medically unnecessary technology uses has generally been supported. Containing costs by establishing relationships with selected or preferred medical technology providers, however, has been more tentative because of its obvious intrusion on freedom of choice. Regardless, programs employing selected or preferred providers are experiencing significant growth.

With future demands to contain health-care costs likely to continue, increasing pressure will be placed on payers to exclude costly medical technologies as insured benefits under general coverage provisions. Rather, these costly technologies will be considered special coverage issues requiring special funding solutions. One extreme solution is individual funding; another extreme solution is society funding. Both are associated with problems. With individual funding, access will be determined by affluence. With society funding, access will be achieved by compromising our current economic system. To avoid each of these problems and yet achieve equitable medical technology access, the challenge to medical technology manufacturers and providers of services is succinct: to develop and deliver the most cost-effective and cost-beneficial technologies possible. Savings achieved by eliminating technologies that are not cost effective or cost beneficial will considerably enhance a payer's ability to cover costly medical technology services under general provisions.

35

The Private Insurer Response to Advanced Health Care Technology

The Case of Organ Transplants

JOEL E. MILLER

1. INTRODUCTION

With advances in medical skill and technology inevitably accompanied by a blur of media attention, organ transplants are increasingly regarded as accepted therapeutic interventions for a variety of degenerative diseases. Although the number of the nation's transplant operations remains relatively small, enough are being performed, and long waiting lists indicate considerably more could be performed, to warrant classification of many as therapeutic and no longer experimental. For insurers and all health-care consumers, the critical question here is: Who will pay?

Public pressure has been mounting for private insurers, Blue Cross/Blue Shield organizations, and government entitlement programs to cover the costs of extrarenal transplants. This pressure is being exerted despite the growing complaint that health-care costs are out of balance.

The next big question then is: Can we afford to provide U. S. citizens with equal access to the benefit of transplantation technology? If not, will a two-tier health care system evolve with access to transplantation available only to the wealthy and the employed-insured, and not to the elderly-retiree and the poor? Resolving the problem of organ scarcity and determining how equitably to provide transplants to those who can most benefit are key issues posed by this new technology.

2. ORGANIZATION OF PRIVATE HEALTH INSURANCE

Insurers provide a wide range of coverages to protect individuals from the financial consequences of sickness or injury. By the end of the 1970s, an estimated 9 in 10 Americans under age 65 had some form of private health insurance. The major source of this protection is the more

JOEL E. MILLER • Insurance, Managed Care, and Provider Relations Division, Health Insurance Association of America, Washington, D. C. 20036.

than 1200 commercial insurance companies that wrote individual and/or group health insurance covering more than 100 million persons at year-end 1985 (Health Insurance Association of America, 1987).

These insurers consist of legal-reserve life insurance companies, casualty insurance companies, and separately organized health insurance companies. They are organized for profit on either a stock or mutual basis. A legal reserve company is an insurance company operating under state insurance laws specifying the minimum basis for the reserves the company must maintain on its policies. Casualty insurance refers to automobile, liability, aviation, Workers' Compensation insurance, and other plans. Health insurance companies provide various types of insurance such as accident insurance, disability income insurance, medical and hospital expense insurance, accidental death insurance, and dismemberment insurance.

A stock life insurance company's goal is to make a profit for its stockholders. Policies are referred to as nonparticipating if the policyowner shares neither in any savings or profits nor in any losses that might arise in the operation of the business. Since policyholders will not receive dividends, their fixed premiums represent both the initial and the final cost to them for their insurance coverage. Stock companies sometimes issue participating policies, on which dividends may be paid to policyowners, as well as nonparticipating policies (Huebner and Black, 1982).

A mutual life insurance company is also a corporation, but it has no capital stock and no stockholders. The mutual is organized and owned by its policyowners, from whom all its resources are derived. The policyowner in a mutual company is both a "customer" and, in a sense, an "owner"; by contrast, the stock company policyowner is a "customer" only (Huebner and Black, 1982).

There are approximately 132 mutual companies and 1963 stock companies. Although less than 10% are mutual, they are important. For example, they possess almost two thirds of life insurance industry's total assets and account for about one half the total amount of life and health insurance in force in the United States (American Council of Life Insurance, 1984).

Policies issued by insurance companies provide for payment directly to the insured or, if assigned by the insured, to the provider of services for reimbursement of expenses incurred. Insurance company health insurance coverage can be divided into two basic categories: medical expense insurance and disability income insurance. Medical expense is reimbursement type coverage, providing benefits that can cover virtually all expenses connected with hospital and medical care and related services. Disability income insurance provides periodic payments when the insured is unable to work because of sickness or injury.

The Blue Cross and Blue Shield Association coordinates the Blue Cross and Blue Shield plans of the nation. The nonprofit member plans service statewide and other geographical areas, offering individual and group coverage. Blue Cross plans provide hospital care benefits on essentially a "service type" basis, under which the organization, through a separate contract with member hospitals, reimburses a hospital for covered services provided to the insured. Blue Shield plans provide benefits for physician surgical and medical services.

Some 60% of insurance group coverage is estimated to be represented by administrative service only (ASO) arrangements and minimum premium plans (MPPs). Under these systems, corporations and other organizations establish self-funded health plans. Insurance carriers or private organizations are paid a fee by the self-funding group to process claims and benefits paperwork.

At the end of 1985, 181 million persons were covered for hospital expenses by private health insurance, the most common type of medical expense coverage. This coverage provides specific benefits for daily hospital room and board and usual hospital services and supplies during hospital confinement (HIAA, 1987).

Also, at the end of 1983, 179 million persons had insurance protection against the cost of surgical procedures performed as a result of an accident or sickness. Benefits of this form of insurance might be paid according to a schedule of surgical procedures, with the policy listing the maximum benefit for each type of operation covered. An increasing number of insurance plans offer surgical benefits for the physician's fee up to the "reasonable and customary" charge for the procedure performed. At year-end 1983, 173 million persons had physician expense coverage (HIAA, 1985b). This form of health insurance provides benefits to help pay physicians' fees for nonsurgical care in the hospital, home or doctor's office.

Major medical expense insurance has grown rapidly. By year-end 1985, some 160 million persons under 65 years of age had this coverage through insurance company policies, Blue Cross–Blue Shield, HMOs, and other independent plans (HIAA, 1987). Major medical coverage provides broad protection for large, unpredictable medical expenses. It covers a wide range of medical charges with a few internal limits and a high overall maximum benefit. Basically, there are two types of major medical plans: one supplements basic hospital-surgical/physicians expense insurance programs; the other provides comprehensive protection for both basic coverage and extended health care benefits.

3. HEALTH INSURANCE ASSOCIATION OF AMERICA (HIAA)

The Health Insurance Association of America is the health insurance industry's leading trade association. It is composed of some 350 U. S. and Canadian insurance companies responsible for about 85% of the U. S. and 90% of the Canadian health insurance business written by private commercial insurance companies. Its purpose is to promote the development of voluntary health insurance that provides sound protection against loss of income and other financial burdens resulting from sickness or accidental injury.

3.1. Policy

A board of directors determines the policy of HIAA and directs its activities. This board, composed of executives of member insurance companies, is elected by the membership. Committees of member insurance company officers furnish guidance to the board and to the association's professional and administrative staff.

3.2. Legislation

HIAA studies federal and state legislation and reports to its membership the effects on the health insurance business. It also presents its members' views on proposed legislation and regulation before legislative, administrative, and other government bodies.

3.3. Insurance, Managed Care, and Provider Relations

HIAA works on issues pertaining to group, individual, and disability insurance and furnishes information and technical assistance to national, and local organizations of doctors, hospitals, dentists, and other providers of health care, as well as to consumer organizations concerned with the delivery and quality of health care. These efforts are designed to:

1. Stabilize health care costs
2. Improve the quality of health care by participation in programs under hospital, medical, and community leadership
3. Improve communications among private health insurers, health-care professionals, and consumer organizations

In addition to providing health insurance information and technical assistance to relevant groups, HIAA supports a wide variety of programs developed under voluntary or legislative sponsorship to achieve specific objectives. These include hospital prospective payment systems, health care management information systems, technology assessment, hospital utilization review, quality assurance, and capital resource allocation for needed facilities and services.

HIAA also works to improve communications between private health insurers and the health care professions and consumer groups involved in the financing, delivery, and quality of health care. Among other activities, HIAA improves communication by publishing releases for member company's home office and field staffs on significant developments in the health care management arena, including technology assessment and organ transplantation.

3.4. Research and Statistics

HIAA conducts a variety of regular and special actuarial and statistical studies. They include an annual report of the number of lives insured for health care expenses and disability income, a quarterly survey of health insurance benefit payments, a semiannual survey of prevailing surgical and dental care charges, and a semiannual survey of hospital charges. In addition, specific studies on health insurance and health economics are undertaken. Long-range planning and research are conducted to help companies respond to the changing health-care environment.

3.5. Insurance Education

A comprehensive program of formal study courses in health insurance is sponsored by HIAA for company personnel and others interested in learning the health insurance business.

HIAA is vitally interested in the emergence of organ transplants as a means of treatment for various life-threatening illnesses and conditions. With 350 member companies writing 85% of the private health insurance business in the United States, the cost and method of health care delivery have a major impact on the viability of these companies. Because organ transplantation is expensive and its frequency is likely to increase, it has become a critical issue for commercial health insurers.

4. COVERAGE-DETERMINATION PROCESS

To start, it should be recognized that any decision an insurance company reaches on a procedure, specifically organ transplantation, it is not dictated by the HIAA. As a trade organization for highly competitive health insurers, the HIAA does not set policy for its member companies. Rather, each member company makes its own decision on coverage issues.

Still, two key questions must be resolved before an insurance company can approve payment for any medical technology or specifically organ transplantation. First, is the treatment experimental? Here, medical societies are often in conflict, with one group insisting a procedure is experimental, and the other saying it is safe and effective. Second, if the technology is not considered experimental, how much does the company pay for the procedure, and under what circumstances (e.g. only at designated centers). There are some cases in which an insurer will exclude coverage because of medical appropriateness, even if the procedure is not considered experimental.

4.1. Contractual Provisions

An informal association survey covering the use of medical appropriateness in health insurance contracts found that some companies defined a "covered expense" as services or supplies that are "reasonably necessary" in the treatment of an accidental bodily injury or diagnosed illness.

Furthermore, from an administrative viewpoint, for a service or supply to be considered "reasonably necessary," it must be (1) ordered by a physician, and (2) commonly and customarily recognized by the physician and medical profession as appropriate in the treatment of the patient's diagnosed sickness or injury.

The survey also found that some companies use the term "medically necessary" to mean any confinement, treatment, or service, i.e., prescribed by a physician; considered by a majority of the medical profession to be necessary, appropriate and nonexperimental; and considered not in conflict with accepted medical standards. Other analogous provisions used by companies responding to this survey included "usual and necessary medical care" and "generally accepted medical practice."

4.2. Reviewing New Procedures

Aside from contractual language considerations, a standard policy or procedure for review of a technology, device or procedure, specifically an organ transplant procedure, is present in most insurance organizations. This policy consists of medical society approval, internal medical review, and policyholder interest. We found a low rate of acceptance by insurers of Medicare guidelines as a key determinant for coverage of a technology. By contrast, policyholder interest and preference plays a critical role in determining the coverage of a particular technology. For transplant procedures, there may be a difference in coverage between different insurance contracts within the same company.

Insurers also review current medical literature and attend major medical conferences in which new technologies are discussed. At the same time, they consult with medical researchers in large teaching hospitals and at universities on medical appropriateness issues, as well as with leading medical technology assessment organizations.

Meanwhile, many insurers are developing a formalized process to make intelligent decisions on organ transplants. Aside from contractual language considerations, each company's review process may include the following queries:

1. Is the evaluation of risk factors related to the transplant?
2. Is the procedure considered safe and effective by medical technology assessment organizations?
3. Does the patient meet the medical criteria established by the transplanting facility?
4. What physical or medical status is the patient presently in?
5. What other courses of treatment have been pursued?

After contractual provisions are reviewed and it is determined that the procedure is normally covered, subject to the remaining contractual provisions, a patient's physician may be contacted for a current medical history, physical status and confirmation of the proposed procedure. Next, the transplanting coordinator for the transplanting facility is contacted for medical criteria particular to the transplant proposed. When appropriate, additional information is obtained from medical and industry resources, and then the decision is made as to whether a specific claim will be allowed.

Several companies have begun developing committees or teams composed of senior officers in marketing, actuary, underwriting, claims, policy design, and computer data services to make decisions on coverage/payment precedents. In this way, all disciplines in the consideration of this activity are used throughout the company.

4.3. Cost Effectiveness

Third-party payors are attempting to focus more on the cost effectiveness of new procedures and reviewing general cost/benefit principles on which to evaluate the effect of one procedure as an alternative to other surgical or medical procedures. This occurs not only because of cost considerations, but because of the increased tendency of insurers to become providers themselves. Still, most private insurers have not included cost-effectiveness considerations in their reimbursement decisions on new medical procedures.

5. TECHNOLOGY-ASSESSMENT ORGANIZATIONS

5.1. Private-Sector Organizations

To determine what procedures are experimental, investigational or safe and effective, health insurers often consult with leading medical technology assessment organizations. Such private sector programs include the following:

The Clinical Efficacy Assessment Project (CEAP)—a medical technology evaluation program of the American College of Physicians. It evaluates medical tests, procedures and therapeutic interventions within the purview of internal medicine and/or certified subspecialities, e.g., gastroenterology, cardiology, and oncology.

The American Hospital Association—has initiated the Hospital Technology Series Program. This program is a health-care technology evaluation and information dissemination program targeted to the hospital administrator.

The American Medical Association Diagnostic and Therapeutic Technology Assessment (DATTA) Program—attempts to answer questions that might arise about the safety, effectiveness and level of acceptance in clinical practice of medical technologies. It responds briefly and promptly, primarily assessing diagnostic and therapeutic procedures and technologies.

The Council of Medical Specialty Societies (CMSS)—handles questions from insurers regarding the clinical appropriateness of possibly outdated or unnecessary procedures, as well as new and emerging procedures and technologies.

5.2. Public-Sector Organizations

There are several public-sector medical technology assessment programs from which commercial insurers seek assistance on the safety, efficacy, effectiveness and cost-effectiveness of procedures and technologies:

The Office of Health Technology Assessment of the National Center for Health Services Research and Health Care Technology Assessment. The Office has the direct responsibility for conducting technology evaluations to make recommendations in response to HCFA requests.

The Office of Medical Applications of Research of the National Institutes of Health. A Consensus Development Program is offered that evaluates, in a public forum, scientific information concerning biomedical technologies and arrives at consensus statements useful to both health care providers and the public.

5.3. Institute of Medicine's Council on Health Care Technology

Commercial health insurers recognize that the gradations between "experimental" and "investigational" and "generally accepted medical practice," are, in some instances, not as distinct in practice as they are, perhaps, in concept. Consequently, although certain surgeries or procedures are still investigational to a greater or lesser degree, there are no hard and fast rules to indicate that, say, after a given number of clinical trials with humans, a procedure will move out of the investigational phase in its development to become a generally accepted medical practice. Furthermore, reasonable medical experts sometimes reach different opinions on medical acceptability of various procedures.

In an attempt to resolve this problem, the HIAA supported the establishment of the Institute of Medicine's Council on Health Care Technology. This joint public/private sector entity's purpose is to assess technology used in medical care. The council was formed in 1986 and is now fully operational. It will initially set up a clearinghouse of technology assessment information and has published a *Medical Technology Assessment Directory* that includes profiles of technology assessment organizations and over 3000 reports by these organizations. One of its objectives is to stimulate, coordinate, and commission assessments. The council is focusing on assessing medical technologies within the context of clinical practice. It has developed a set of criteria for identifying medical technologies as candidates for assessment. Using these criteria, the council has generated a list of clinical issues for initial consideration for assessment.

6. REIMBURSEMENT

If a decision is made to cover a particular organ transplant operation, hospital days, surgery, and drugs would be covered in most instances. Actual payment would depend on the type of contract that covers that individual. Under a hospital basic medical care expense benefits policy, coverage would include hospital expense benefits, surgical expense benefits, physician visits, expense benefits, and diagnostic radiographic and laboratory examinations.

These benefits could also be provided under major medical expensive plans in which covered expenses could be provided in one of two ways. One way would be to insure certain expenses through a basic plan of hospital–surgical–medical benefits, leaving the balance for major medical reimbursement. (These are called supplemental major medical expense insurance plans.) The second way would be to have an overall reimbursement formula apply against the total covered expenses without distinguishing between those expenses that normally would be considered eligible for basic plan type benefits and major medical type benefits. (This approach is known as a comprehensive major medical expense insurance plan.)

Two important issues are donor and transportation costs. The HIAA has adopted a statement on human organ or tissue transplants. Basically, it endorses the principle that the donation by a live donor of a healthy organ or tissue, except for cosmetic or elective surgery, should be considered as a valid "non occupational disease or disability" of the donor. It urges insurers to adopt this principle in designing and revising health care expense contracts and disability income contracts.

The HIAA also recommends that the insurer of the recipient adopt or expand the practice of reimbursing the medical expenses of a live donor to the extent that benefits remain, and are available under the recipient's plan after benefits for the recipient's own expenses have been paid. Benefit payments as to the charge for securing the organ from a cadaver donor should also be considered for adoption by insurers.

With regard to covering transportation for the patient and the family to the transplant facility, several insurers said they had no experience at all. Most plans indicated they would consider covering transportation for the patient on a case-by-case basis if medically necessary but would not assume responsibility for covering the family's transportation costs. Regarding the donor cost issue, several insurers indicated they would cover all benefits except the search and evaluation of the donor organ. Policyholder preference will also play a key role in determining whether these expenses are covered.

We also recognize that despite cost or complexities, many procedures or devices are gaining wider medical acceptance and, as technological advancements continue, competitive considerations will become more important to insurers in their formulation of coverage decisions.

Health insurers do not want to be unresponsive to the demands of their existing policyholders, nor do they want to alienate potential policyholders. Specifically, many companies have adopted the philosophy that organ transplant experience should not be given any special consideration in either pricing or dividend treatment.

7. COVERAGE MECHANISMS

To the extent that transplant expenses, along with any other expenses, cause an individual or aggregate stop loss point to be exceeded, claims are forgiven and a pool charge assessed in its place. Otherwise, no specific pooling or reinsurance is associated with organ transplant procedures. Claims experience under a group policy are subject to chance fluctuations. For example, claims on one individual may approach $1 million for some medical care expense coverages such as major medical. Accordingly, insurers have developed pooling techniques to stabilize the claims charged to the experience account. Through pooling, certain claims are removed from experience charged to each group, and a claim charge representing the average experience under all groups is substituted.

Even insurers with firm policies against coverage for certain transplants will accommodate the needs of the policyholder or employer, as long as the policyholder is willing to pay for such nonstandard coverage. Employers want to provide this type of coverage, but are concerned about whether they can afford it. Should an employer have to specifically purchase transplant coverage, or should it simply be added as part of the basic group policy at no additional cost? Companies defend their rider policies by arguing that coverage for risky transplants should be separate from routine medical coverage to keep the employer's loss experience in line. To date, insurer's experience with transplant procedures has not been significant enough to measure a potential financial impact on their general experience, nor is there sufficient information for each type of transplant to project future risk.

When reviewing for risk of transplants, industry statistics as well as actual data obtained from potential or incurred claims are taken into consideration. There may be a growing demand by employers and other insurers for reinsurance/risk pooling to decrease the cost of transplants to a specific carrier.

Reinsurance represents a mechanism for protecting an insurer from large losses. For example, a health insurer will have insurance up to a certain dollar level, but it might choose to have reinsurance for particularly expensive technologies such as organ transplantation. Several insurers are now offering this reinsurance coverage to health insurers. The insurance company issuing the policy to a group is called the ceding company and the other insurance company that agrees to accept a part of the risk is called the reinsurer.

8. HIAA SURVEY OF REIMBURSEMENT ISSUES

In response to the highly publicized events that occurred during the early 1980s, private insurers began to approach the transplant coverage issue in a systematic manner. They sought information that would enable them to tailor transplant policies to meet the needs of the policyholders. While the information available was at best scanty, they still attempted to fashion what they believed were realistic policies. In June 1983, the HIAA conducted a survey of leading insurance company writers of group health insurance about organ transplant coverage. Thirty-three companies, accounting for 57% of group health insurance premiums written by companies

TABLE I. Transplant Reimbursement Practices of 65 Insurance Companies

Type of transplant	Conditions under which company will pay			Company will not pay	Paying companies as percentage of group business[b] (%)
	Request of policyholder only	Standard practice	Case-by-case basis		
Kidney	—	57	6	2	71.5
Heart	—	37	18	10	70.5
Heart–lung	—	26	19	20	64.7
Pancreas	—	21	16	28	37.0
Cornea	—	54	11	—	72.4
Bone marrow	1	51[a]	14	—	72.4
Bone	—	45	·15	5	72.0
Skin	—	49	14	2	72.1
Liver	—	33	19	13	71.0

[a]One company will pay on either basis, depending on whether the transplant is autogenous or nonautogenous.
[b]Percentage of group health insurance business of insurance companies in the United States.

in the United States in 1982, replied. Of those that responded, 82.1% indicated they had reimbursed for heart transplants. By mid-1984, most private insurers were covering heart transplants on a routine basis. The association conducted a survey in early 1985 to solicit information on the practices of the entire HIAA membership in covering various types of transplants under group comprehensive and major medical expense plans (HIAA, 1985b). Of the 65 companies that responded (accounting for 72% of the group health insurance business of insurance companies in the United States), this is what we found:

As shown in Table I, reimbursement as a standard practice is common for kidney transplants (88% of companies), followed by cornea (83%), bone marrow (78%), and skin transplants (75%). It is least common for transplant of the pancreas (32%).

All 65 companies were at least willing to consider payment for corneal and bone marrow transplants. Sixty-three companies (97% of respondents) said they would reimburse for kidney and skin transplants. For a bone transplant, the percentage was 92% and for heart 85%, for liver 80%, and for heart–lung transplants 69%.

8.1. Immunosuppressive Drugs

Table II presents data on the extent to which companies pay for hospital care, physician services and immunosuppressive drug therapy, such as cyclosporine, on an outpatient basis. Where a transplant is covered, all companies reimburse for hospital and physician expenses. The percentage of companies that pay for immunosuppressive drug therapy ranges from 86% for a cornea transplant to 100% for heart–lung and pancreas transplants.

8.2. Reimbursement Criteria

The third issue the survey addressed was reimbursement criteria. The vast majority of companies use the "medically necessary" language of the group contract in deciding whether or not a particular organ or tissue transplant is covered. Accordingly, to the extent that a treatment is investigational or experimental and not commonly or customarily recognized by the medical profession as appropriate treatment for a condition, it is not reimbursable.

TABLE II. Type of Service and Drugs Reimbursed by the 65 Insurance Companies

Type of transplant	No. of companies			Immunosuppressive drug therapy (e.g., cyclosporin) on an outpatient basis	
	Company will pay	Hospital	Physician	No. of companies	Percentage of companies (%)
Kidney	63	63	63	61	96.8
Heart	55	55	55	54	98.2
Heart–lung	45	45	45	45	100.0
Pancreas	37	37	37	37	100.0
Cornea	65	65	65	56	86.2
Bone marrow	64	64	64	58	90.6
Bone	60	60	60	53	88.3
Skin	63	63	63	55	87.3
Liver	52	52	52	50	96.2

In addition to the "medically necessary" language, some companies also require (1) medical documentation that conventional treatment would be unsatisfactory, unavailable, and/or more hazardous than the transplant; (2) that the patient's condition is life-threatening; and (3) that the patient is legally required to pay for the transplant procedure. Only a few companies have a specific exclusion for experimental and/or investigational procedures in one or more of their contracts.

8.3. Patient and Provider Selection Criteria

Companies were asked to describe any criteria they might have established for the selection of the patient or provider. In the main they said they had not established specific criteria for such selection, other than that which normally applies to claims reimbursement in general. A few indicated that for reimbursement purposes, the hospital must be recognized and certified to perform transplant surgery and the physician must be recognized as being a specialist in the area of transplants. With respect to the patient, several companies said that the patient should be relatively free of any other disease and should have a high risk of death if the transplant were not performed.

8.4. Source of Information

Carriers say they use various sources of health-care technology assessment information, both within the public and private sectors, many of which were reviewed earlier.

8.5. Basis of Payment

Of the 65 responding companies, 63 pay benefits for transplant recipients on the same basis as any other illness, with no special restrictions. For 57 of those companies, that practice applies to all plans and to all types of transplants. The remaining six cover transplants as a separate benefit, with their own internal limits for certain transplants or group cases.

9. IMPLEMENTATION OF COVERAGE

Commercial insurers pay hospital charges as long as those charges do not exceed usual, customary, and reasonable (UCR) or cost-containment guidelines. Some policies specify dollar amounts for specific procedures, while others may impose a maximum amount for a hospital stay. Commercial insurers have not set up diagnosis-related group (DRG) systems for organ transplantation, but are about to experiment with the concept within benefit programs they are offering their policyholders.

The private health insurance industry is in the midst of a revolution. Whereas in the past private insurers played a relatively passive role of simply paying claims, today many are actively trying to affect both the quality of care and the cost of health services for their beneficiaries. This "managed care" involves coordination of new strategies and processes in the coverage of medical services, in the reimbursement for those services, and in utilization review and quality assurance. The result for many insurers is an organized policy to moderate costs and improve the quality of care for policyholders.

The emphasis of managed care is medical efficiency: reduced hospitalization, appropriate use of ancillary services, and "primary care gatekeeping." Many analysts predict one or another form of managed care entities (HMOs, integrated hospital/insurer systems) or a subset of entities (the so-called "supermeds") will dominate medicine by the next century.

The accuracy of any particular structural forecast, however, is irrelevant to the issue at hand. Managed care is in full blossom, and it will continue to grow regardless of the size or affiliation of those who might capture the market. For medical innovation, this scenario implies some specific market hurdles and a new group of decision-makers helping to shape the patterns of technology use.

9.1. Traditional Insurance/Managed Care Conflict

One issue that has arisen is the technology coverage discrepancy that many insurers see between their traditional and managed insurance/provider policies, e.g., health maintenance organizations (HMOs), individual practice associations (IPAs), preferred provider organizations (PPOs). There are clear ethical and legal implications, not only for this discrepancy in general, but particularly when this discrepancy exists within the same insurance/provider. This type of discrepancy may have particular impact on physicians in an IPA arrangement, which may be a predominant mode of prepaid practice. A physician working in an IPA, for example, may be placed in a particularly difficult ethical and legal situation because part of his or her practice may be covered under a traditional health insurance contract, while the other half will be in an IPA arrangement. There are many other implications for discrepancy coverage between HMOs and traditional private insurance. Among the issues is adverse selection.

10. CENTERS OF EXCELLENCE

Recognition of transplant surgery as accepted practice poses an important problem for all payors of health care: private insurers, Blue Cross, Medicare, Medicaid, and individual patients. Excess hospital capacity and growing physician supply in many areas of the country have generated strong competition for patients among hospitals and physicians. Widespread insurance coverage for transplant surgery may encourage hospitals to assemble transplant capability and liberalize medical indications for the surgery as a way to use existing capacity and attract preferred physicians and medical students. The emergence of redundant hospital capability, or the performance of marginally beneficial transplants, would accelerate health care costs and affect medical outcomes.

With these issues in mind, HIAA advocates the use of the "qualified medical center" or "designated center" approach. We favor this approach because we believe it minimizes misclassification of experimental transplant procedures and assures that those transplant procedures that are in transition from the investigational to the generally accepted phase of development are performed only at certain specialized institutions.

We see two distinct advantages in using these centers. First, when only a few institutions perform a high volume of transplant procedures, the quality of outcomes is likely to improve and thereby minimize the risk of death or serious complications for transplant patients. Second, the designation of only specific institutions as qualified institutions for performance of transplantation will prevent unnecessary duplication of investment in transplant capacity and thus help contain health care costs.

Private-sector payors are concerned that restricting reimbursement to selected centers will raise antitrust considerations and that supporting or implementing the designated center approach will make them vulnerable to charges of restraint of trade. With the federal government limiting Medicare reimbursement for transplants to designated centers, some private-sector payors believe that the antitrust implications may be minimized, if not eliminated.

In June 1986, the Department of Health and Human Services (HHS) announced that Medicare would cover heart transplantations at specified centers. The approval of facilities will be based on an institution's experience and expertise as well as on its commitment to the heart transplant program. The criteria outlined in the regulations are similar to recommendations developed by the HHS Task Force on Organ Transplantation to establish qualified transplant centers. Criteria that must be met address facility requirements, staff experience, training requirements, volume of transplants to be performed each year, and minimum patient and graft survival rates.

Although probably less than 10% of all recipients of heart transplants will be covered by Medicare, the designation of specialized centers will have implications beyond the immediate regulatory action, since decisions made by HHS may be weighed heavily by third-party payors. These other payors of health care costs may reimburse only federally designated centers for cardiac transplantation. The inference may be that cardiac transplantation in a nondesignated center is experimental, more costly, or performed by less qualified physicians.

11. MANDATED BENEFITS

Since 1975, the HIAA has taken the position that it favors the preservation of a system that allows the prospective purchaser of health insurance free choice of which risks he or she wishes to cover from among the various coverages offered by competing insurance carriers. We also believe that the choice of how the policyholder spends what funds are available for health insurance should be free of government decree. Our reasoning is that mandated benefits produce adverse market displacements for commercial health insurers. To provide additional mandated benefits, insurers must raise their premiums.

In response, larger firms and organizations may choose to self-insure through an employee benefit plan subject to the Employee Retirement Insurance Security Act (ERISA). Such plans are not subject to state insurance laws covering employee benefit plans. Hence, they are not required to offer state mandated benefits. Similarly, smaller firms and organizations may decide to no longer provide group coverage to their employees.

The result is a decreasing insured base under which the mandated benefit would apply. The introduction, at the national or state level, of the various mandated benefit approaches as possible legislative responses to the demand for transplant coverage should be closely examined, given the net effect of these proposals on the availability of such coverage.

12. ACCESS/COST/TECHNOLOGY TUG-OF-WAR

The most critical determinant of the future of transplantation is donor supply. It determines total number of transplants performed; survival of transplant recipients; total expenditures associated with transplantation; legal and ethical issues related to transplants; number of transplant programs needed to maximize use of donor organs; and the role of viable mechanical alternatives.

Yet, this picture could change depending on the supply of donor organs during the next few years. If the number of organs does increase, the financial implications of transplantation, specifically heart transplantation, could be much greater than estimated. This issue, as well as the issue of selective contracting with hospitals to perform transplants, will be driving forces dictating reimbursement and overall health-care expenditures in this area.

In addition, the future of organ transplant coverage will be determined by two major factors: (1) the technological imperative for increased use, as improved surgical techniques and additional immunosuppressive drugs are developed; as well as (2) the cost-containment imperative for decreased use, as policyholders demand increased insurer vigilance. The fear is that without a reasonable and effective mechanism for controlled expansion of technology, the conflict between technological advancement and health care cost containment in all areas will become even more difficult to resolve in the future. That is why HIAA has supported not only the designated center approach but also systemwide reform to truly contain health-care costs. HIAA believes prospective payment programs would provide the financial incentives to encourage hospitals to specialize. It follows that under prospective payment systems, those hospitals that can perform transplants economically would be rewarded. Most important, the patient will receive the best care possible in the most appropriate setting. Our greatest challenge is the practical integration of proven procedures at a reasonable cost to all consumers.

REFERENCES

American Council of Life Insurance, 1984, *Life Insurance Fact Book,* HIAA, Washington, D.C.

Health Insurance Association of America, 1985a, *Organ Transplants and Their Implications for the Health Insurance Industry,* Public Relations Division, HIAA, Washington, D.C.

Health Insurance Association of America, 1985b, *Source Book of Health Insurance Data,* 1984–1985, HIAA Public Relations Division, HIAA, Washington, D.C.

Health Insurance Association of America, 1985c, *HIAA Survey of Coverage for Organ and Tissue Transplant Recipients Under Group Comprehensive and Major Medical Expense Plans, Other Than Collectively Bargained Plans,* HIAA Research and Statistical Bulletin No. 2–85, HIAA, New York.

Health Insurance Association of America, 1987, *Source Book of Health Insurance Data,* 1986–1987, HIAA Public Relations Division, HIAA, Washington, D.C.

Huebner, S. S., and Black, K., Jr., 1982, *Life Insurance,* Prentice-Hall, Englewood Cliffs, New Jersey.

36

FEDERAL EFFORTS TO IMPROVE THE ORGAN PROCUREMENT SYSTEM

DAVID N. SUNDWALL and LINDA D. SHEAFFER

1. INTRODUCTION

It is always a pleasure to be able to tell our side of the story when it comes to federal efforts to improve the organ procurement system. We believe the federal government has been treated rather unfairly by some members of Congress and in the media. We have been blamed for foot dragging in implementing the National Organ Transplant Act and even blamed for the death of very young children because donors were not found in time to save their lives. In the end, transplant patients, their families and the general public have been misled into believing that the organ procurement system is in total disarray and without continued direct federal involvement and intervention will come tumbling down around us.

This is not to say that there is no basis for the criticism. The National Organ Transplant Act was signed into law on October 19, 1984, and a couple of the mandated tasks are just getting under way. The agency moved very quickly to get the Task Force on Organ Transplantation started, but the transplant community wanted and expected the Executive Branch to move quickly to implement the entire law. We believe that the transplant community and transplant patients have benefitted in the long run by our waiting until the task force completed its work and made specific recommendations on programs mandated by the law before moving to implement the rest of the law. We simply did not want to get started on a program without the benefit of advice from the experts on the task force. We describe the history of federal involvement in transplantation, how we have handled implementation of the new law, and the progress we have made.

The federal government first became involved in organ transplantation by supporting biomedical researchers in their quest to diagnose, prevent and treat end-stage organ diseases, and more recently by providing researchers with support to perfect surgical procedures required in transplantation. For example, clinical research done by Starzl and Shumway to perfect liver and heart transplantation has been supported by the National Institutes of Health (NIH).

DAVID N. SUNDWALL • U.S. Department of Health and Human Services, Rockville, Maryland 20857.   LINDA D. SHEAFFER • Office of Organ Transplantation, Bureau of Resources Development, Health Resources and Services Administration, Rockville, Maryland 20857.

For kidney transplantation, researchers had mastered both the artificial kidney (dialysis) and kidney transplantation by the mid-1950s. But the costs associated with the procedures prohibited many kidney patients from benefitting from the new technology. For individuals with end-stage renal disease (ESRD), life and death came down to a question of money. To assist these patients, Congress passed the Social Security Act Amendments in 1972, which created a special entitlement under Medicare for dialysis and kidney transplants. Thus, dialysis and kidney transplantation became widely available to practically all residents of the United States, regardless of their ability to pay.

The ESRD program cost $140 million in 1972; it served between 5000 and 7000 patients. The program now costs taxpayers more than $2.4 billion annually and serves 80,000 patients nationwide. As organ transplantation has become more medically acceptable (i.e., nonexperimental in nature), the federal government has been called upon to pick up the tab for additional procedures and to expand the population group eligible to receive this benefit. Procedures no longer considered experimental include bone marrow transplants for lukemia and aplastic anemia, corneal transplants, liver transplants for children with biliary atresia, and heart transplants. In addition, Congress recently directed the federal government to begin covering the first year costs of immunosuppressive drug therapy for all Medicare covered transplants.

Thus, our early involvement focused on perfecting the technology so that more people could benefit from it, and paying for transplant procedures for ESRD patients. In doing so, a new problem emerged because the demand for donor organs exceeded the supply. The federal government was once again looked to for assistance.

2. INCREASING THE SUPPLY OF SOLID ORGANS FOR TRANSPLANTATION

The federal government's role in improving the organ procurement system actually had its genesis in early 1983. In an article that appeared in the November–December 1983 issue of *Public Health Reports,* the Surgeon General described his efforts this way: Recent successes in the transplantation of solid organs have made it obvious that more organs are going to be needed than are being donated. Kidneys have been in short supply since the advent of the transplant era. However, dialysis is available for patients with renal failure. Unfortunately, there is no temporizing mechanism such as a dialysis procedure, available for someone being considered as a candidate for heart or liver transplantation. The plight of parents seeking donated livers for children, many suffering from biliary atresia, who would otherwise die without a transplant operation, is perhaps the most recent dramatic manifestation of the dilemmas created by this major accomplishment of modern medicine. Following appeals to the White House for several of these children, the Public Health Service was asked by President and Mrs. Reagan to convene a group of experts to discuss ways to increase the supply of organs for transplantation. Forty-two people—many representing national organizations interested in transplantation—were invited to participate in a Surgeon General's workshop at Project HOPE headquarters, near Winchester, Virginia, June 7–9, 1983 (Koop, 1983).

It was at this early workshop that Surgeon General Koop encouraged the participants not to seek a strong federal role in trying to "fix" the system; that it was simply not necessary for the government to be involved in every problem or part of the solution of every problem facing our country. After this initial meeting, Dr. Koop agreed to an eight-point action plan that included a commitment to host another workgroup session to help refine the major recommendation of the first workgroup, that is, to address the formation of a federation of those organizations with an interest in transplantation.

The workgroup met at Project HOPE September 21–22, 1983 and formed the American Council on Transplantation (ACT). At the end of this workshop, Dr. Koop concluded that the present voluntary system of organ donation should continue and that responsibility for organ procurement should continue in the private sector. However, he adopted a statement of one of the workgroups and concluded that ''Individuals and organizations should continue their specialized efforts but need now to identify common interests and unite in the pursuit of goals that are beyond the ability of any one person or group to accomplish'' (Koop, 1983).

Congress agreed that the problem cried out for national attention and in 1983 began holding hearings on the issue of the shortage of organs for transplantation. In October 1984, Congress passed and the President signed the National Organ Transplant Act which accomplished the following:

1. Authorized a national Task Force on Organ Transplantation to study the economic, medical, legal, ethical and social issues presented by organ transplantation
2. Authorized grants to organ procurement organizations for planning, establishment, initial operation and expansion of their activities
3. Required the establishment of a national organ procurement and transplantation network (OPTN)
4. Required the establishment of a scientific registry of organ transplant recipients
5. Authorized the establishment of an entity in the Public Health Service to administer the law
6. Prohibited the buying and selling of human organs. (This last provision is not under our purview, so it is not addressed in this chapter.)

2.1. Task Force on Organ Transplantation

The Secretary established the Task Force on Organ Transplantation on January 24, 1985. The task force was unique in that it was the first of its kind on a national level to carry out a comprehensive study of the major issues in the field of transplantation. The group was composed of physicians and scientists in medical specialties related to human organ transplantation; organ procurement coordinators; individuals with expertise in law, theology, ethics, health-care financing, and the social and behavioral sciences; health insurance representatives; members of the general public, and ex-officio members representing the director of the NIH, the Commissioner of the Food and Drug Administration (FDA), the Administrator of the Health Care Financing Administration, and the Surgeon General.

Over a period of 15 months, the task force met publicly nine times and held two public hearings. During this time, the task force heard testimony from all the participants of the transplant community—physicians and surgeons, patients, families, organ procurement coordinators, tissue and eye personnel, national medical associations, voluntary health organizations, organ-sharing systems, and many other professional organizations.

The task force produced two reports: Task Force on Organ Transplantation, Report to the Secretary and the Congress on Immunosuppressive Therapies, Department of Health and Human Services (October 1985), and Organ Transplantation: Issues and Recommendations, Report of the Task Force on Organ Transplantation (April 1986). These two reports contain more than 70 recommendations which address some of the major concerns of Congress, including such issues as increasing organ donation, improving organ procurement, and ensuring equitable access to organs. In addition to carrying out its mandated tasks, the task force proved to be of enormous help in assisting our agency to develop the specifications for a National Organ Procurement and Transplantation Network, and to set our priorities for funding organ procurement organizations.

2.2. Grants to Organ Procurement Organizations

The National Organ Transplant Act authorizes a grant program for organ procurement organizations (OPOs). Currently, there are 72 OPOs, including hospital-based and independent programs. In 1986, the federal government spent an estimated $102 million for kidney acquisition costs, much of which supported the salaries and expenses of OPOs. Congress appropriated $2.4 million for grants to organ procurement organizations in its fiscal year 1986 budget for the Department of Health and Human Services.

Concurrent with this congressional action, in January 1986, the Task Force on Organ Transplantation gave us its recommendations regarding our grant program. The task force recommended the following priorities: The first priority would be for applications that propose to consolidate and coordinate organ procurement efforts where multiple programs currently exist. The second priority would be for applications that propose new approaches to improve the efficiency and effectiveness of an existing program so as to increase the number of organ donors within a service area, e.g., professional education. The third priority would be for applications that propose to expand present efforts to increase the number of organ donors within a service area, e.g., satellite programs, computerization of data, expanding services to serve dispersed rural populations (Recommendations of the Task Force on Organ Transplantation, Jan. 1986).

The agency received 47 applications for the fiscal year 1986 grant cycle. All applications were reviewed by a peer review committee. Eighteen of the 47 applicants were funded with grants totaling about $1.9 million.

In fiscal year 1987, we continued to give highest priority to organizations intending to consolidate multiple programs. However, the greatest number of applicants requested funding for professional and public education activities. A total of 18 projects were funded, totaling $2.7 million. By the time of grant awards for fiscal year 1988, all 73 OPOs formally designated by HCFA were established and operating entities and consolidation grants were no longer necessary. As in the previous two years, 18 OPOs received grants totaling $1.3 million, and like fiscal year 1987, most grant activities were in the area of professional and public education.

2.3. National Organ Procurement and Transplantation Network

An underlying concept in our society is that every person should have equal access to a basic minimum of health care. This concept gets rather complicated in organ transplantation because the demand for donor organs exceeds the supply. As long as the imbalance in supply–demand continues, methods used to allocate organs among potential recipients will continue to be an issue.

According to the task force report, the principle that donated cadaveric organs are a national resource implies that "any citizen or resident of the U. S. in need of a transplant should be considered as a potential recipient of each retrieved organ on a basis equal to that of a patient who lives in the area where the organs or tissues are retrieved. Organs and tissues ought to be distributed on the basis of objective priority, and not on the basis of accidents of geography" (Hunsicker, 1985).

The Task Force on Organ Transplantation spent a great deal of time on this issue of organ sharing, and it was probably one of the most controversial issues it discussed over its 15-month tenure. Not everyone agrees with the concept of organ sharing, certainly not on a national level or even at a regional level. The task force did, however, conclude that organ sharing did have some benefits:

1. Organ sharing increases access (especially for highly sensitized patients and pediatric patients) to organ transplantation.
2. Organ sharing improves HLA matching (kidneys only).
3. Organ sharing means fewer kidneys will be discarded or sent abroad.

There is a down side to organ sharing that really amounts to some rather practical and technical limitations. For example, the costs and risks of transportation, the decline of interest by the surgical team because they are unable to transplant an organ they have procured, and delayed function of kidneys because of longer ischemic times are all potential disadvantages of organ sharing. There are programmatic problems as well, such as the concern that more effective organ procurement organizations will be supporting the less effective ones; OPOs will be unable to provide organs to meet the needs of the programs that they have traditionally served; more organs will be shared through the network, but perhaps at a higher cost. These are all valid concerns.

The law was rather specific in terms of national organ sharing. Congress mandated that the two well-established organ sharing networks be merged into one national Organ Procurement and Transplantation Network (OPTN) and that we provide a contract to establish the OPTN. In September 1986, we contracted with the United Network for Organ Sharing (UNOS) of Richmond for this purpose. Initially, we awarded $379,000 and another $1.2 million was awarded in September 1987. Under this contract, the two existing voluntary national networks consolidated to create the computer hardware necessary for a single unified network. The principal functions of the OPTN are to maintain a computerized waiting list of individuals needing renal and extra-renal organs; assist in matching available organs with potential recipients on the list using medical criteria; provide transplant centers and organ procurement organizations with 24-hour telephone access to the waiting list and matching system; and develop and maintain a national data base on organ procurement and transplantation.

UNOS has elected a Board of Directors meeting our contract requirements to oversee development of the network. Its 31-member Board has broad geographic representation. It includes representatives of transplant physicians and surgeons, tissue typers, transplant coordinators, independent organ procurement agencies, and voluntary health organizations. It also has five public members. The membership of the network itself will include all transplant centers, OPOs, and histocompatibility laboratories, so all its users comprise its membership.

We are enthusiastic about the future of the OPTN. UNOS is making the changes required in the contract and is moving toward assuring that the network truly becomes what it is intended to be: a system that serves all transplant centers and procurement agencies in the United States, and a system that ensures that patients who need and can benefit from transplants have access to donor organs in the fairest and most equitable manner possible. We want to stress, however, that the network will only be as successful and fair as its members want it to be. Without active and committed participation, the network will fail.

2.4. Scientific Registry

The National Organ Transplant Act requires the Secretary to establish a scientific registry of transplant recipients to assess the clinical and scientific status of transplantation. In September 1987 we awarded a separate contract to UNOS to establish a comprehensive registry covering all types of the organ transplants. Under this contract, data collection from existing single organ registries will be coordinated. The first year of the contract was used to design the data system, and the second year will be used for implementation and operation of the data base. Data will be maintained on all types of transplantation procedures. We expect it will facilitate research on short-term and long-term outcomes of transplants and on the medical and other factors that affect transplant outcomes. It will be the first time that national data will be available from the same source on all organs. We view it as an important step forward in transplantation.

3. RECENT LEGISLATIVE ACTIONS AFFECTING TRANSPLANTATION

The Congress, in its Omnibus Budget Reconciliation Act of 1986, took several steps that will help insure appropriate organ donation and strengthen the organ procurement system. These include:

1. Hospitals participating in Medicare and Medicaid must establish written protocols for encouraging organ and tissue donation and for identifying potential donors.

2. Participating hospitals are also required to notify an organ procurement agency, when a potential donor is identified.
3. Hospitals that perform transplants must be members of the national organ procurement and transplantation network and must comply with its rules if they wish to receive Medicare and Medicaid reimbursement.
4. All organ procurement organizations must be federally designated in order to receive Medicare and Medicaid reimbursements, and only one procurement agency can be designated in each service area. To become designated, organ procurement organizations must meet performance standards prescribed by the Secretary (Omnibus Budget Reconciliation Act, 1986).

4. FUTURE DIRECTIONS

The Health Resources and Services Administration intends to continue its efforts to encourage awareness of organ donation through public information programs. We now are in the process of building up the staff of our Office of Organ Transplantation to meet these and other responsibilities.

There is much that remains to be done. We, as a nation, must continue to strive to reach our maximum potential in getting more donors to meet the increasing demand. However, we must continue to find better methods to preserve organs for longer periods of time as well as improved ways to suppress the immune system.

The Health Resources and Services Administration's role is one of partnership with the transplant community. Although our roles are very different, they complement each other. Together, we can contribute to making the miracle of organ donation and transplantation available to more people in need of this life-saving technology. It is an exciting and promising field, and we are pleased to be part of it.

REFERENCES

Hunsicker, L. G., 1985, Public Hearings. Task Force on Organ Transplantation, Chicago, Illinois, May 22, 1985.
Koop, C. E., 1983, Increasing the supply of solid organs for transplantation, *Public Health Rep.* 98:566–572.
National Organ Transplant Act, P.L. 98–507.
Omnibus Budget Reconciliation Act of 1986, Section 9318, P.L. 99–509, October 21, 1986.
Recommendations of the Task Force on Organ Transplantation on the Organ Procurement Organization Grant Program, Adopted January 9, 1986, Office of Organ Transplantation, Rockville, Maryland.
Report of the Task Force on Organ Transplantation, 1986, Organ Transplantation: Issues and Recommendations. U. S. Department of Health and Human Services, Public Health Service, Office of Organ Transplantation, April 1986.
Task Force on Organ Transplantation, 1985, Report to the Secretary and the Congress on Immunosuppressive Therapies, Department of Health and Human Services, October 1985.

Index